Dr. Aisha Hill-Hart

The Practical Science of Herbs

An Evidence-Backed Guide to 50 Therapeutic Herbs and How to Use Them

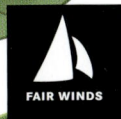

FAIR WINDS

Quarto.com

© 2026 Quarto Publishing
Text © 2026 Aisha Hill-Hart

First Published in 2026 by Fair Winds Press, an imprint of The Quarto Group,
100 Cummings Center, Suite 265-D, Beverly, MA 01915, USA.
T (978) 282-9590 F (978) 283-2742

EEA Representation, WTS Tax d.o.o.,
Žanova ulica 3, 4000 Kranj, Slovenia.
www.wts-tax.si

Fair Winds Press titles are also available at discount for retail, wholesale, promotional, and bulk purchase. For details, contact the Special Sales Manager by email at specialsales@quarto.com or by mail at The Quarto Group, Attn: Special Sales Manager, 100 Cummings Center, Suite 265-D, Beverly, MA 01915, USA.

30 29 28 27 26   1 2 3 4 5

ISBN: 978-0-7603-9878-4

Digital edition published in 2026
eISBN: 978-0-7603-9879-1

Library of Congress Cataloging-in-Publication Data available.

Design and page layout: Studio Quarante Douze Inc.
Cover and illustrations: Studio Quarante Douze Inc.
Photography: Madelynne Grace @Bitesandbevsmedia

Printed in Guangdong, China TT092025

The information in this book is for educational purposes only. It is not intended to replace the advice of a physician or medical practitioner. Please see your health-care provider before beginning any new health program.

For Sheldon—
My steady flame and fiercest cheer.
Your love is the soil where all my dreams took root.
Thank you for lifting me, lighting me, and believing in the magic before it bloomed.
—Love, Your Favorite Potion

Contents

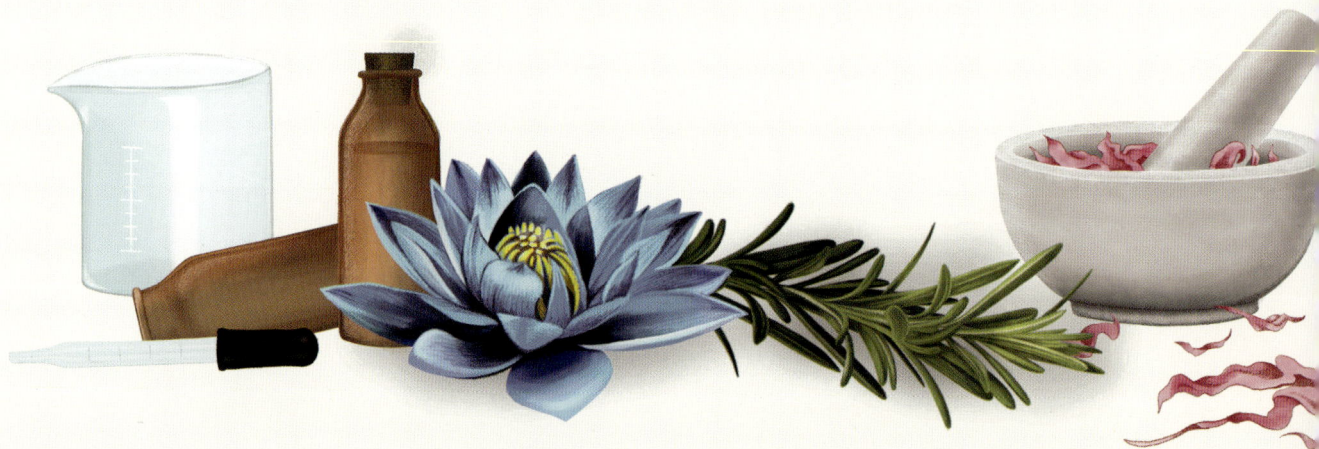

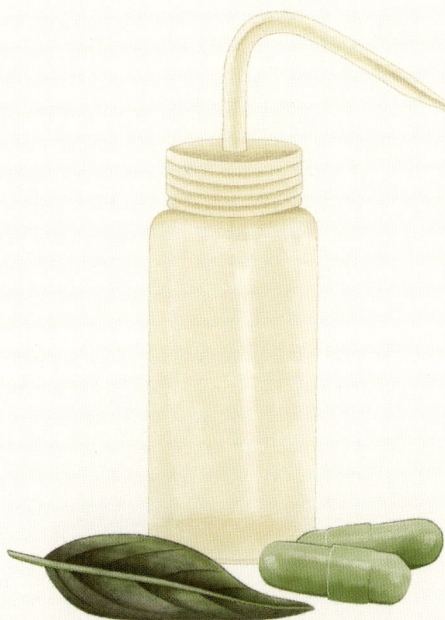

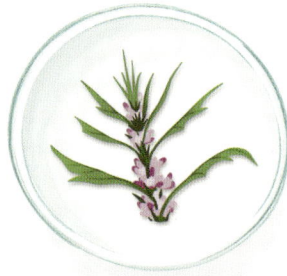

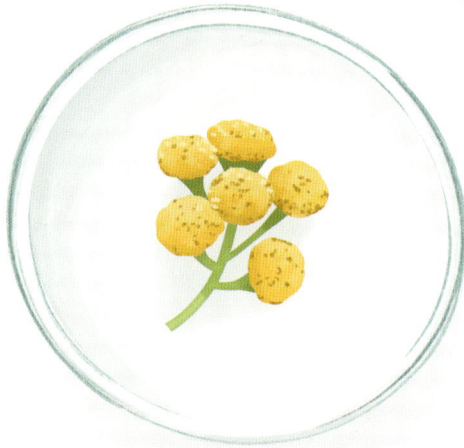

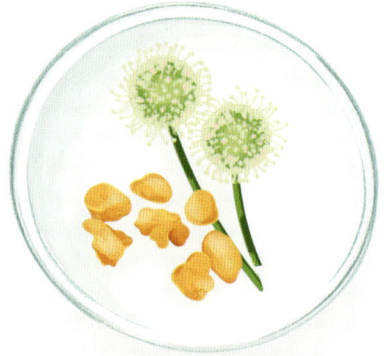

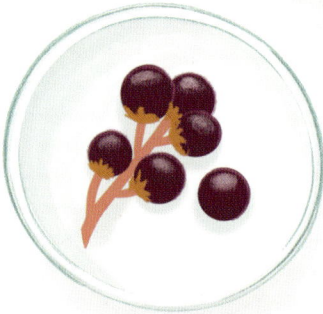

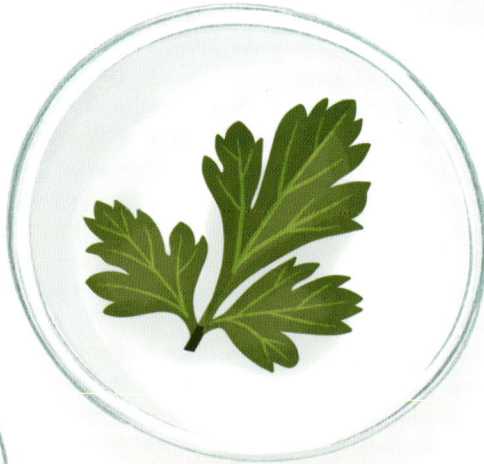

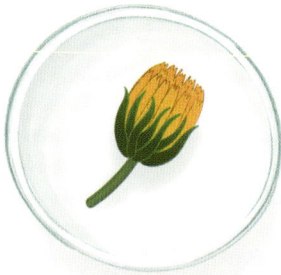

Introduction

Welcome to *The Practical Science of Herbs*, your trusted guide to evidence-based herbalism. This book is for those who love herbs, whether you're a home herbalist, a wellness enthusiast, or a practitioner seeking a solid foundation in scientifically studied botanicals.

First, let me introduce myself. I'm Dr. Aisha Hill-Hart, a plant scientist and health researcher with a deep passion for merging tradition with science. My background spans biotechnology, immunology, epidemiology, and medicinal plant research, and I've spent years studying how herbs interact with the body on a cellular level. Beyond the lab, I'm also someone who finds joy in crafting tinctures in my kitchen, growing herbs in my garden, and helping my community reconnect with the healing power of plants. I wrote this book to bridge the gap between traditional herbal knowledge and modern scientific research, ensuring that every herb discussed has been rigorously studied and supported by peer-reviewed evidence.

Herbalism has been practiced for centuries, with countless traditions passing down wisdom about plants' healing properties. However, in today's world, separating fact from fiction is more important than ever. That's where evidence-based herbalism comes in— it allows us to appreciate traditional uses while grounding our knowledge in scientific validation. This book ensures that you have access to both perspectives, helping you make informed decisions about incorporating herbs into your health and wellness routine.

In a world where misinformation spreads rapidly, having access to reliable, research-backed herbal knowledge is invaluable. Evidence-based herbalism doesn't mean rejecting traditional wisdom; it means enhancing it with scientific corroboration. By examining studies on herbal constituents, mechanisms of action, and clinical efficacy, we can make informed decisions about how to use plants safely and effectively.

Many herbs have been extensively studied in pharmacological research, yet much of this information doesn't always reach the general public. This book seeks to bridge that gap. Whether you're using herbs for everyday wellness or addressing specific concerns, knowing what science says about their effects can help maximize benefits while avoiding potential risks.

I'm so excited to guide you through this blend of tradition and science—where every plant has a story and every chapter brings us closer to understanding the true power of herbs.

How to Use This Book: Your Guide to Evidence-Based Herbalism

This book takes a scientific yet accessible approach to herbalism. You don't need a background in science to benefit from the information, because all of the research findings are written in a way that's easy to understand. Many of the studies will also help you understand just how these plants work within the body.

This book is designed to be both educational and practical. Each herb is presented in a structured format, covering its background, history, active constituents, studied uses, indications, contraindications, and interactions. To make this book a valuable reference, herbs are categorized by body systems, ensuring that you can easily find relevant information based on specific health needs. My personal insights as a scientist and herbalist are woven throughout. Herbalism is not just about knowing what an herb does; it's also about understanding how to integrate it into daily life in a way that supports overall health and well-being.

Beyond presenting scientific data, this book also offers insights into traditional applications, helping you appreciate how historical use aligns—or in some cases, differs—from modern findings. This book is not about replacing professional medical advice but about empowering you with knowledge to use herbs safely and effectively.

Each chapter also includes a practical recipe, whether it be a tincture, infusion, extract, or another herbal preparation, so you can apply the information directly. Whether you're new to herbalism or an experienced practitioner, this book will guide you through the exciting world of evidence-based plant medicine.

A glossary is included in this book to clarify terminology, ensuring that scientific and herbal terms are easily understood. Words that appear in **bold** throughout the text are featured in the glossary, so please consult it whenever you need to. References—most of which are peer-reviewed—are provided for further exploration, allowing you to dive deeper into the research behind these herbs.

Herbalism is a deeply personal and empowering journey. With the right knowledge, you can cultivate a practice that supports health in a meaningful, informed way. This book serves as a reliable companion, guiding a deeper understanding of plants and their potential in a wellness routine.

Let's explore the fascinating world of scientifically studied herbs.

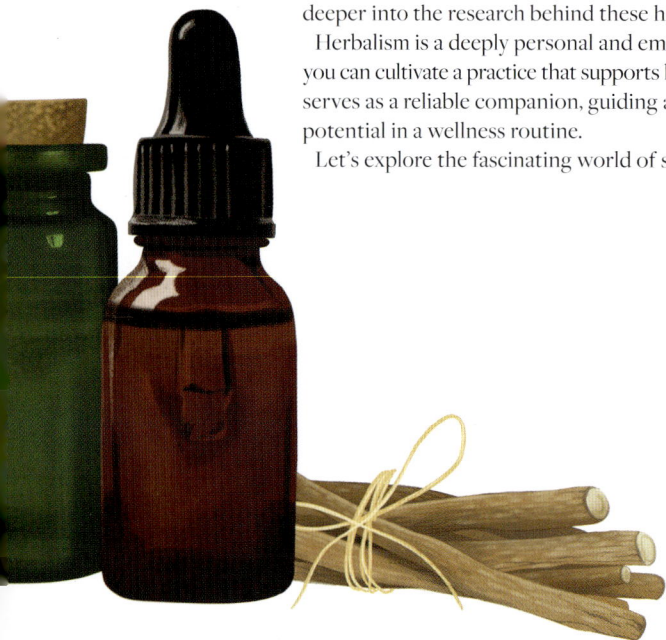

The Practical Science of Herbs

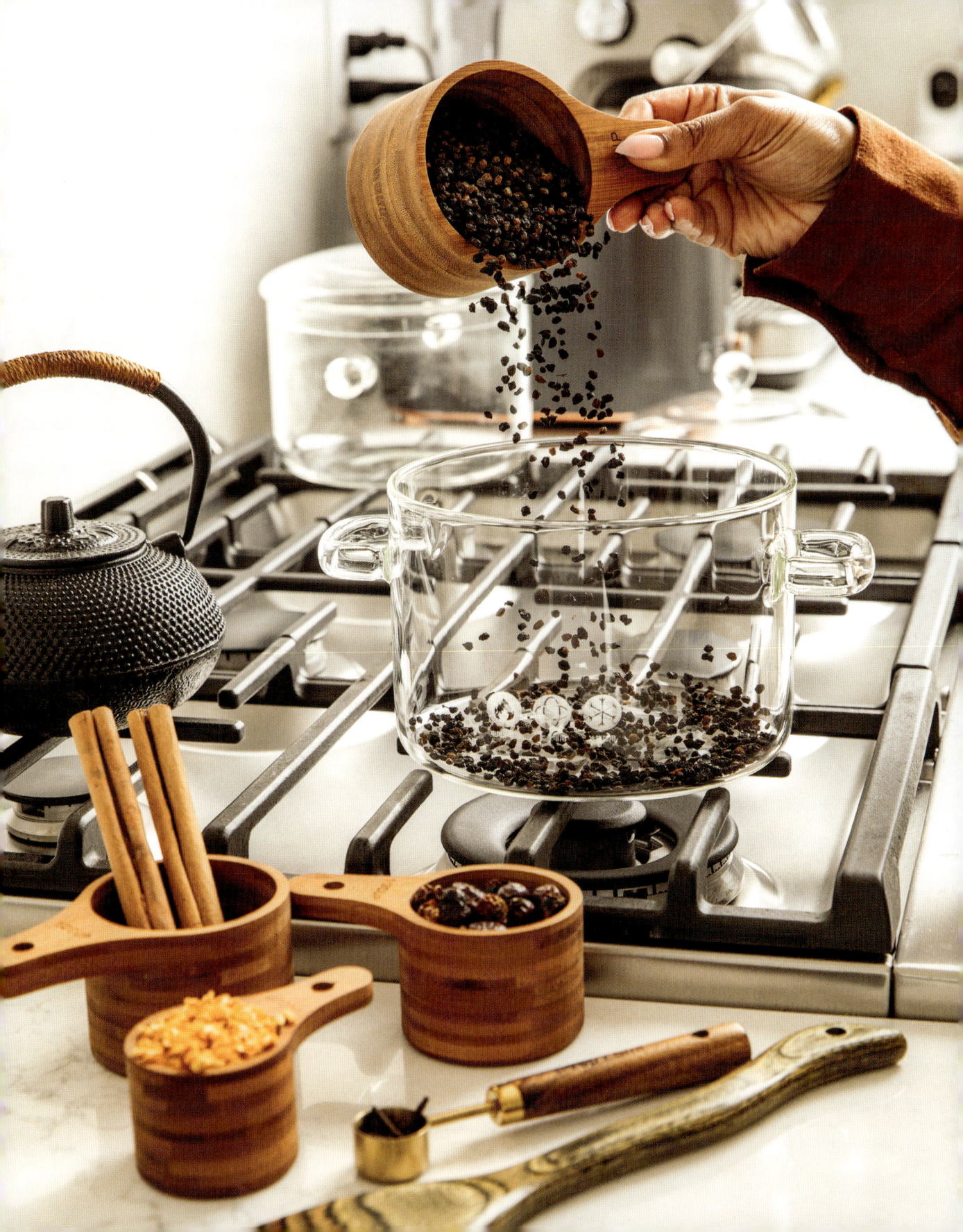

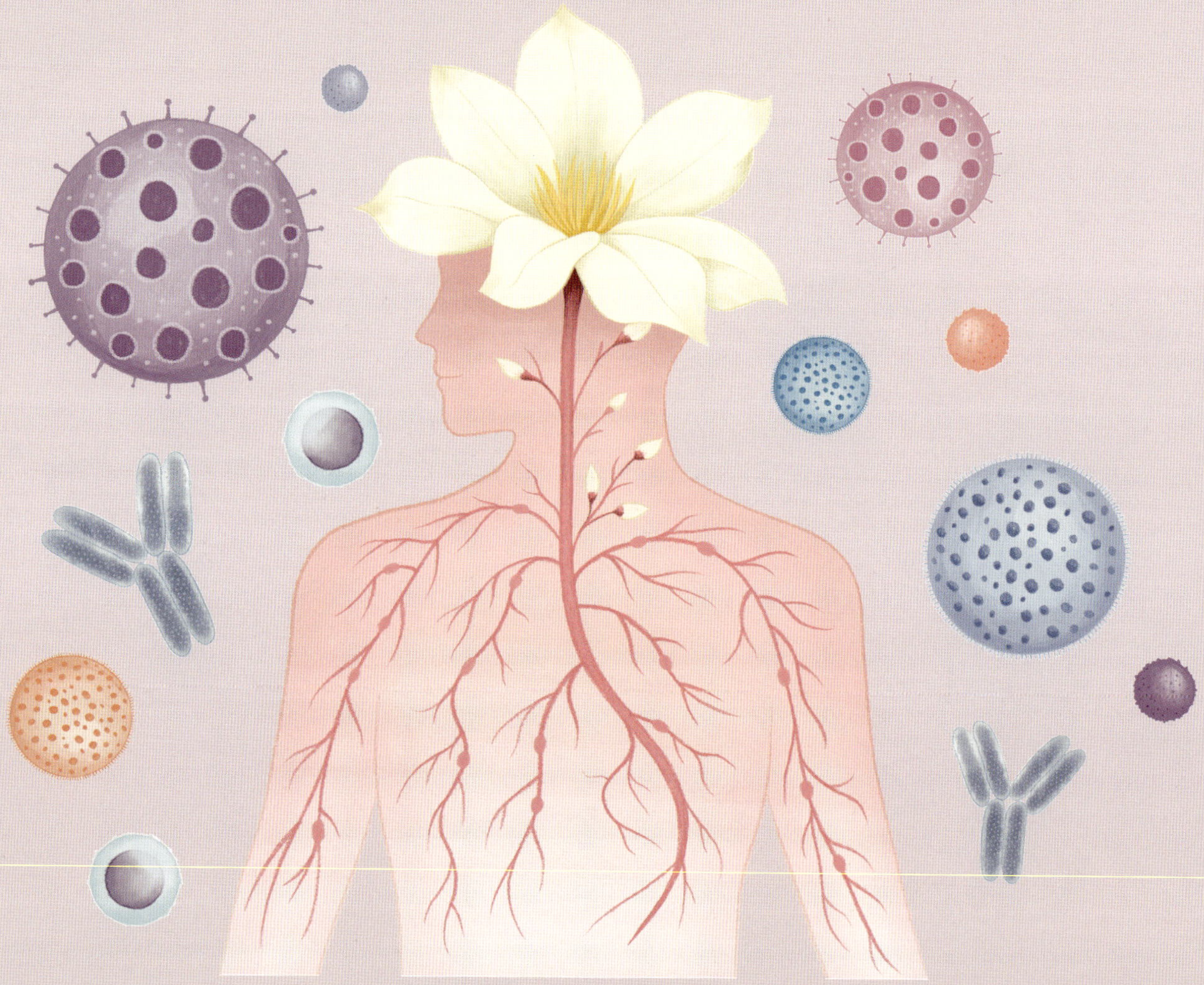

Chapter 1

Defense Squad:
Herbs for Immune Support

Welcome to the front line of your body's defenses! Imagine your immune system as a well-organized neighborhood watch, a network of cells, tissues, and organs working tirelessly to protect you. At its core, it's like a security team, with specialized roles designed to detect and neutralize "intruders" such as viruses and bacteria. From the skin cells acting as a physical barrier against damage to the white blood cells patrolling your bloodstream for foreign bodies, every part of this system plays a vital role.

Even with its impressive capabilities, the immune system sometimes needs extra support—especially during times of stress, lack of sleep, or seasonal changes. That's where herbs come in. These plant allies are nature's way of reinforcing your immune defenses, enhancing specific aspects of your body's response.

When it comes to strengthening your immune system, a few herbs truly rise to the occasion. Echinacea helps activate immune responses at the first sign of imbalance. Elderberry offers antiviral support wrapped in antioxidant-rich sweetness. Garlic brings heat and antimicrobial power, while Andrographis—though bitter—packs a potent punch during acute illness.

In this chapter, we'll explore simple, science-backed ways to invite these herbs into your life. Picture sipping a warming elderberry syrup or crafting a classic echinacea tincture with edible glitter for fun. These recipes are effective, enjoyable, and designed to build your defenses over time.

Let's dive in!

Elderberry (*Sambucus nigra*)
A Natural Cold and Flu Remedy

Native to Europe, North Africa, and parts of Asia, elderberry has a rich and ancient history in traditional medicine and has been used for thousands of years to ward off colds, flu, and other respiratory ailments. Hippocrates, the "father of medicine," referred to elderberry as his "medicine chest" thanks to its vast range of applications. Indigenous peoples of North America utilized elderberry for its medicinal properties, using the berries and flowers to make syrups, teas, and poultices for fevers and infections. During the Middle Ages, elderberry was a common remedy for respiratory ailments, and its popularity persisted through the nineteenth and twentieth centuries. Today it remains a staple in modern herbalism, prized for its immune-boosting properties and its ability to fight off viral infections during cold and flu season.

What the Science Says
Elderberry (*Sambucus nigra*), a small deciduous tree or shrub, produces clusters of tiny white flowers that mature into deep purple berries. Both the flowers and berries have medicinal uses, but the latter are particularly valued for their antiviral and immune-supporting properties. This is because the berries contain high levels of **anthocyanins**, **flavonoids** that are responsible for the berries' rich color and have a potent antioxidant effect. In addition to protecting immune cells from oxidative damage, anthocyanins reduce inflammation that can ease symptoms like congestion and body aches, while strengthening the body's natural defenses and, in turn, speeding recovery.

The berries also contain flavonoids such as quercetin and rutin that inhibit viral replication and prevent viruses from entering cells and spreading. This inhibition slows viral spread, allowing the immune system more time to respond effectively. Flavonoids also stimulate cytokine production, which alerts the body to invading pathogens and help stop them. Research confirms this. A 2016 study in *Nutrients* showed the effectiveness of the proprietary formula sambucus elderberry in reducing cold duration and severity in air travelers, thanks to its high concentration of bioactive compounds that enhance immune response and inhibit viral replication.

Elderberries also contain small amounts of vitamin C, a well-known immune booster, along with vitamin A, potassium, and iron, contributing to overall health. **Phenolic acids** add an extra layer of antimicrobial protection by inhibiting the growth of bacteria and fungi.

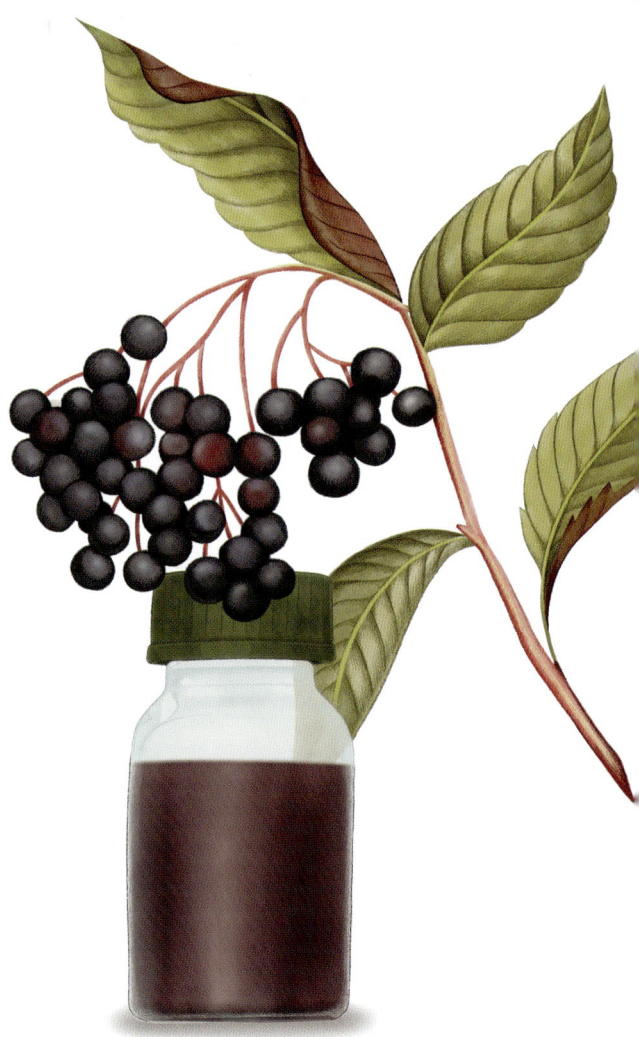

A randomized, double-blind, placebo-controlled study published in *The Journal of International Medical Research* (2004) found that participants who took elderberry extract recovered four days earlier on average compared to the placebo group. These findings further reinforce elderberry's reliable science-backed role in respiratory health.

Uses and Indications
Elderberry is a smart choice for anyone looking to prevent and manage cold and flu symptoms. Taken at the first sign of illness, it can reduce the duration and severity of symptoms such as fever, cough, sore throat, and congestion. The flowers of the elderberry plant are often used in herbal preparations for their diaphoretic properties, meaning they help promote sweating during fevers.

Research supports the use of elderberry as a preventive measure, particularly during the winter months or times of heightened viral activity (or year-round for people frequently exposed to illnesses, such as teachers and healthcare workers, or those with school-age children).

Interactions and Safety

Elderberry is generally safe for most people when used as directed. However, the raw berries, leaves, and bark of the plant contain cyanogenic glycosides, compounds that can release cyanide, a toxic chemical that interferes with cellular respiration when metabolized. Consuming raw elderberries or improperly prepared products may lead to digestive upset, including nausea, vomiting, and diarrhea. While not typically life-threatening, it's important to note that proper preparation—such as cooking—renders elderberry safe for consumption.

If you take immunosuppressive medications, consult a healthcare provider before using elderberry, because its immune-boosting properties could potentially interfere with the intended effects of these drugs.

While elderberry is considered safe for short-term use, its effects during pregnancy and breastfeeding are not well studied. As with any herbal remedy, it's best to seek professional advice before you use it.

Growing and Harvesting Elderberry

Elderberry is a fast-growing shrub that thrives in temperate climates, preferring moist, well-drained soil and full to partial sunlight. It can grow up to 10 feet (3 m) tall and produces clusters of small, fragrant flowers in late spring, followed by dark purple berries in late summer.

For medicinal use, the berries should be harvested when they are fully ripe, as unripe berries may contain higher levels of cyanogenic glycosides. The flowers can be harvested earlier in the season and dried for later use. Proper drying and storage are essential to preserve the herb's medicinal properties.

Elderberry's ability to attract pollinators like bees and butterflies adds ecological value to its cultivation. Elderberry also serves as a habitat and food source for birds, making it an excellent choice for sustainable gardening practices.

Fun Fact

In European folk medicine, elderberry trees were considered sacred and often planted for their protective properties to ward off evil spirits and illness. Cutting down an elder tree without permission from these spirits was thought to bring misfortune.

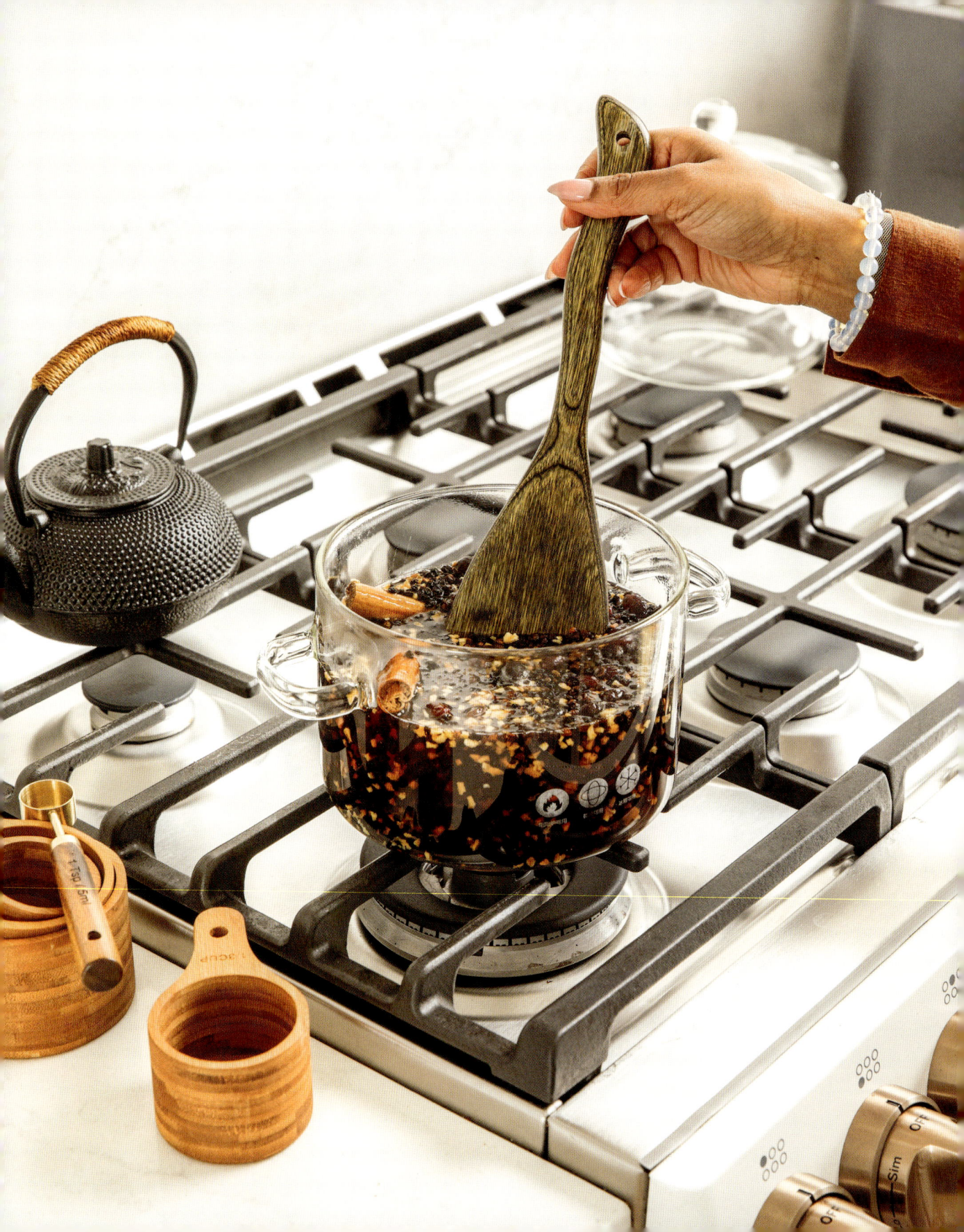

Elderberry Syrup for Cold and Flu Prevention

Elderberry syrup is a trusted natural remedy to help boost immunity and keep colds and flu at bay. Packed with antioxidants and vitamins, this syrup is a delicious way to support your body during the colder months or whenever your immune system needs a little extra care. With its warm, spiced flavor, it's perfect for the whole family (*just omit honey for children under one year old, as infants should not consume honey*).

Preparation

Combine the dried elderberries, water, cinnamon stick, cloves, orange peel, and rosehips in a large pot. Bring the mixture to a gentle simmer over low heat, stirring occasionally to ensure the ingredients are evenly distributed and to prevent them from sticking to the bottom of the pot. Simmer for 30 to 45 minutes, allowing the liquid to reduce by half. Stir every 10 to 15 minutes for consistent extraction. Remove from the heat and let the decoction cool to room temperature.

Strain the mixture through a fine strainer or cheesecloth into a clean bowl, discarding the solids. Stir in the honey, adjusting to taste, until fully dissolved. Pour the syrup into an airtight glass jar or bottle and store it in the refrigerator.

Yield: 4 to 5 cups (1 to 1.2 L)

1 cup (56.5 g) dried elderberries

2 quarts (1.9 L) water

1 cinnamon stick

3 or 4 cloves

2 tablespoons (16 g) dried orange peel

2 tablespoons (16 g) dried rosehips

1 cup (240 ml) raw honey (adjust to taste)

How to Use

Take 1 tablespoon (15 ml) daily as a preventive measure. When symptomatic, take up to three times daily to support recovery.

Andrographis *(Andrographis paniculata)*
The Immune Activator

Andrographis *(Andrographis paniculata)*, known as the "king of bitters," has been a cornerstone of traditional medicine in South and Southeast Asia for centuries. This herb is widely used in Ayurveda and Traditional Chinese Medicine (TCM) to treat fevers, respiratory infections, and digestive issues. Its Sanskrit name, *Kalmegh*, translates to "dark cloud," referring to both its intensely bitter taste and its ability to dispel illness, much like a rain cloud clears the air.

In Ayurvedic medicine, Andrographis is classified as a cooling herb, ideal for managing heat-related conditions such as fever and inflammation. In TCM, Andrographis is used to "clear heat and detoxify," often prescribed for respiratory infections, fevers, and gastrointestinal disturbances.

During the 1919 influenza pandemic, Andrographis gained attention in India for its ability to reduce mortality rates and manage flu symptoms effectively. Modern herbalists regard it as one of the most powerful immune-supporting herbs, particularly for managing respiratory illnesses and inflammation. Its reputation as a natural antibiotic and immune activator has led to its widespread use in both traditional and contemporary herbal medicine.

What the Science Says

Andrographis *(Andrographis paniculata)* is widely recognized for its immune-boosting, antiviral, and anti-inflammatory properties. These are primarily derived from its stems and leaves, which contain andrographolides, compounds that belong to a group of **diterpene lactones** responsible for both its bitter taste and its medicinal potency.

These bioactive compounds have been studied for their ability to slow the spread of infections like the common cold and flu. Research published in *Pharmaceuticals* in 2021 showed that andrographolides interfere with viral replication, suggesting potential applications for respiratory infections beyond the common cold.

At the same time, Andrographis activates macrophages and natural killer (NK) cells, which work to eliminate harmful bacteria, viruses, and infected cells. A 1999 study in *Phytomedicine* found that Andrographis extract significantly reduced cold symptom severity and duration, especially when taken at the first signs of illness. Its immune-modulating effects ensure that the body responds effectively to infections and prevents excessive immune reactions that could cause further inflammation.

These anti-inflammatory properties also help regulate pro-inflammatory cytokines that contribute to fever, congestion, and body aches, which alleviates symptoms and speeds recovery. A 2022 study in *Frontiers in Pharmacology* underscored this herb's ability to suppress excessive inflammation, making it useful not just for acute infections but also for managing chronic inflammatory conditions.

In addition, Andrographis stimulates B cells and T cells, which improves antibody production and strengthens immune memory, which can help prevent future infections.

Andrographis also provides antioxidant protection through its **flavonoids** and **phenolic acids**, which help neutralize free radicals that can weaken immune defenses. By reducing oxidative stress, these compounds contribute to immune resilience and overall cellular health.

Uses and Indications

You can use Andrographis to both support the immune system and reduce the severity and duration of colds, flu, and sinusitis. Research shows that Andrographis can alleviate symptoms such as sore throat, cough, nasal congestion, and fever.

You may also find this herb useful when it comes to digestive complaints, including diarrhea, dysentery, and indigestion, especially when these issues are caused by infections or inflammation. Its ability to "clear heat" in TCM terms makes it effective for managing conditions associated with excessive internal heat, such as fevers and inflammatory bowel diseases.

Andrographis can help you prevent a cold or the flu when you're exposed to pathogens or have increased stress. It's also an excellent choice if you have recurrent infections and want to strengthen your immune defenses during cold and flu season.

You can also use this herb to help manage inflammatory conditions such as arthritis. It can help alleviate joint pain and stiffness, supporting mobility and overall quality of life.

Interactions and Safety

Andrographis is generally safe for short-term use, but because it activates the immune system it can potentially exacerbate symptoms if you have an autoimmune condition such as lupus or rheumatoid arthritis.

Prolonged use of Andrographis may cause mild gastrointestinal discomfort, such as nausea or diarrhea, particularly if you have a sensitive stomach. To minimize these effects, take this herb with food or as directed by a healthcare provider.

If you're pregnant or breastfeeding, avoid Andrographis, as its safety during these stages has not been well studied. If you're taking immunosuppressive medications or anticoagulants, consult a healthcare provider before using Andrographis, because it may interact with these treatments.

Andrographis Herbal Decoction

This herbal decoction uses a traditional method to extract the full medicinal potential of Andrographis, perfect for strengthening your immune system during cold and flu season or supporting overall wellness. Note that this recipe is for a single-use decoction. For regular use, prepare fresh daily to maximize potency.

> *Yield: Approximately 2 cups (480 ml)*

2 teaspoons (10 g) dried Andrographis leaves

1 teaspoon (2 g) dried ginger or 3 slices fresh ginger

1 cinnamon stick

3 cups (720 ml) water

Preparation

Combine the Andrographis leaves, ginger, and cinnamon stick in a small saucepan. Add the water and bring the mixture to a boil over medium heat. Reduce the heat to low and let the mixture simmer gently for 20 to 30 minutes, stirring occasionally to ensure the herbs are evenly infused, until the liquid is reduced to approximately 2 cups (480 ml). Remove from the heat and let the decoction cool slightly. Strain the liquid through a fine strainer or cheesecloth into a mug or thermos, discarding the solids.

How to Use

Drink ½ cup (120 ml) of the decoction warm, two or three times a day, during cold and flu season to strengthen immunity. (You can sweeten the decoction with raw honey or a splash of lemon juice, if needed, to overcome the bitter taste.) Use as a preventive measure or at the onset of symptoms to reduce severity and duration.

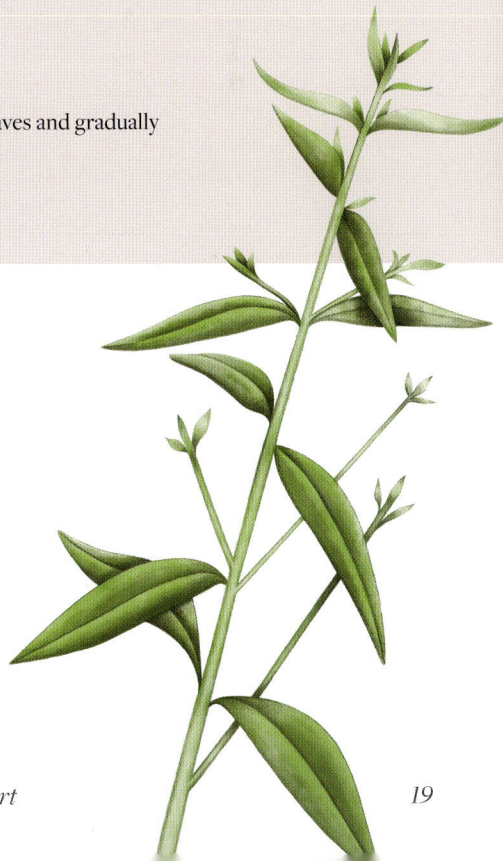

Tip

If the bitterness is too intense, start with 1 teaspoon (5 g) of Andrographis leaves and gradually increase to the full amount as you adjust to the taste.

Growing and Harvesting Andrographis

Andrographis is a hardy annual that thrives in tropical and sub-tropical climates. It prefers well-drained soil and full sunlight and is found in regions with warm, humid conditions, such as India, Sri Lanka, Thailand, China, and other parts of Southeast Asia.

The aerial parts of the plant are harvested when the plant reaches maturity, typically during the flowering stage. Leaves and stems are dried and processed into powders, extracts, or capsules for medicinal use. Proper drying and storage are essential to preserve the herb's bioactive compounds and ensure its potency.

Echinacea *(Echinacea purpurea)*
The Immune Defender

Echinacea, commonly known as the "purple coneflower," holds a long-standing reputation as one of the most important herbs for immune support. Indigenous peoples of North America, including the Lakota, Cheyenne, and Pawnee, understood the medicinal power of echinacea and used it as a versatile remedy for treating both injuries like wounds and snakebites, and ailments like infections and toothaches.

The herb's name comes from the Greek word *echinos*, meaning "hedgehog," a nod to the spiny seed head that resembles the protective quills of a hedgehog. In the nineteenth century, it became a staple of Eclectic medicine, a branch of Western herbalism, and was used to combat infectious diseases, septic wounds, and other ailments, making it one of the most widely used herbs of the time.

With the advent of synthetic antibiotics in the mid-twentieth century, the use of echinacea waned. However, its popularity surged again in the 1980s as the natural health movement grew. Today echinacea is used worldwide for its immune-modulating properties and remains a trusted herb for maintaining health during cold and flu season.

What the Science Says

Echinacea *(Echinacea purpurea)* is chock-full of bioactive compounds that can support your immune health. Echinacea's leaves, flowers, and roots all offer unique benefits. The roots are rich in **alkamides**, lipid-based molecules that are highly bioavailable, meaning they're easily absorbed by the body. These help regulate immune function and reduce inflammation

The aerial parts (leaves and flowers) contain **polysaccharides**, which stimulate macrophages and natural killer cells, and strengthen the body's defense against infections. Both contain **caffeic acid derivatives** like echinacoside and chicoric acid that act as antioxidants, which means they protect immune cells from oxidative stress, while promoting hyaluronic acid production, a key player in tissue repair and immune defense. **Flavonoids**—plant-based antioxidants known for protecting cells and calming inflammation—are present throughout the plant, further contributing to echinacea's antioxidant and anti-inflammatory benefits and amplifying its overall effectiveness.

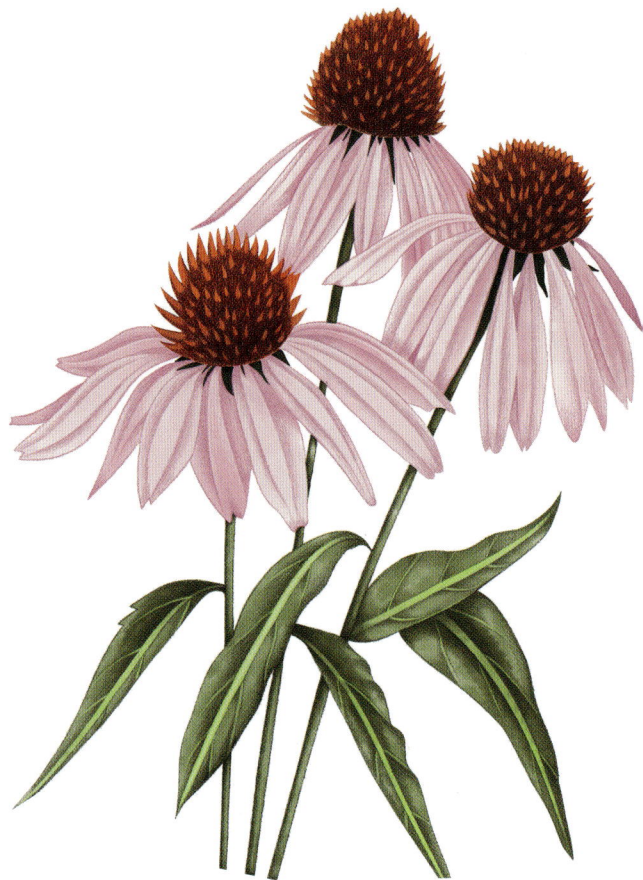

Echinacea also activates phagocytes, which engulf and destroy harmful microbes, and stimulates cytokine production to boost immune function. In addition, this herb boosts T cell and B cell activity, which improves the body's ability to recognize and target pathogens, making it beneficial for both acute infections and long-term immune support.

Clinical studies support echinacea's use as a potent tool to fight colds and flu. In 2007, a meta-analysis in *The Lancet Infectious Diseases* found it reduced the risk of developing a cold by 58 percent and shortened its duration by 1.4 days. Another 2004 study in *Phytomedicine* indicated that echinacea works best when taken at the onset of symptoms, something to keep in mind should you choose to take advantage of this potent herbal ally.

Uses and Indications

Keep echinacea on hand to support immunity during cold and flu season. Take it at the first sign of symptoms to reduce the severity and duration of illnesses.

You can also use echinacea to support immune function if you feel stressed, are undergoing seasonal changes, or are in contact with someone who is sick. You can also tap into its anti-inflammatory properties to support wound healing and address minor infections.

Echinacea's adaptogenic qualities—its ability to help the body adapt to stress and restore balance—further enhance its value. You can use it effectively to support homeostasis, the body's natural state of internal stability, and aid recovery from immune challenges.

Interactions and Safety

Echinacea is generally safe for short-term use, but there are a few precautions to consider. Since it stimulates the immune system, it may not be suitable for individuals with autoimmune conditions such as lupus, multiple sclerosis, or rheumatoid arthritis because it can potentially exacerbate symptoms.

If you're allergic to plants in the Asteraceae family, such as ragweed or daisies, use caution when trying echinacea, as allergic reactions are possible. Symptoms may include itching, swelling, or respiratory discomfort.

Echinacea may interact with certain medications, like immunosuppressants or drugs metabolized by the liver. Pregnant or breastfeeding individuals should consult their healthcare provider before using echinacea, as research on its safety in these populations is limited.

Growing and Harvesting Echinacea

Echinacea is a hardy, low-maintenance perennial that thrives in temperate climates with well-drained soil and full sunlight. The bright flowers bloom from early summer to late fall, providing both aesthetic and ecological benefits.

For medicinal use, the roots are typically harvested in the fall, after the plant has gone dormant and concentrated its energy underground. Leaves and flowers can be harvested throughout the growing season and dried for later use. Proper storage in an airtight container helps preserve the herb's potency.

Echinacea's ability to attract pollinators, such as bees and butterflies, makes it an excellent choice for sustainable gardening practices.

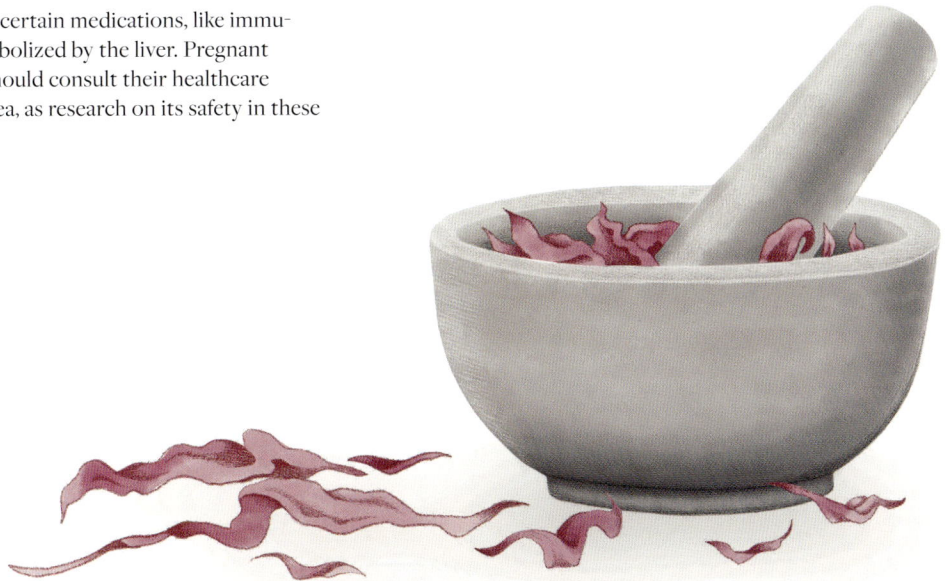

Recipe

Immune-Boosting Echinacea Tincture

This tincture is a concentrated extract of echinacea root combined with warming lemon peel and star anise, making it a potent and convenient remedy to have on hand during cold and flu season.

Preparation

Add the dried echinacea root, lemon peel, and star anise to an airtight glass jar. Pour the vodka or brandy over the herbs, ensuring they are fully submerged. Leave about ½ inch (1 cm) of liquid above the herbs to account for swelling. Seal the jar tightly and place it in a cool, dark place. Let the mixture steep for 4 to 6 weeks, shaking the jar gently every few days to encourage extraction.

After steeping, strain the mixture through a fine strainer or cheesecloth into a clean bowl. Discard the solids. Transfer the tincture into a dropper bottle for easy use.

> Yield: Approximately 1 cup (240 ml)

2 tablespoons (10 g) dried echinacea root

1 tablespoon (3 g) dried lemon peel

2 star anise

1 cup (240 ml) vodka or brandy

How to Use

Take 1 to 2 droppers full (about 1 to 2 ml) at the onset of cold symptoms, up to three times daily.

For preventive use, take 1 dropper full daily during cold and flu season to support overall immune health.

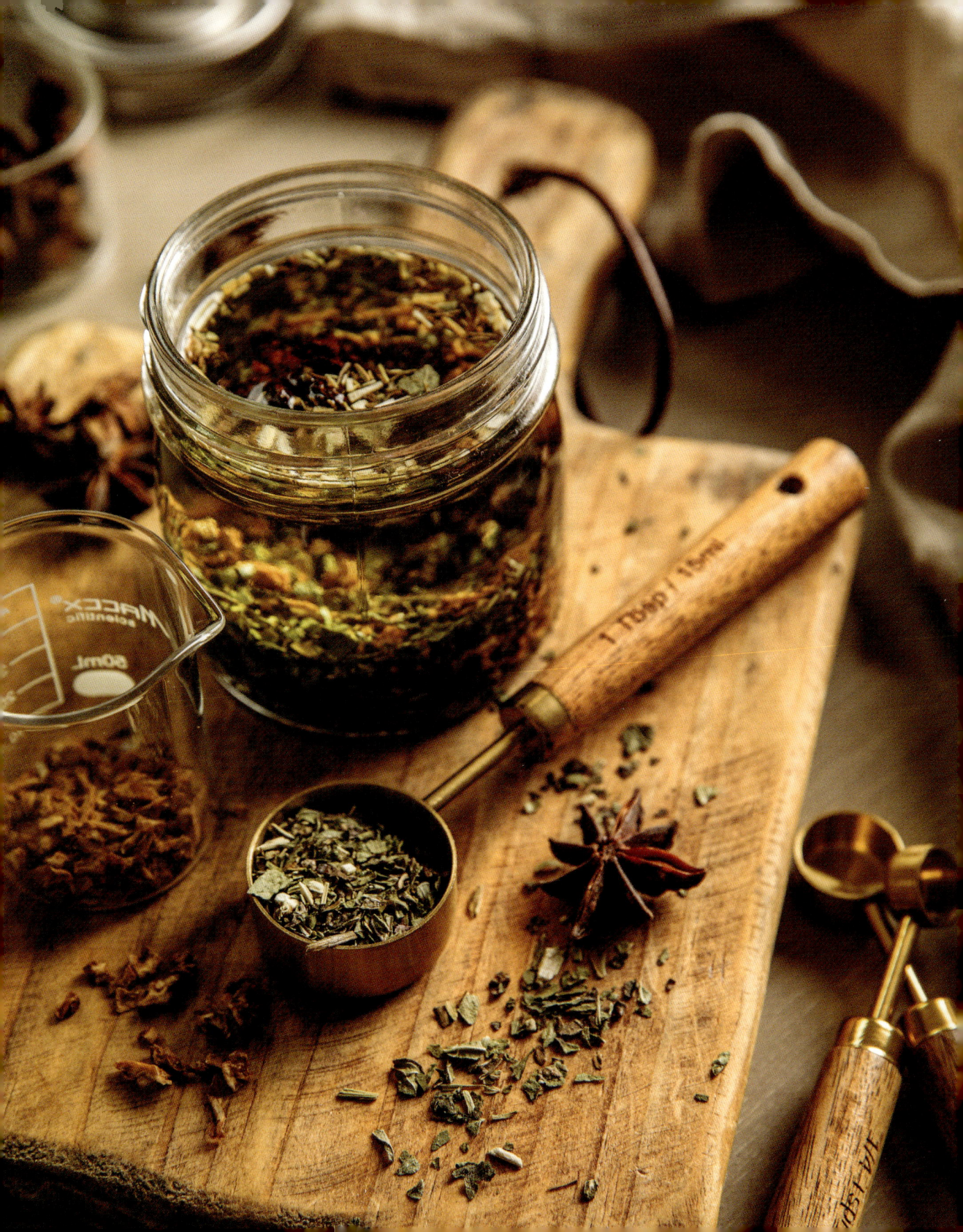

Garlic (*Allium sativum*)
The Antimicrobial Powerhouse

Native to Central Asia, garlic was one of the first cultivated plants and has been used for over five thousand years as a medicinal herb.

Ancient Egyptians used garlic to boost stamina and prevent infections and prescribed it for ailments such as heart disease and intestinal parasites. It was so prized that the cloves were included in pharaohs' tombs for use in the afterlife.

In ancient Greece, Hippocrates prescribed garlic for respiratory and digestive issues, while Roman soldiers used it to improve endurance.

In the Middle Ages, garlic was used throughout Europe to protect against the plague and other infectious diseases. During World War II, it earned the nickname "Russian penicillin" for its use as an antimicrobial when antibiotics were scarce.

Today garlic is a cornerstone of natural medicine, celebrated for its immune-boosting and cardiovascular benefits. One of the most researched medicinal plants, garlic is used worldwide for its ability to combat infections and support overall health.

What the Science Says

Garlic (*Allium sativum*) is one of the most powerful medicinal plants, and its bulb—composed of multiple cloves—serves as the most bioactive part. Its primary active compound, allicin, is formed once the bulb is crushed or chopped. In turn, allicin rapidly breaks down into other sulfur-based compounds such as ajoene, diallyl disulfide, and S-allyl cysteine, all of which have antimicrobial, antioxidant, and anti-inflammatory properties.

Garlic also contains **flavonoids** like quercetin and selenium, which act as antioxidants, protecting immune cells from oxidative damage. **Polysulfides**, another key group of **sulfur compounds**, support cardiovascular health by improving blood flow and relaxing blood vessels. Nutrients such as vitamins C and B_6 and manganese improve garlic's immune-boosting and overall health-supporting effects. You can see why this combination of compounds makes garlic one of the most versatile and widely used natural remedies.

The three most significant therapeutic effects of garlic are its ability to combat pathogens, enhance immune function, and protect cells from oxidative stress. Allicin acts as a potent antimicrobial agent. It disrupts the lipid membranes of bacteria, fungi, and viruses, which leads to their destruction. Allicin also inhibits enzymes essential for pathogen replication, making it particularly effective against antibiotic-resistant bacteria like Methicillin-resistant *Staphylococcus aureus* (MRSA) and fungal infections such as *Candida albicans*.

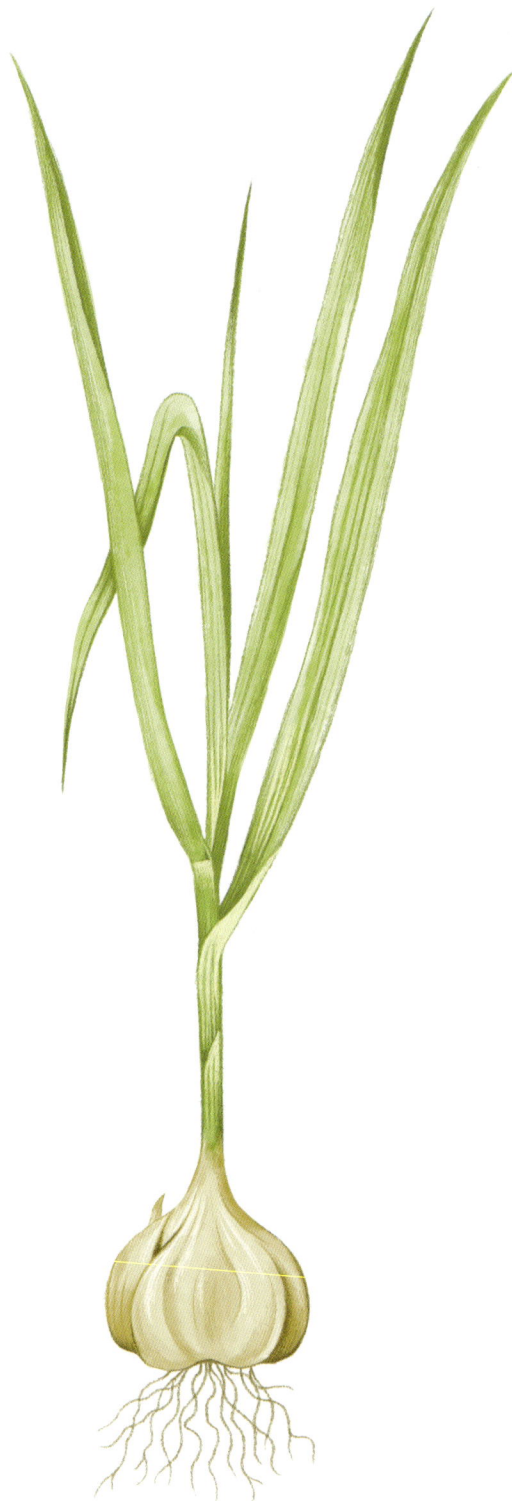

Garlic's antiviral properties prevent viruses from attaching to host cells, helping to stop infections like the common cold and influenza before they can spread. It also enhances immune function by stimulating macrophages and natural killer (NK) cells, which help identify and destroy pathogens. By increasing cytokine production, garlic improves immune cell communication, ensuring a coordinated and efficient response to infections.

The antioxidants in garlic protect immune cells from oxidative stress, which preserves their function and boosts the body's resilience against illness. By promoting production of **hydrogen sulfide (H_2S)**, garlic improves cardiovascular health by relaxing blood vessels and improving circulation. This allows immune cells to speed to areas of infection or injury more quickly.

Scientific research supports garlic's role in immune and cardiovascular health. A double-blind, placebo-controlled study published in *Advances in Therapy* in 2001 found that daily garlic supplementation significantly reduced the incidence and severity of colds. Participants who regularly took aged garlic extract had fewer sick days and recovered faster from upper respiratory infections compared to the placebo group. Another study from 2020 published in *The Journal of Nutrition* confirmed garlic's ability to lower blood pressure and improve cholesterol levels. These findings reinforce garlic's traditional use in immune support and heart health, validating its role as a scientifically backed medicinal herb.

This multifaceted activity makes garlic both a direct antimicrobial and a powerful immune system booster, reinforcing its place as a comprehensive natural remedy.

Uses and Indications

Garlic is most commonly used to support immune function and fight infections. It is especially effective against bacteria, viruses, and fungi, making it a useful remedy during cold and flu season. Its antimicrobial properties help shorten the duration of respiratory illnesses while promoting recovery.

You can also use garlic to support heart health. Regular consumption has been shown to help lower blood pressure, improve cholesterol levels, and enhance circulation, reducing inflammation that can contribute to cardiovascular issues.

Garlic's antifungal and digestive benefits also make it a helpful herb for maintaining gut health, balancing the microbiome, and addressing concerns like Candida overgrowth.

Interactions and Safety

While dietary amounts of garlic are usually safe, medicinal doses require caution. That's because its blood-thinning properties may interact with any anticoagulant medications, such as warfarin, that you may be taking, thus increasing the risk of bleeding. Garlic can also enhance the effects of antihypertensive drugs, potentially leading to low blood pressure.

You may experience digestive discomfort, heartburn, or gas when consuming raw garlic. Cooking garlic can reduce these effects while preserving many of its health benefits.

If you're pregnant or breastfeeding, consult a healthcare provider before using garlic supplements, as research on its safety in these populations is limited.

Growing and Harvesting Garlic

Garlic is a hardy plant that thrives in a variety of climates and is typically planted in the fall and harvested in the summer when the leaves turn brown. Keep in mind that proper curing is essential to preserve the bulb's medicinal properties. After harvesting, dry garlic in a cool, dark, and well-ventilated area for several weeks. Once cured, you can store garlic for months without losing its potency. For home gardeners and herbalists alike, garlic provides both culinary and medicinal benefits year-round.

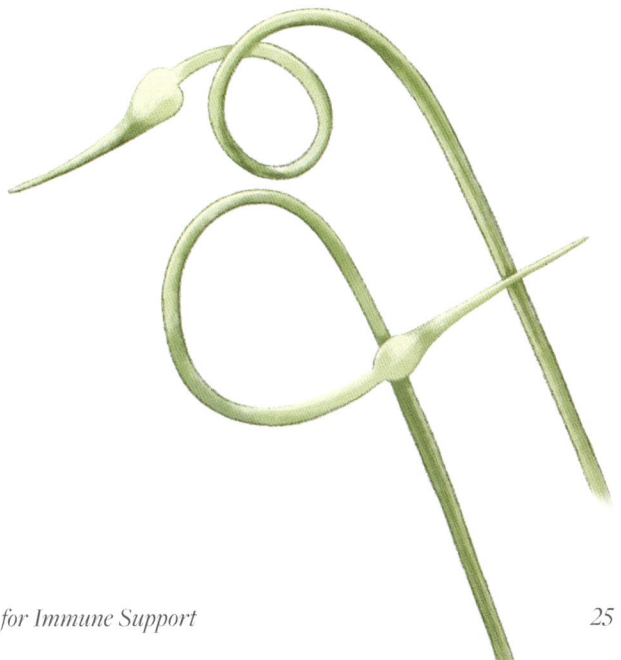

Immune-Boosting Garlic Syrup

This recipe combines the medicinal properties of raw garlic with the soothing sweetness of raw honey, which provides antimicrobial properties. The apple cider vinegar adds immune-supporting and digestive benefits while balancing the syrup's flavor. Note: *This syrup is not recommended for children under one year old, as infants should not consume honey.*

10 to 12 cloves fresh garlic, peeled
½ cup (120 ml) water
½ cup (120 ml) apple cider vinegar
1 cup (240 ml) raw honey

Preparation

Lightly crush the garlic cloves with the flat side of a knife or the bottom of a jar to release their bioactive compounds, such as allicin.

In a small saucepan, combine the water and apple cider vinegar. Add the crushed garlic cloves and bring the mixture to a gentle simmer over low heat, stirring occasionally. Simmer for 10 minutes, keeping the heat low to preserve the garlic's medicinal properties while allowing the flavors to meld. Remove from the heat and let the garlic mixture cool to room temperature.

Pour the mixture through a fine strainer or cheesecloth into a clean bowl, pressing the garlic gently to extract all the liquid. Stir the raw honey into the cooled garlic mixture until fully dissolved. Transfer the garlic syrup to a clean mason jar or airtight glass container and store it in the refrigerator for up to 2 months.

How to Use

Take 1 tablespoon (15 ml) daily during cold and flu season to boost immunity. During illness, take 1 to 2 tablespoons (15 to 30 ml) every 3 to 4 hours to help fight infections and soothe symptoms.

Tip

For a milder garlic flavor, reduce the simmering time or increase the honey.

Herbalism as Self-Care

Herbs have been used for centuries not only as medicine but also as a way to maintain long-term wellness. Ancient cultures wove herbal knowledge into their daily lives, ensuring that food, healing, and self-care were deeply connected. From the Ayurvedic practice of sipping spiced teas to maintain digestive fire to the European tradition of bitters before meals, herbalism has always been a seamless part of daily routines. Yet, in modern times, many of these traditions have been lost in favor of synthetic, quick-fix solutions.

Reintegrating herbs into daily life brings us back to a more balanced, natural way of supporting health. Rest assured, this doesn't have to be overwhelming or time-consuming. Small, intentional steps create meaningful routines that provide long-term benefits. A simple cup of ginseng or matcha tea in the morning offers a smooth, sustained lift, while a few drops of echinacea tincture in water fortify the immune system. Digestive allies like peppermint and ginger can be sipped after lunch to ease bloating and enhance nutrient absorption. In the evening, a calming ritual with lemon balm, chamomile, or lavender can help transition the body into a restful state, whether infused into tea, added to a warm bath, or diffused as an essential oil.

These small acts of herbal self-care accumulate, building a rhythm that supports overall well-being. The key is consistency—allowing herbs to work gradually and synergistically with the body. Over time, these practices evolve, responding to the seasons, personal needs, and shifting priorities, making herbalism a deeply personal, ever-changing journey.

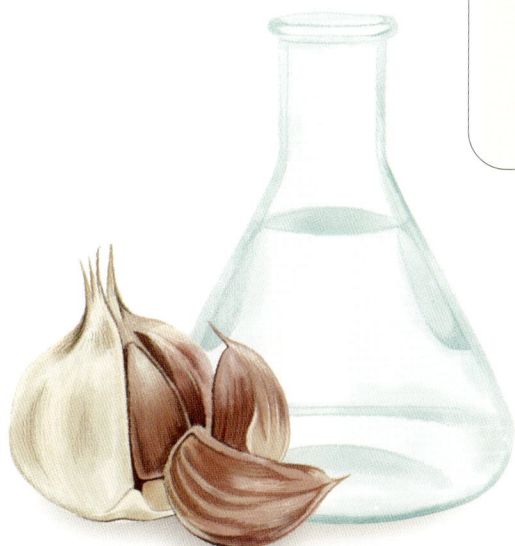

Chapter 2

Breathe Easy:
Herbs for the Respiratory System

Breathing—it's the one thing we do every moment of every day, yet it often goes unnoticed. Our respiratory system is a life-sustaining powerhouse. From the instant air enters through the nose or mouth, this system works tirelessly to filter, warm, and deliver oxygen to the bloodstream, all while keeping out unwelcome guests like dust and pathogens.

At the cellular level, the respiratory system is both a provider and a protector. Airways are lined with mucus and cilia that trap debris and sweep it out, while immune cells act as vigilant guards against deeper threats. However, modern challenges such as pollution, allergens, and seasonal shifts can put additional strain on our lungs, leaving them in need of extra support.

That's where herbs come in, offering gentle yet effective ways to bolster respiratory health. Mullein, with its soothing properties, eases irritation in dry or scratchy lungs. Elecampane acts as a gentle expectorant, helping the body clear mucus naturally. Licorice root provides anti-inflammatory support to the respiratory lining, while thyme's antimicrobial properties make it a powerful ally against respiratory infections.

In this chapter, we'll explore recipes like a Mullein-Elecampane Respiratory Cordial for when your lungs need extra care, and a Licorice and Thyme Steam for Sinuses for a spa-like experience for your airways. Let's ensure your breath—the foundation of life—remains smooth, clear, and deeply supported.

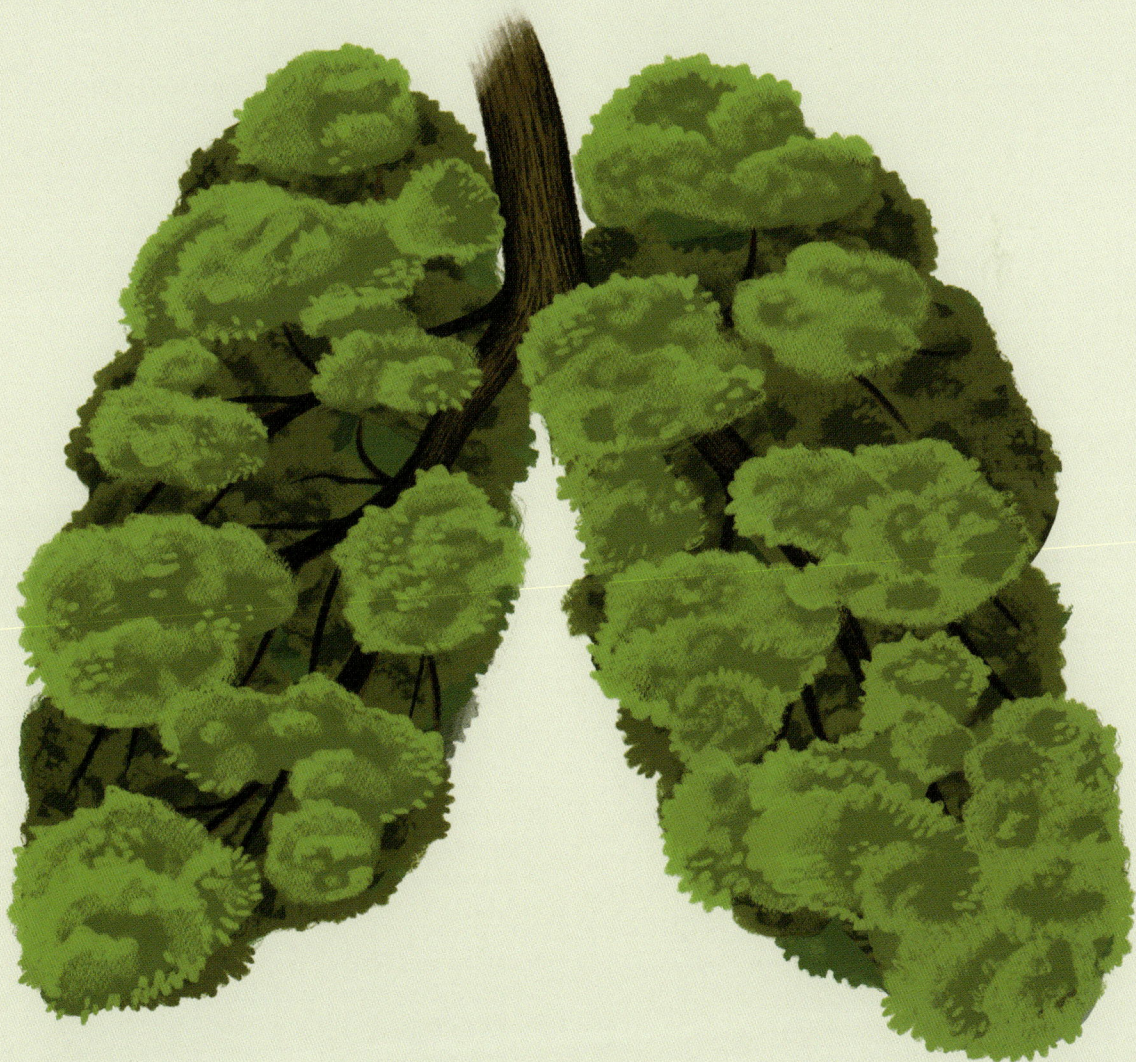

Licorice Root *(Glycyrrhiza glabra)*
The Lung's Anti-Inflammatory Ally

Licorice root, derived from the perennial legume *Glycyrrhiza glabra*, is among the most ancient and versatile medicinal herbs. Over four thousand years ago, ancient Egyptians referred to it as "sweet root" and incorporated it into healing balms and elixirs for respiratory and digestive complaints. Licorice root was found in King Tutankhamun's tomb, signifying its importance to both life and the afterlife.

Hippocrates recommended licorice for respiratory discomfort, and Dioscorides, in his *Materia Medica*, highlighted its ability to ease coughs and hoarseness. In Traditional Chinese Medicine (TCM), *Gan Cao* ("licorice root") is considered a harmonizing herb, balancing the effects of other herbs and supporting the body's energy, or *qi*.

By the twentieth century, its therapeutic potential gained wide-spread recognition in modern herbalism and pharmacology. Today licorice remains a trusted ally for respiratory and inflammatory health, celebrated for its gentle yet powerful support.

What the Science Says

Licorice (*Glycyrrhiza glabra*) root contains a variety of bioactive compounds that produce comprehensive therapeutic effects for respiratory health. To start, glycyrrhizin, a naturally occurring **triterpenoid saponin** (soap-like compounds found in plants) that is responsible for licorice's sweet taste, has anti-inflammatory, antiviral, and mucoprotective properties. It suppresses pro-inflammatory cytokines, helping to calm inflammation in the airways, and stimulates mucus production, coating and soothing irritated tissues and promoting healing in the throat and lungs. Research supports these findings. A 2020 study in *The Journal of Ethnopharmacology* found that glycyrrhizin significantly reduced inflammation in chronic respiratory diseases, and a 2018 study in *Evidence-Based Complementary and Alternative Medicine* demonstrated its ability to soothe coughs and protect mucosal membranes.

As an antiviral, glycyrrhizin prevents viruses from attaching to host cells, blocking reproduction. Research in *Phytomedicine* in 2003 supported this, demonstrating glycyrrhizin's ability to inhibit respiratory viruses, including influenza and coronaviruses.

But that's just one compound. Licorice also includes **flavonoids** like liquiritin and isoliquiritigenin that neutralize free radicals, protecting lung tissue from oxidative stress, and **polysaccharides** that activate macrophages and natural killer (NK) cells, improving the body's ability to fight infections. Additional compounds such as **coumarins** improve circulation and reduce inflammation, while **phytoestrogens** mimic estrogen, aiding hormonal balance.

Together, these constituents soothe irritation, modulate immune responses, and support respiratory health, with glycyrrhizin playing a central role in protecting mucosal linings.

Uses and Indications

Licorice root is a versatile herb for respiratory health, and its gentle and multifaceted actions make it suitable for both acute and long-term use. Licorice is good to have on hand during cold and flu season to improve immunity and combat respiratory infections. You can use it to soothe dry or irritated coughs, reduce lung inflammation, and support recovery from bronchitis, asthma, or pneumonia. It is also beneficial for adrenal health, because it reduces cortisol breakdown, which eases chronic stress or fatigue. Finally, it can also be a supportive herb for digestive health, treating ulcers, gastritis, and acid reflux by protecting and repairing the stomach lining.

Interactions and Safety

While licorice is generally safe for short-term use, you'll want to observe certain precautions. Glycyrrhizin can cause sodium retention and potassium loss, which can lead to elevated blood pressure and edema. If you have hypertension, you should limit use or opt for deglycyrrhizinated licorice (DGL), which removes glycyrrhizin to reduce these risks. While this process alters some of licorice's therapeutic properties, DGL still retains benefits for digestive health, particularly in soothing acid reflux, ulcers, and indigestion without the concerns of elevated blood pressure.

Licorice may interact with diuretics, corticosteroids, or medications for heart conditions. Its hormonal effects make it unsuitable during pregnancy without professional guidance. Prolonged use of glycyrrhizin-containing licorice is discouraged, and DGL is recommended for extended use. Consult a healthcare professional before using licorice if you have underlying conditions or are taking medications.

Growing and Harvesting Licorice

Licorice is a hardy perennial that thrives in sandy, well-drained soil and warm, temperate climates. It can grow up to 5 feet (60 cm) tall and requires full sunlight. The roots, the primary medicinal part, are typically harvested in the autumn of the plant's second or third year. After harvesting, the roots are carefully cleaned, dried, and stored in airtight containers to preserve their medicinal properties. In addition to its therapeutic value, licorice enriches soil by fixing nitrogen, making it a valuable crop for sustainable gardening practices.

Licorice and Thyme Steam for Sinuses

This herbal steam combines the anti-inflammatory properties of licorice with the antimicrobial benefits of thyme (see page 38), providing a natural remedy to ease sinus congestion and respiratory discomfort.

Preparation

Place the dried licorice root and thyme in a heatproof bowl. Pour the boiling water over the herbs and steep for 5 to 10 minutes.

Yield: Approximately 4 cups (1 L)

1 tablespoon (8 g) dried licorice root

1 tablespoon (5 g) dried thyme

4 cups (1 L) boiling water

How to Use

Once the herbs have steeped, cover your head with a towel and lean over the bowl, maintaining a safe distance to avoid burns.

Inhale deeply for about 10 minutes, letting the steam soothe your sinuses and reduce inflammation.

This steam can be used once or twice daily during colds or sinus infections to ease breathing and promote relief.

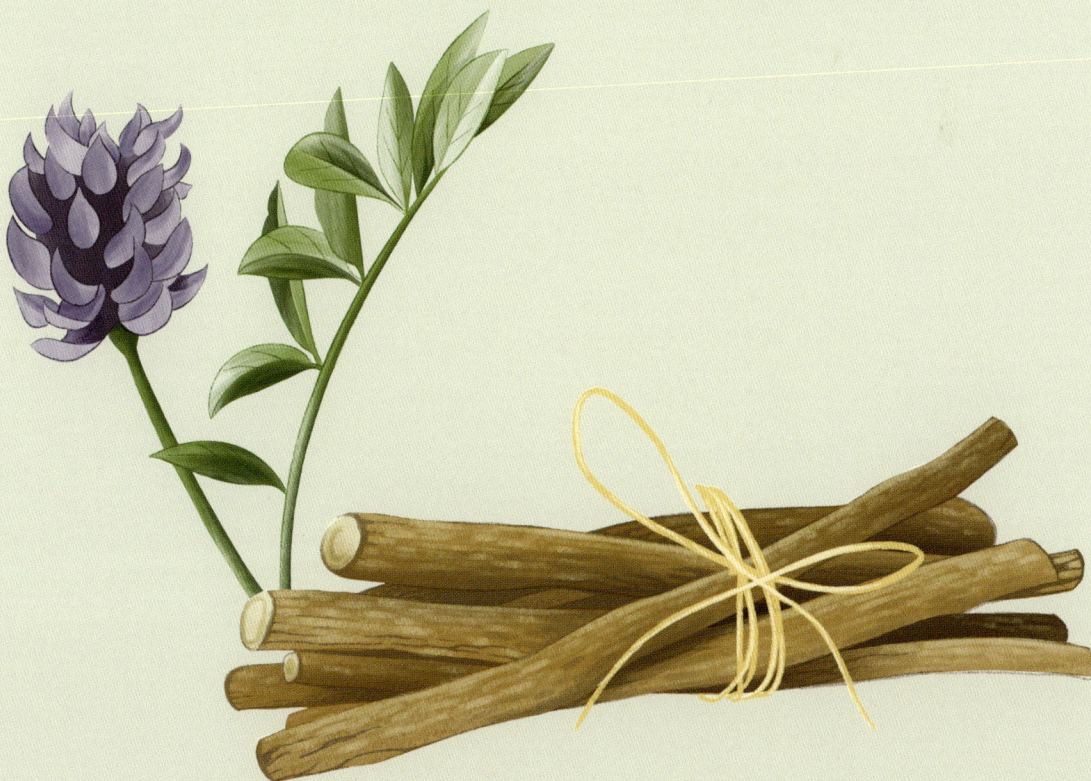

Elecampane (*Inula helenium*)
The Lung Soother

Elecampane, *Inula helenium*, is a towering herb with golden-yellow flowers that was first found in Europe and Asia and has been cherished for centuries as a remedy for respiratory health. Its name is linked to Helen of Troy. Legend says the plant emerged from her tears, so the Romans called it "helena campana," or "Helen's plant."

The ancient Greeks and Romans used elecampane as a treatment for ailments such as coughs and asthma. Dioscorides, a famed Greek physician, used the root to expel phlegm and ease breathing. Elecampane later became a staple in the apothecaries of medieval Europe, addressing conditions such as tuberculosis. It was also used as a flavoring in sweetmeats and liqueurs.

By the nineteenth century, elecampane was commonly used in the United States for its expectorant properties to ease bronchitis, pneumonia, and persistent coughs. Today it remains a staple in herbal medicine, valued for its ability to support lung health and ease respiratory symptoms.

What the Science Says

The thick, aromatic roots of elecampane (*Inula helenium*) contain a range of bioactive compounds that make it a powerful respiratory remedy. This includes **sesquiterpene lactones** such as alantolactone and isoalantolactone—a class of naturally occurring plant compounds known for their antimicrobial, anti-inflammatory, and expectorant properties. These lactones stimulate tiny hair-like structures (cilia) in the respiratory tract, aiding in mucus expulsion and congestion relief. Research in *Molecules* (2022) supports this, confirming that elecampane helped people with chronic bronchitis expel mucus more easily.

Alantolactone and isoalantolactone also combat bacteria, fungi, and even some parasites, helping to clear certain kinds of respiratory infections. Another study published in *Pathogens* in 2020 showed alantolactone effectively fights bacteria that cause infections, including staph bacteria and pneumonia-related microbes.

In addition to these two powerful lactones, elecampane's essential oils, which contain helenin, a natural mixture primarily made up of alantolactone and isoalantolactone, have lung-supportive and antiseptic effects. **Flavonoids** like quercetin offer antioxidant protection for lung tissue, while mucilage, a gel-like compound, soothes and coats irritated mucous membranes in the throat, reducing dry cough discomfort.

The root's properties also calm inflammation in the airways to ease wheezing and chest tightness, which makes breathing more comfortable. In 2020, a study in the *NFS Journal* confirmed the effect of its anti-inflammatory compounds, which can provide asthma relief.

Inulin, another key compound found in elecampane, is a prebiotic **polysaccharide**—a type of indigestible carbohydrate that feeds beneficial gut bacteria. This supports gut health and indirectly strengthen immune function. As a bitter tonic, this herb also supports digestion, which plays a crucial role in nutrient absorption and overall immune health.

Uses and Indications

Elecampane's dual actions as a lung soother and digestive aid make it a versatile herbal remedy. You can use elecampane to clear mucus and reduce inflammation if you have a chronic cough, bronchitis, asthma, a sinus infection, or pneumonia. Taking this herb can also improve your resistance to new infections by soothing inflamed tissues and combating pathogens. The carminative properties of the herb—meaning its ability to relieve gas and soothe the digestive tract—can be helpful in easing bloating, gas, and indigestion. You can also use it to support your gut health thanks to its prebiotic inulin.

Interactions and Safety

Taking elecampane is considered safe, but use caution if you're sensitive to Asteraceae family plants (e.g., ragweed, chamomile). Due to limited research, elecampane is not recommended during pregnancy and breastfeeding without professional guidance. In rare cases, elecampane can cause nausea or diarrhea, so start with a small dose to avoid this. If you're taking diuretics or blood pressure medications, consult a healthcare provider before taking elecampane, which may interact with those medications.

Growing and Harvesting Elecampane

Elecampane thrives as a hardy perennial in well-drained soil with full sunlight. It can grow up to 6 feet (2 m) tall, making it a striking addition to gardens. Its lance-shaped leaves and bright yellow flowers attract pollinators, supporting biodiversity. Plant seeds in early spring or propagate via root division in the fall. Roots are best harvested in the plant's second or third year, after foliage dies back in autumn. Clean and dry the roots thoroughly to preserve their medicinal qualities. Store dried roots in airtight containers away from light and moisture to maintain potency.

Mullein-Elecampane Respiratory Cordial

This cordial blends the soothing qualities of mullein with elecampane's respiratory benefits, creating a warming remedy for lung support. Note: *This syrup is not recommended for children under one year old, as infants should not consume honey.*

> *Yield: About 2 cups (480 ml)*

2 tablespoons (10 g) dried elecampane root

2 tablespoons (18 g) dried mullein leaves

1 cinnamon stick

3 slices fresh ginger

2 cups (480 ml) water

1 cup (240 ml) raw honey

1 cup (240 ml) brandy or vodka (optional, for preservation)

Preparation

Combine the elecampane root, mullein leaves, cinnamon stick, ginger, and water in a saucepan. Simmer gently over low heat for 30 minutes, stirring occasionally. Remove the mixture from the heat and allow it to cool slightly. Strain through a fine strainer or cheesecloth into a clean bowl. Stir in the raw honey until fully dissolved. For extended shelf life, add the brandy or vodka. Transfer the cordial to an airtight glass bottle and refrigerate for up to 3 months, or longer if alcohol is added.

How to Use

Take 1 to 2 tablespoons (15 to 30 ml) daily during cold and flu season, or up to three times daily at the onset of symptoms to support respiratory recovery. While the cordial's flavor makes it enjoyable, its potency means more isn't necessarily better. Exceeding the recommended dose may lead to excessive mucus release or mild digestive upset. For a milder approach, try diluting it in warm water or tea for a soothing, extended effect.

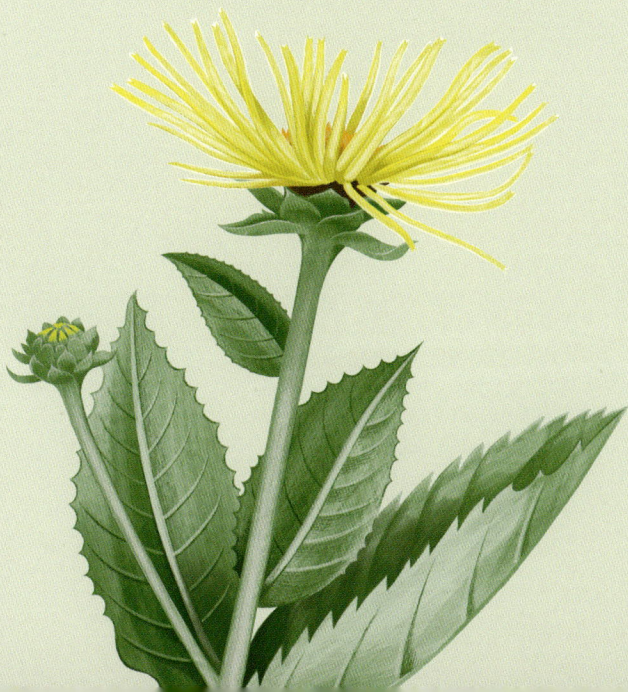

Mullein (*Verbascum thapsus*)
The Gentle Lung Guardian

Mullein, often called the "velvet plant" for its soft, fuzzy leaves, has a rich history rooted in its reputation as a gentle yet powerful remedy for respiratory health. This biennial herb is native to Europe, Asia, and North Africa and has been revered across cultures as a "guardian of the lungs."

Mullein has been used for treating respiratory ailments as far back as ancient Greece and Rome. Native American tribes, including the Cherokee and Iroquois, adopted mullein as a sacred remedy for lung health. Its leaves and flowers were used to create teas, poultices, and smokes for treating coughs, asthma, and bronchial inflammation. The plant's gentle nature made it suitable for a wide range of people, from children to elders.

By the nineteenth century, mullein had become a staple of Western herbalism. Eclectic physicians in North America frequently prescribed it for conditions such as tuberculosis, chronic coughs, and pleurisy, thanks to its ability to soothe inflamed airways and promote healthy mucus production. Mullein has long been a true guardian of health—comforting, versatile, and invaluable to those who have relied on its many gifts.

What the Science Says

The therapeutic effects of mullein (*Verbascum thapsus*) come from its ability to act as both an expectorant (helping the body remove excess mucus) and a soothing agent (protecting irritated tissues). The first effect is thanks to **saponins**, which are **phytocompounds**—plant-derived chemicals—primarily found in the leaves and flowers of the plant that work as natural expectorants. These compounds help loosen and break down mucus, making it easier to expel from the lungs. This supports productive coughs (clearing congestion) and promotes better lung function.

The second effect comes from the leaves, which are rich in mucilage, a gel-like substance that coats and protects the mucous membranes, reducing inflammation and irritation in the respiratory tract. This protective barrier helps soothe dry, scratchy coughs and provides relief for irritated tissues. A 2021 study published in *Biology* found that saponins and mucilage work together to help thin mucus and soothe inflamed tissues, making breathing easier.

Mullein flowers contain **flavonoids** and **iridoid glycosides**, plant compounds known for their anti-inflammatory and antimicrobial effects, such as aucubin, which can help reduce irritation and fight infection. A 2021 study published in *Pharmacognosy Journal* showed mullein's antimicrobial activity against common respiratory pathogens, supporting its traditional use for respiratory infections.

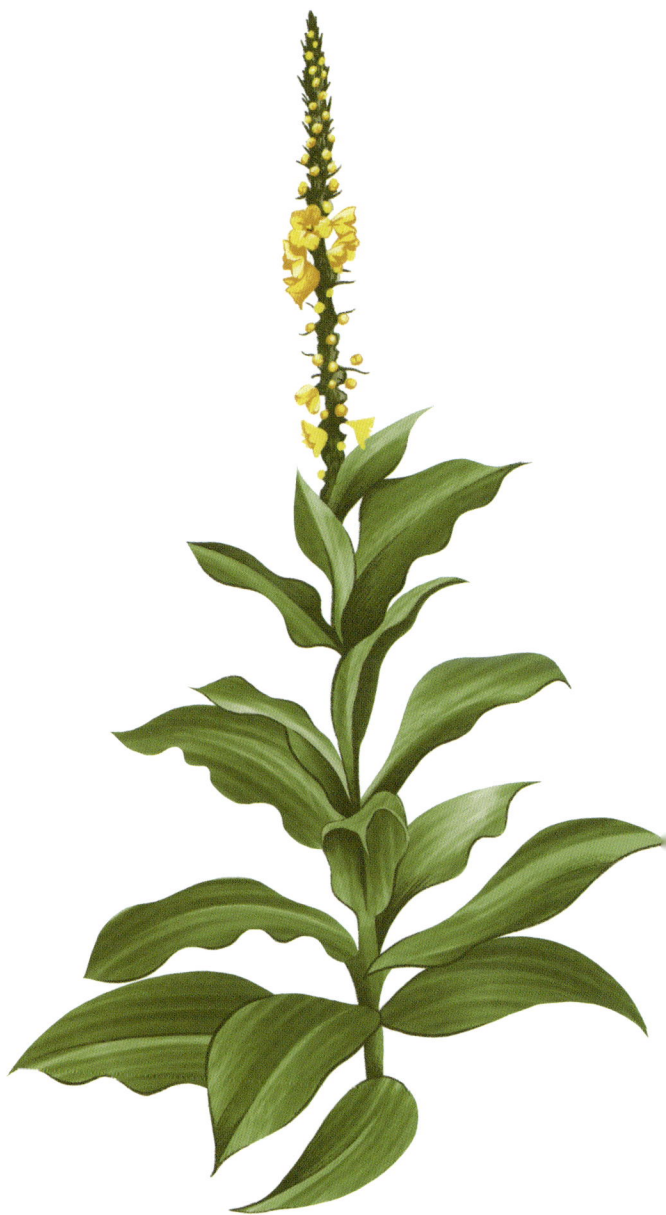

All these compounds work together to support lung health, making mullein a go-to remedy for coughs, congestion, and respiratory discomfort.

Uses and Indications

You can use mullein to treat a variety of respiratory conditions. It can help treat a persistent cough, whether it's dry and irritating or wet and productive. If you have bronchitis, mullein offers relief by thinning mucus and reducing inflammation, helping to restore normal breathing.

If you have asthma, mullein can help calm inflamed airways. By reducing bronchial irritation, the herb can also ease wheezing and improve airflow. If you suffer from seasonal allergies, mullein helps soothe and calm irritated sinuses and reduce congestion.

Mullein is good to keep on hand during cold and flu season as a natural remedy for common respiratory symptoms, including sore throats, nasal congestion, and chest tightness. Traditionally it is also used for smoker's cough, because it helps remove tar and toxins from the lungs while promoting lung repair.

Interactions and Safety

Mullein is safe and well-tolerated by most individuals. However, the fine hairs on mullein leaves can irritate the throat and lungs if inhaled directly, so it is essential to strain any infusions or preparations thoroughly before use.

Allergic reactions to mullein are rare but possible, particularly for individuals with sensitivities to other members of the Scrophulariaceae family, such as figwort (*Scrophularia nodosa*), buddleia (*Buddleja davidii*), or verbascum species. Symptoms may include mild skin irritation or respiratory discomfort. People with severe or chronic lung conditions, such as chronic obstructive pulmonary disease (COPD), should consult a healthcare provider before using mullein to ensure it aligns with their treatment plan.

Quality of mullein can vary, so if you'd like to use it for respiratory health be sure to choose high-quality preparations and consult a healthcare professional, especially if you are pregnant, nursing, or managing chronic respiratory conditions.

Growing and Harvesting

Mullein is a resilient biennial plant that thrives in a wide range of climates and soil types. During its first year, the plant develops a low rosette of soft, woolly leaves. In its second year, it sends up a striking flower stalk, often reaching 6 feet (2 m) or more in height, adorned with yellow blooms.

For medicinal purposes, the leaves are best harvested during the plant's first year when they are at their most potent. The flowers, which bloom in the second year, should be collected on sunny days when they are fully open. Both the leaves and flowers should be dried in a cool, dark, and well-ventilated space to preserve their therapeutic properties. Proper storage in airtight containers will ensure the herb's potency for months to come.

Mullein is also a valuable addition to the ecosystem. Its tall stalks and vibrant flowers attract pollinators like bees and butterflies, while its presence in gardens or wild spaces supports biodiversity.

Fun Fact

Mullein's velvety texture has also earned it the nickname "flannel leaf," a reference to the comforting, wool-like feel of its foliage, which has provided practical uses throughout history. It has been used as makeshift bandages, as linings for shoes to prevent blisters, and been tucked into clothing as a natural insulation layer against the cold, making it a cherished survival plant.

Mullein Extract (Alcohol-Free) for Respiratory Relief

Yield: Approximately 2 cups (480 ml)

This extract is a gentle and alcohol-free preparation, perfect for soothing the lungs and promoting clearer breathing. Its easy-to-use format makes it an excellent choice for respiratory health during cold and flu season or times of congestion.

½ cup (72 g) dried mullein leaves

11 ounces (308 ml) vegetable glycerin

5 ounces (140 ml) very warm distilled water

Preparation

Add the dried mullein leaves to a clean, airtight glass jar. In a separate container, mix the vegetable glycerin and warm distilled water to create the solvent. Pour the solvent over the mullein leaves, ensuring they are fully submerged, leaving about ½ inch (1 cm) of liquid above the herbs to account for swelling.

Seal the jar tightly and store it in a cool, dark place for 4 to 6 weeks, shaking it gently every few days to encourage extraction.

After steeping, strain the mixture through a fine strainer or cheesecloth into a clean bowl, pressing the plant material to extract all the liquid. Transfer the extract to a dark glass dropper bottle and store it in a cool, dark place.

How to Use

Take 1 to 2 droppers full (about 1 to 2 ml) as needed to calm the lungs, ease congestion, and promote clearer breathing. This extract is particularly helpful during cold and flu season or for individuals seeking gentle respiratory support.

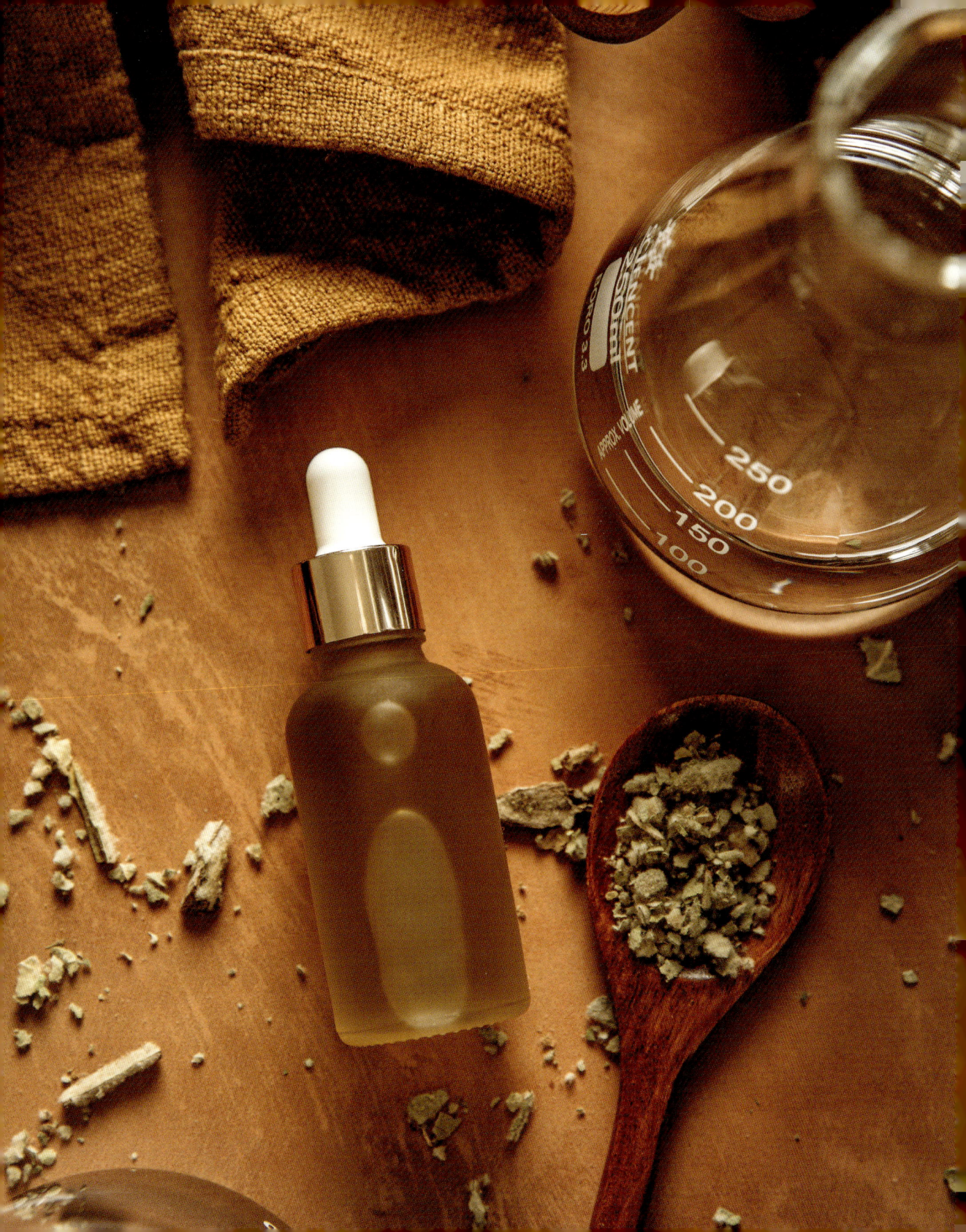

Thyme *(Thymus vulgaris)*
The Antimicrobial Lung Defender

Thyme, a fragrant culinary and medicinal herb native to the Mediterranean region, has been valued for its healing properties for thousands of years. Its use dates back to ancient Egypt, where it was used in embalming practices and as a remedy for respiratory ailments. The Greeks and Romans regarded thyme a symbol of courage and purification and often burned it in sacred spaces, in addition to using it to flavor food. Hippocrates documented thyme's effectiveness in treating respiratory conditions such as coughs and bronchitis. Later, in the Middle Ages, thyme essential oil was applied to wounds to prevent infection and carried as a protective herb to ward off disease.

Today thyme continues to be a staple in herbal medicine, particularly for its ability to support respiratory health and fight infections.

What the Science Says

Thyme *(Thymus vulgaris)* derives its medicinal properties from its aerial parts—the leaves, flowers, and stems support respiratory health by disrupting pathogens, reducing inflammation, and clearing mucus from the lungs. Clinical trials, such as those published in *Arzneimittel-Forschung* in 2006 demonstrated that thyme extracts, when combined with other herbs like ivy leaf (*Hedera helix*), primula root (*Primula veris*), and elderflower (*Sambucus nigra*), can alleviate symptoms of bronchitis and cough and improve respiratory function. This is in large part thanks to its most potent compound: thymol, which is a **phenolic compound**—a plant-based molecule made up of at least one hydroxyl group attached to an aromatic ring—with antimicrobial, antifungal, and antiviral properties.

A 2019 study in *Veterinary Dermatology* found that thymol exhibits strong antimicrobial activity against respiratory pathogens, including *Staphylococcus aureus* and *Streptococcus pneumoniae*. It works in partnership with carvacrol, another compound found in the herb. Carvacrol is a monoterpenoid phenol, a type of small, aromatic plant compound known for its strong antimicrobial activity. Thymol and carvacrol work together to break down the cell membranes of bacteria, fungi, and viruses, effectively neutralizing harmful microbes.

Thyme also contains **flavonoids** and rosmarinic acid, a **polyphenolic compound**—plant-based molecules made up of multiple linked phenol units known for strong antioxidant and anti-inflammatory effects. Both of these compounds provide antioxidant protection for lung tissues and reduce inflammation. Research published in *Phytomedicine* in 2024 confirmed thyme's ability to reduce lung inflammation, thus making it easier to breathe.

Thyme also functions as a natural expectorant, helping to loosen and clear mucus from the lungs, which promotes faster recovery from respiratory infections. This is due in part to its **terpenes**—aromatic plant compounds with antimicrobial and anti-inflammatory properties that help combat pathogens and protect respiratory tissues.

With its broad-spectrum antimicrobial effects, inflammation-reducing properties, and ability to support lung health, thyme remains a powerful herbal remedy for respiratory wellness.

Uses and Indications

You can use thyme to treat respiratory conditions such as bronchitis, asthma, and sinus infections. Not only do its antimicrobial properties make it effective against bacterial, viral, and fungal infections, but its anti-inflammatory and expectorant effects also soothe irritated airways and promote mucus clearance. You can also use thyme used to support digestive health, boost immunity, and enhance overall respiratory function.

Interactions and Safety

Thyme is generally safe when used in culinary or medicinal doses. However, if you have allergies to plants in the Lamiaceae family, such as mint or oregano, you may also be allergic to thyme. If you're pregnant or breastfeeding, you should consult a healthcare professional before using thyme in medicinal amounts.

To prevent skin irritation, thyme's essential oil should always be diluted before being used topically. Excessive use of thyme may cause gastrointestinal discomfort or interact with anticoagulant medications, so caution is advised.

Growing and Harvesting Thyme

Thyme is a hardy perennial herb that thrives in well-drained soil and full sunlight. It is drought-tolerant and requires minimal maintenance, making it an ideal choice for home gardens. Thyme can be propagated from seeds, cuttings, or root divisions and grows best in temperate climates. The aerial parts of the plant should be harvested just before flowering, when the concentration of essential oils is at its peak. After harvesting, thyme can be dried and stored in an airtight container to preserve its potency.

See page 31 for a recipe for a Licorice and Thyme Steam for Sinuses that can be used to relieve sinus congestion and respiratory discomfort.

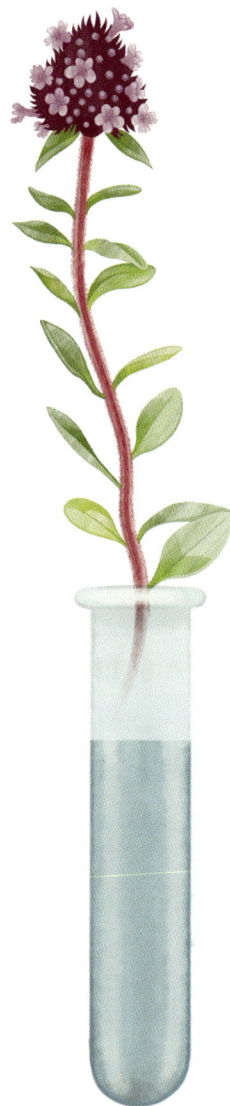

Fun Fact

Thyme was once burned like incense in ancient temples, not just for the heavenly aroma, but because people believed it could "purify" the air. Turns out, they were onto something: Thyme's vapors actually contain compounds that can help clear airborne bacteria and open up your airways. Ancient air freshener *and* a breath of fresh thyme!

Chapter 3

Take Heart: Herbs for the Cardiovascular System

The heart is far more than a pump—it's the rhythm, pulse, and lifeline of our body. As the centerpiece of the cardiovascular system, it works alongside arteries, veins, and capillaries to deliver oxygen, nutrients, and warmth to every cell while removing waste. On a cellular level, the heart drives blood flow through intricate networks of vessels, ensuring each tissue and organ receives the resources it needs to thrive.

Every beat is powered by the flow of ions across cell membranes, triggering contraction and maintaining the rhythm that defines our vitality. However, factors like stress, poor diet, and aging can strain this system, leading to inflammation, high blood pressure, or plaque buildup that disrupts circulation. Fortunately, herbal allies can support cardiovascular health at both cellular and systemic levels, promoting resilience and balance.

Hawthorn, a traditional heart tonic, supports circulation and heart function, gently helping to regulate blood pressure. Motherwort offers calming support, easing stress that can elevate blood pressure. While arjuna is renowned in Ayurvedic medicine for its antioxidant protection of blood vessels, ginkgo simultaneously promotes blood flow by dilating vessels and supporting oxygen delivery to the brain and extremities.

In this chapter you'll find recipes including a heart-strengthening Hawthorn Berry Cordial and a soothing Motherwort and Coleus Tonic for Heart Calm, perfect for moments when life feels overwhelming. Caring for our hearts goes beyond physical health; it nurtures emotional and energetic balance, helping us stay in tune with the rhythm of life. Let's explore how herbs can keep our hearts strong, calm, and connected.

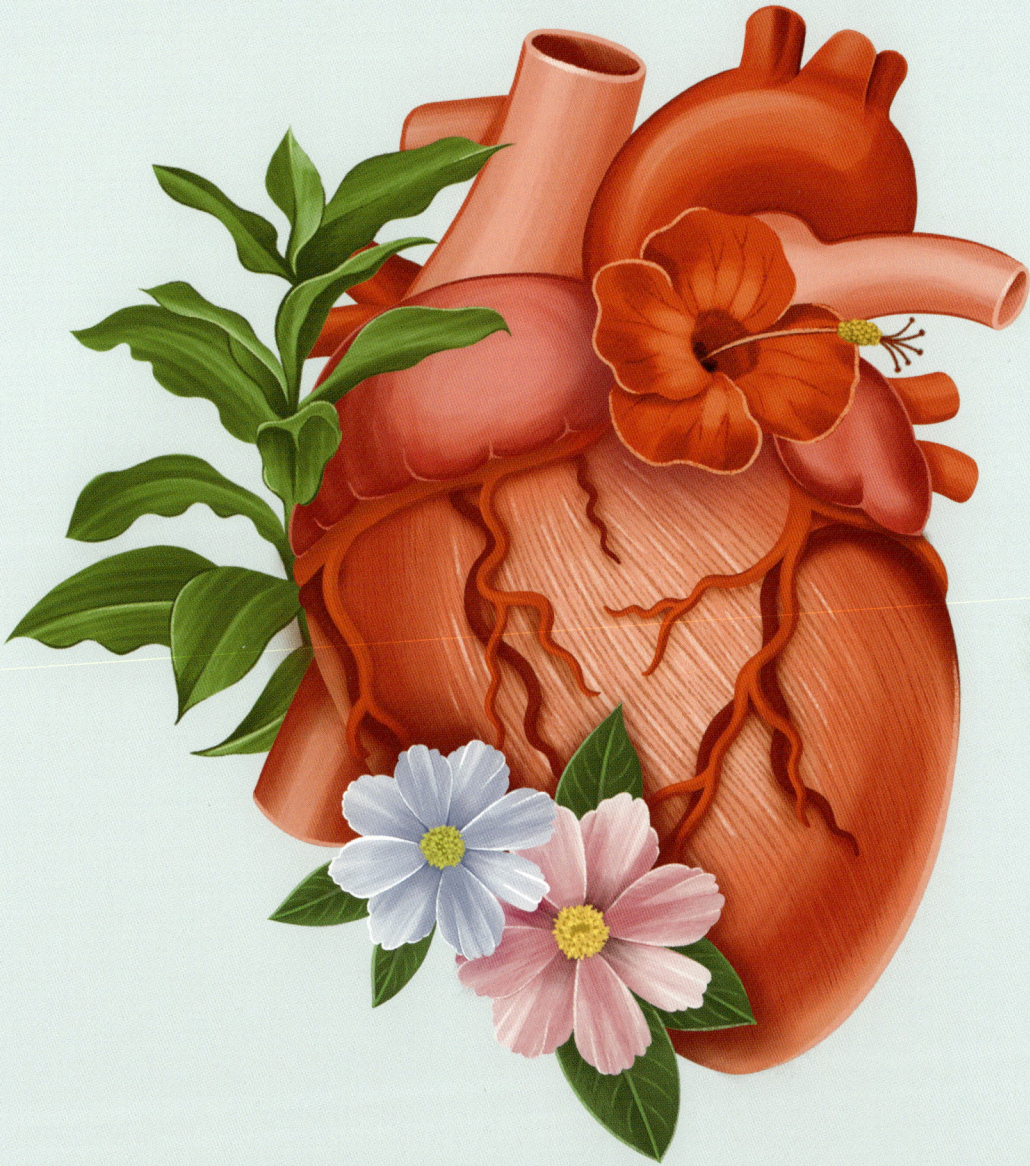

Motherwort (*Leonurus cardiaca*)
The Heart Calmer

Motherwort (*Leonurus cardiaca*) has long been cherished in both European and Chinese medicine for its ability to calm the heart and mind. Historically, it was used to ease heart palpitations, address mild hypertension, promote circulation, and calm anxiety. In fact, European herbalists prepared motherwort tonics not only for cardiovascular health but also as a soothing remedy for nervous tension and restlessness, recognizing its ability to bring balance to both the body and mind.

Motherwort is often closely allied with feminine energy. In medieval Europe, it was used as a remedy for women's reproductive health, earning it the name "mother's herb" for its role in easing menstrual and postpartum discomforts. It plays a similar role in Traditional Chinese Medicine. Known in that tradition as *Yi Mu Cao*, it was revered for its ability to invigorate blood flow, regulate menstruation, and support the heart. It was often prescribed to promote circulation and relieve stagnation, aligning with its Western use for easing mild hypertension and heart palpitations.

By the nineteenth century, motherwort was a staple in Western herbal medicine, frequently recommended by Eclectic physicians for irregular heart rhythms, anxiety, and reproductive health. Today its gentle yet effective properties continue to make it a go-to herb for those seeking natural support for both the heart and hormonal balance. More than just a medicinal plant, motherwort represents resilience, protection, and the deep connection between physical and emotional well-being.

What the Science Says

Motherwort (*Leonurus cardiaca*) is valued for its aerial parts—the leaves, flowers, and stems—which contain a range of bioactive compounds that support both cardiovascular and emotional health. Motherwort's effects on the heart and nervous system stem from its cardiotonic, vasodilating, and nervine properties.

One of its key active compounds is leonurine, an **alkaloid**—a naturally occurring compound often found in medicinal plants with potent physiological effects—that is known for its heart-strengthening (cardiotonic) and mild sedative properties.

Leonurine relaxes smooth muscles in blood vessels, promoting vasodilation, which helps improve blood flow and ease strain on the heart. This makes motherwort useful for mild hypertension and heart palpitations. A 2008 study in *The Cochrane Database of Systematic Reviews* confirmed that leonurine improves heart function by enhancing blood flow and reducing oxidative stress.

Another significant compound, stachydrine, improves circulation and supports uterine health, contributing to motherwort's traditional use in women's reproductive wellness. The herb's **flavonoids** and **phenolic acids** provide antioxidant protection, neutralizing free radicals that could otherwise damage cardiac tissues. **Volatile oils** and phenolic acids add to motherwort's calming and anti-inflammatory effects, reinforcing its ability to soothe both the heart and the mind.

Motherwort's nervine properties act on the central nervous system, helping to ease stress, anxiety, and tension. By calming the fight-or-flight response, motherwort promotes emotional resilience and relaxation, which reinforces its reputation as a "heart calmer" for both physical and emotional well-being. A 2011 study in *Phytotherapy Research* confirmed motherwort's mild sedative effects and its ability to reduce anxiety-related symptoms.

With its unique combination of heart-supporting, stress-reducing, and circulation-enhancing properties, motherwort remains a trusted herbal ally for cardiovascular and nervous system health.

Uses and Indications

You can use versatile motherwort for heart palpitations, mild hypertension, and stress-related cardiovascular symptoms. It is particularly beneficial if you experience irregular heartbeats or anxiety-induced heart discomfort. In fact, motherwort is generally effective for reducing stress and promoting emotional balance due to its calming effect on the nervous system. For people who menstruate, motherwort supports reproductive health by easing menstrual cramps, regulating cycles, and alleviating postpartum discomfort.

Interactions and Safety

Motherwort is generally safe when used appropriately, though it should be avoided during pregnancy, as its uterine-stimulating properties may increase the risk of miscarriage. If you're on blood-thinning or heart medications such as beta-blockers, talk to your healthcare provider before using motherwort to avoid potential interactions. Mild side effects, such as gastrointestinal discomfort or drowsiness, are rare but possible, particularly at higher doses. For optimal safety, it's best to use motherwort under the guidance of a qualified professional, especially if you have a pre-existing heart condition.

Growing and Harvesting

Motherwort is a hardy perennial that thrives in a variety of climates, preferring well-drained soil and full to partial sunlight. It is commonly found in meadows, along roadsides, and in gardens, where its tall, spiky stems and clusters of small purple flowers attract pollinators. The aerial parts of the plant are harvested during its flowering stage in late spring or early summer, when its medicinal compounds are most concentrated. After harvesting, the plant material should be dried in a well-ventilated area away from direct sunlight to preserve its potency. Proper storage in an airtight container ensures the herb's therapeutic properties remain intact for months.

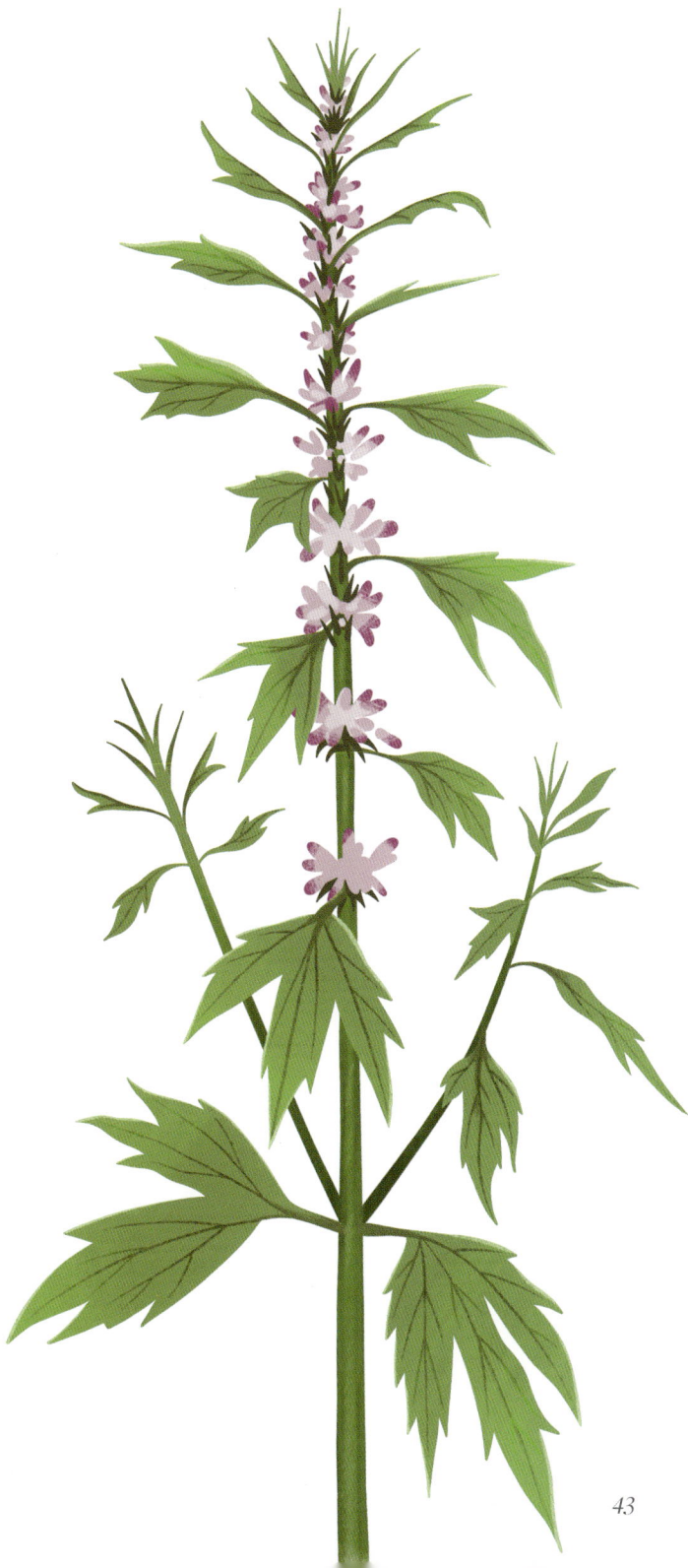

Motherwort and Coleus Tonic for Heart Calm

This soothing tonic combines the calming properties of motherwort with the circulatory benefits of coleus (see page 172), creating a heart-supportive remedy that is both effective and enjoyable. Note: *This syrup is not recommended for children under one year old, as infants should not consume honey.*

Yield: About 2 cups (480 ml)

2 tablespoons (28 g) dried motherwort

1 tablespoon (3 g) dried coleus leaves

1 cinnamon stick

1 teaspoon (0.66 g) dried lemon balm

2 cups (480 ml) water

1 cup (240 ml) raw honey

1 cup (240 ml) brandy or vodka (optional, for preservation)

Preparation

Combine the dried motherwort, coleus leaves, cinnamon stick, lemon balm, and water in a medium saucepan. Simmer gently over low heat for 20 to 30 minutes, stirring occasionally to extract the herbs' medicinal properties. Remove the mixture from the heat to cool it slightly. Strain the liquid through a fine strainer or cheesecloth into a clean bowl, pressing the solids to extract as much liquid as possible. Stir in the raw honey until fully dissolved, and if desired, add brandy or vodka to extend the tonic's shelf life. Transfer the prepared tonic to an airtight glass bottle and refrigerate for up to 3 months (or longer if alcohol is included).

How to Use

Take 1 to 2 tablespoons (15 to 30 ml) daily as a heart tonic or up to three times daily during periods of heightened stress or heart discomfort. The tonic can be enjoyed on its own, but for a more soothing drink, try adding 1 to 2 tablespoons (15 to 30 ml) to warm water or herbal tea. It also pairs well with sparkling water and a squeeze of lemon for a refreshing, heart-supportive beverage.

Fun Fact

Motherwort's Latin name, *Leonurus cardiaca*, translates to "lion-hearted," symbolizing courage and strength while reflecting its use in cardiovascular health. In medieval Europe, it was believed to instill courage and resilience, with warriors using it to steady their nerves before battle.

Three Common Herbal Myths and Misconceptions

Despite the growing popularity of herbalism, misconceptions persist, often preventing people from embracing the full potential of plant medicine. First, one of the most common myths is that "natural always means safe." While herbs offer powerful health benefits, they must still be used with knowledge and respect. Some herbs interact with medications, and certain plants can be toxic in high doses. Understanding proper usage and contraindications is key to using herbs safely and effectively.

The second widespread misconception is that herbs work instantly, similar to pharmaceutical drugs. Herbalism focuses on long-term support and restoring balance, rather than offering a quick fix. While some herbs, such as valerian or peppermint, can provide immediate relief, most herbal remedies work gradually, strengthening the body's systems over time. Consistency and patience are essential when working with plant medicine.

Third, there's a common belief that herbalism should replace conventional medicine. In reality, herbs work best when integrated into a holistic lifestyle that includes proper nutrition, exercise or movement, and, when necessary, conventional medical care. Herbal medicine and modern medicine are not mutually exclusive; they can complement each other, enhancing overall well-being.

By dispelling these myths, we can foster a more informed and empowered approach to herbalism—one that values both tradition and scientific understanding.

Arjuna *(Terminalia arjuna)*
The Heart's Guardian

Arjuna *(Terminalia arjuna)* is a revered herb in Ayurvedic medicine, renowned for thousands of years for its role as a protector of heart health. Often referred to as "the guardian of the heart" in India, this herb has been used traditionally to strengthen the heart, improve circulation, and promote longevity. Ancient texts, including the *Charaka Samhita* and *Sushruta Samhita*, document arjuna's use in treating heart ailments and supporting overall vitality. Beyond its physical benefits, arjuna was also valued for its ability to calm the mind and uplift the spirit, making it a holistic remedy for both the body and the soul.

In addition to its cardiovascular benefits, Ayurvedic practitioners turned to arjuna for its cooling and stabilizing effects on the nervous system, using it to ease stress, regulate blood pressure, and bring emotional balance. It was commonly prepared as a decoction, infused in milk or water, and sometimes combined with warming spices like cinnamon to enhance its absorption and synergy with the body.

By the time Ayurveda spread beyond India, arjuna gained global recognition for its potent effects on heart health. Modern research continues to validate its traditional uses, highlighting its role in supporting cardiac function, improving circulation, and promoting arterial strength.

What the Science Says

The bark of the arjuna tree *(Terminalia arjuna)* is its most medicinally active part, containing a variety of bioactive compounds that support heart health. Among these are compounds that function similarly to coenzyme Q10, a nutrient vital for cellular energy production, helping to strengthen the heart muscle and improve its pumping efficiency. This can improve cardiovascular endurance. In fact, a 1994 study published in the *Journal of the Association of Physicians of India* found that arjuna extract significantly reduced the frequency of angina episodes and improved cardiac performance.

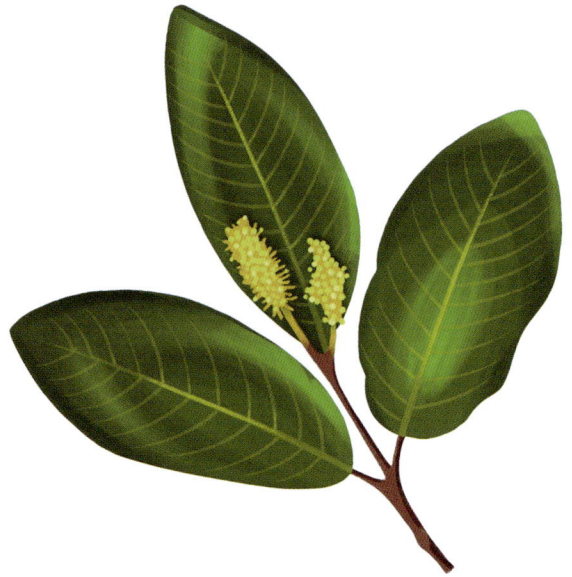

Arjuna also offers potent antioxidant protection through **flavonoids** such as quercetin. These shield the cardiovascular system from oxidative stress and reduce the risk of heart disease. **Tannins**—plant-based **polyphenols** with astringent properties—fortify blood vessel walls, improving their elasticity and structural integrity. Together, these compounds protect blood vessels from oxidative damage, maintaining their integrity and reducing the risk of plaque buildup. A 2014 study published in *Cardiology Research and Practice* highlighted these antioxidant effects, showing that it protected against ischemic heart damage, a condition caused by reduced blood flow and oxygen to the heart muscle, often due to arterial blockages.

Arjuna also promotes healthy cholesterol metabolism via **saponins**—naturally occurring plant glycosides known for their ability to bind to cholesterol and fats in the digestive tract. These saponins aid in the breakdown of LDL ("bad") cholesterol and triglycerides. This is supported by a 2021 study published in *Plant Archives*, which showed that arjuna lowered total cholesterol and LDL levels, supporting heart health.

In addition, calcium and magnesium found in arjuna bark play a role in regulating heart rhythm and muscle contractions. Its mild diuretic effect also helps reduce fluid retention, which can alleviate symptoms of hypertension and heart failure. Anti-inflammatory properties further ease stress on the cardiovascular system, making it a valuable remedy for chronic heart conditions.

With its heart-strengthening, cholesterol-regulating, and circulation-enhancing properties, arjuna remains one of the most trusted botanical remedies for long-term cardiovascular support.

Uses and Indications

You can use arjuna to support heart function, promote healthy blood pressure, and improve circulation. This is especially helpful if you have a mild to moderate heart condition, such as angina, arrhythmias, or hypertension. Arjuna's ability to strengthen the heart muscle makes it an excellent choice if you are recovering from a cardiac event or want to prevent cardiovascular disease. Beyond its cardiovascular benefits, arjuna supports stress management by calming the nervous system and promoting emotional resilience. Its holistic approach to heart health makes it a valuable addition to any wellness routine.

Interactions and Safety

For optimal safety, use this herb under the guidance of a qualified professional, especially if you have a pre-existing heart condition. Arjuna is generally safe when used appropriately. But it may enhance the effects of certain heart medications, such as beta-blockers or calcium channel blockers, so if you're taking these drugs talk to your doctor first. Avoid arjuna if you're pregnant or breastfeeding, as there is limited research on its safety in these populations. Mild side effects, such as gastrointestinal discomfort, are rare but possible if taken in high doses.

Growing and Harvesting

Arjuna is a fast-growing tree native to the Indian subcontinent, thriving in well-drained soils near riverbanks and wetlands. The tree can reach heights of up to 65 feet (20 m), with smooth gray bark that is harvested for medicinal use. The bark is typically collected in the spring or fall, using sustainable methods that allow the tree to regenerate. After harvesting, the bark is dried in a well-ventilated area away from direct sunlight to preserve its active compounds. Once fully dried, it can be broken into smaller pieces and ground into a fine powder using a mortar and pestle or a spice grinder for ease of use in teas and formulations. Proper storage in airtight containers ensures its potency for months to come.

Fun Fact

In ancient Indian mythology, the arjuna tree is named after the heroic warrior Arjuna from the *Mahabharata*, symbolizing strength, resilience, and the ability to overcome challenges. This connection reflects the herb's role as a protector of the heart and a source of vitality for those who use it.

Arjuna Heart-Strengthening Tea

This warming tea combines the benefits of arjuna bark with the cardiovascular support of hibiscus and cinnamon, creating a soothing remedy for heart health.

Yield: 1 cup (240 ml)

1 cup (240 ml) water

1 teaspoon (3 g) arjuna bark powder

½ teaspoon (0.88 g) dried hibiscus flowers (optional, for added cardiovascular support)

¼ teaspoon (0.65 g) ground cinnamon (optional, for flavor and heart health)

Raw honey or maple syrup to taste (optional)

Preparation

Bring the water to a boil in a small pot or kettle. Add the arjuna bark powder, along with the hibiscus and cinnamon if desired. Reduce the heat and let the mixture simmer gently for 10 to 15 minutes, allowing the medicinal compounds to infuse. Strain the tea into a mug using a fine-mesh or tea strainer. Sweeten with raw honey or maple syrup if desired, and sip warm to support heart health and circulation.

How to Use

Drink 1 cup (240 ml) daily as a heart tonic or enjoy during times of stress to promote relaxation and cardiovascular support.

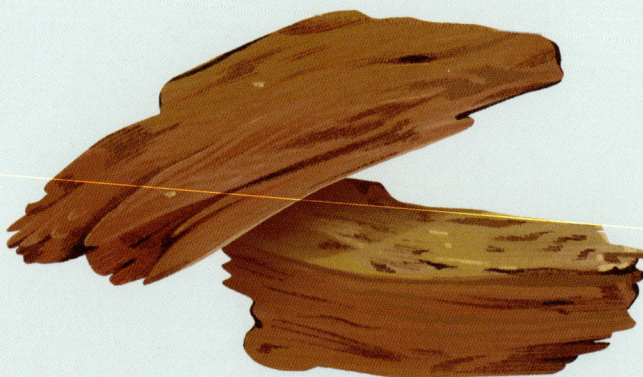

Ginkgo (*Ginkgo biloba*)
The Circulation Enhancer

Known as one of the oldest living tree species, ginkgo (*Ginko biloba*) has been thriving since the time of the dinosaurs and holds a revered place in Traditional Chinese Medicine. Ancient Chinese practitioners prescribed ginkgo for circulatory health and cognitive support, often emphasizing its value in aging populations. Beyond China, ginkgo found its way into Japanese and Korean traditions, where it was planted at Shinto shrines and used in herbal preparations for memory and vitality.

By the eighteenth century, ginkgo made its way to Europe, where its resilience and striking foliage captured the attention of botanists. Western herbalists quickly adopted its use, intrigued by its potential to enhance blood flow and cognitive function. Today ginkgo remains one of the most extensively studied medicinal plants, bridging ancient wisdom with modern scientific research in the fields of neuroprotection, vascular health, and overall longevity.

What the Science Says

The medicinal power of ginkgo (*Ginkgo biloba*) resides primarily in its leaves, which are rich in **terpenoids**—bioactive compounds that improve blood flow and protect nerve cells—and **flavonoids**. Together, these bioactive compounds work in synergy, supporting both vascular integrity and cognitive function, making ginkgo an exceptional remedy for circulatory and neurological health.

Terpenoids, including ginkgolides and bilobalides, promote better circulation by reducing blood viscosity, inhibiting platelet aggregation, and dilating blood vessels. This reduces the risk of blood clots and improves overall blood flow. A 2015 study in *Integrative Medicine International* showed that ginkgo enhanced peripheral circulation, reduced symptoms of claudication (poor circulation), and improved walking distance in patients.

At the molecular level, terpenoids improve blood vessel elasticity and stimulate the production of nitric oxide, which helps relax blood vessels and promotes healthy circulation. This improved circulation benefits the brain and extremities by ensuring a consistent supply of oxygen and nutrients.

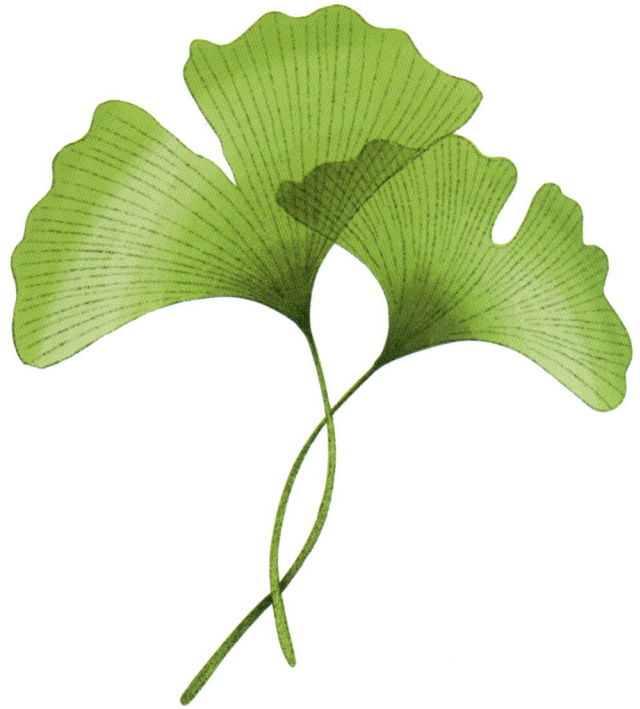

Ginko's flavonoids, which include quercetin and kaempferol, add an extra layer of protection by neutralizing free radicals, preventing oxidative damage to blood vessels and brain cells. Research published in the *Journal of the American Society for Experimental NeuroTherapeutics* (2019) confirmed these protective effects for both the brain and the cardiovascular system.

This dual action—improving circulation and protecting against oxidative stress—makes ginkgo a powerful tool for both vascular health and mental clarity. A 2020 study published in *Neurotherapeutics* found that ginkgo extract improved cognitive function and memory in individuals with mild cognitive impairment. Whether used to sharpen the mind, enhance circulation, or maintain overall vitality, ginkgo continues to prove why it has remained a staple in herbal medicine for centuries.

Uses and Indications

You can use ginkgo to improve circulation, support cognitive function, and reduce symptoms associated with poor blood flow, such as cold or pain in the extremities. It is particularly beneficial if you seek to boost blood flow to the brain, improve focus and mental clarity, or manage age-related cognitive decline. You can also use ginkgo as a supportive remedy for tinnitus, vertigo, and other conditions linked to vascular insufficiency. Its holistic approach to circulation and brain health makes it an essential herb if you're looking to remain vital as you age.

Interactions and Safety

Ginkgo is considered safe for most people. But since it reduces platelet aggregation in blood vessels, it may enhance the effects of blood-thinning medications, such as warfarin or aspirin, increasing the risk of bleeding. If you have a bleeding disorder or are scheduled for surgery, avoid ginkgo or consult a healthcare provider beforehand. Mild side effects, such as gastrointestinal discomfort or headaches, are rare but possible. If you're pregnant or breastfeeding, use ginkgo with caution as there is limited safety data in these populations. For optimal results, ginkgo should be used under professional guidance, especially when combined with other medications.

Growing and Harvesting

Ginkgo trees are remarkably hardy and thrive in a variety of climates. They prefer well-drained soil and full sunlight but are adaptable to urban environments, often found lining streets and parks. The trees can grow up to 130 feet (40 m) tall and are resistant to pests and diseases, making them a low-maintenance addition to gardens. Ginkgo leaves are typically harvested in late summer or early fall, when their concentration of bioactive compounds is highest. After harvesting, the leaves are dried in a cool, dark, and well-ventilated area to preserve their potency. Proper storage in airtight containers ensures their medicinal value is retained.

Fun Fact

Ginkgo trees are often referred to as "living fossils" because they have remained virtually unchanged for over 200 million years. Remarkably, ginkgo trees were among the few living plants to survive the atomic bombing of Hiroshima, symbolizing resilience and longevity—qualities reflected in the herb's medicinal benefits.

Ginkgo Leaf Extract

This gentle, alcohol-free preparation captures the therapeutic properties of ginkgo leaves, making it a convenient remedy for promoting circulation and mental clarity.

Yield: About 1 cup (240 ml)

½ cup (25 g) dried ginkgo leaves

¾ cup (180 ml) vegetable glycerin (food-grade)

¼ cup (60 ml) distilled water

Preparation

In a clean, airtight glass jar, combine the dried ginkgo leaves with the vegetable glycerin and distilled water. Seal the jar tightly and shake to mix thoroughly. Store the jar in a cool, dark place for 4 to 6 weeks, shaking it gently every few days to encourage extraction. After the steeping period, strain the mixture through a fine strainer or cheesecloth into a clean bowl, pressing the leaves to extract all liquid. Transfer the extract to a dark glass dropper bottle for storage.

How to Use

Take 1 to 2 droppers full (1 to 2 ml) daily to support circulation and cognitive health. This extract is particularly beneficial during times of mental fatigue or when enhanced focus is needed.

Hawthorn (*Crataegus monogyna*)
The Heart Strengthener

Hawthorn, a beloved heart herb with bright red berries, is a centuries-old remedy that bolsters heart health and fortifies and supports longevity. In Traditional Chinese Medicine (TCM), it was used to calm the spirit, aid digestion, improve circulation, and regulate the heartbeat. Practitioners of European folk medicine not only used it to ward off heart ailments but also infused it into wines and tonics, recognizing the berries' ability to fortify the body and provide steady, lasting energy.

By the nineteenth century, scientific interest in hawthorn's cardiovascular benefits grew, with Eclectic physicians in the United States recommending it for arrhythmias, high blood pressure, and nervous tension. Today hawthorn remains a widely studied herb, valued for its ability to promote healthy circulation, strengthen arterial walls, and help the heart adapt to stress.

What the Science Says

Hawthorn (*Crataegus* spp.) is a well-known cardiovascular herb, with its berries, leaves, and flowers containing an array of bioactive compounds that support heart health. **Flavonoids** such as quercetin and vitexin act as vasodilators, widening blood vessels to improve blood flow, ensuring the heart muscle receives adequate oxygen and nutrients. This reduces strain on the heart, allowing it to function more efficiently. Flavonoids also function as antioxidants, protecting cardiac cells from free radical damage that can contribute to heart disease.

In addition to its powerful flavonoids, hawthorn contains oligomeric procyanidins (OPCs), potent antioxidant compounds that support vascular integrity, reduce oxidative stress, and enhance overall cardiovascular function. These compounds reinforce the structure of blood vessels, strengthening collagen fibers and maintaining vascular elasticity. This further helps protect the heart from damage caused by oxidative stress. Hawthorn also has an anti-inflammatory effect due to **triterpene acids**—naturally occurring plant compounds known for their ability to modulate immune responses and reduce inflammatory signaling—like ursolic and oleanolic acid. Systemic inflammation is a major contributor to chronic heart conditions. By countering it, these acids help reduce stress on the heart and blood vessels.

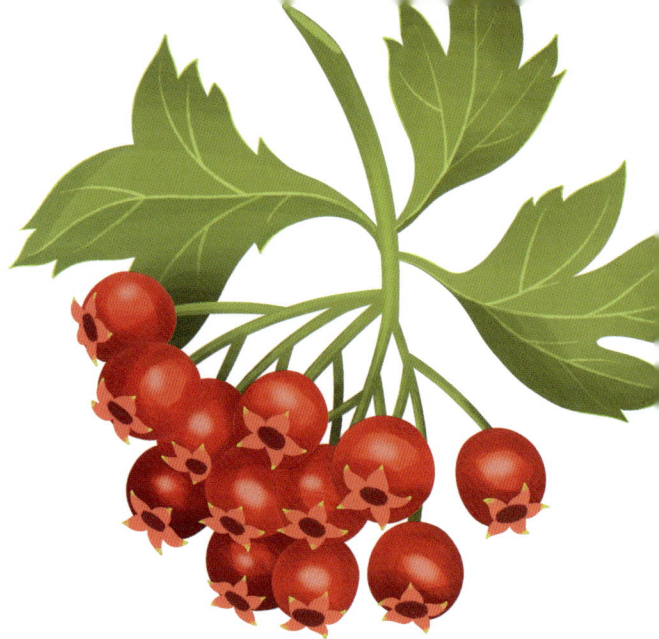

Finally, hawthorn inhibits angiotensin-converting enzymes (ACEs), which help relax blood vessels. This helps maintain healthy circulation and supports optimal blood pressure levels. Research in 2020 in *Frontiers in Pharmacology* highlighted hawthorn's ability to regulate blood pressure and reduce cholesterol levels, reinforcing its historic use as a heart tonic.

A 2003 meta-analysis in the *American Journal of Medicine* found that hawthorn extract significantly improved heart function and reduced symptoms in individuals with chronic heart failure. With its vasodilating, antioxidant, and anti-inflammatory effects, hawthorn remains one of the most trusted herbs for cardiovascular well-being, offering both preventive and therapeutic benefits for heart health.

Uses and Indications

You can use hawthorn to support overall cardiovascular health, regulate blood pressure, and provide gentle yet effective relief for mild heart conditions. It is particularly beneficial if you experience occasional heart palpitations, high blood pressure, or angina, because it helps normalize heart rhythm and relaxes blood vessels for easier circulation.

Beyond heart health, hawthorn can also help promote emotional balance, reduce anxiety, and foster a sense of calm, reflecting its traditional role as a heart-centered remedy. Its adaptogenic qualities further enhance its value, supporting resilience during times of physical or emotional stress.

Interactions and Safety

Hawthorn is generally safe and well-tolerated, but it can enhance the effect of certain heart medications like beta-blockers, calcium channel blockers, and antihypertensive drugs. Be sure to consult your healthcare provider before taking hawthorn if you're taking one of these drugs. Although rare, mild side effects like dizziness, nausea, or gastrointestinal discomfort may occur, particularly if you take high doses. Due to limited research on its safety during pregnancy and breastfeeding, avoid taking hawthorn at these times unless your doctor approves its use.

Growing and Harvesting

Hawthorn is a hardy, deciduous shrub that thrives in temperate climates, preferring well-drained soil and full sunlight. It is often planted as a hedgerow or ornamental tree, producing delicate white flowers in the spring and vibrant red berries in the fall. The berries, leaves, and flowers are all harvested for medicinal use. Flowers and leaves should be collected in the spring when blooms are at their peak, while berries are best harvested in late autumn, once fully ripened. Proper drying and storage in airtight containers protect the herb's potency, ensuring its therapeutic benefits remain intact.

Fun Fact

Hawthorn's rich history extends beyond medicine. In Celtic lore, the tree was considered sacred, and cutting down a hawthorn was thought to bring misfortune. In medieval Europe, hawthorn was planted near homes and woven into charms to ward off malevolent forces, reinforcing its reputation as a guardian of well-being.

Hawthorn Berry Cordial

This delicious cordial combines hawthorn berries with warming spices, creating a heart-supportive remedy that is both therapeutic and enjoyable.
Note: *This syrup is not recommended for children under one year old, as infants should not consume honey.*

Yield: About 2 cups (480 ml)

1 cup fresh (200 g) or dried (48 g) hawthorn berries

1 cinnamon stick

3 whole cloves

1-inch (2.5 cm) piece fresh ginger, sliced

2 cups (480 ml) water

1 cup (240 ml) raw honey

1 cup (240 ml) brandy or vodka (optional, for preservation)

Preparation

In a medium saucepan, combine hawthorn berries, cinnamon stick, cloves, ginger, and water. Simmer gently over low heat for 30 minutes, stirring occasionally to ensure even extraction of flavors and medicinal properties. Remove the mixture from the heat to allow it to cool slightly. Strain the liquid through a fine strainer or cheesecloth into a clean bowl, pressing the solids to extract as much liquid as possible. Stir the raw honey into the strained liquid until fully dissolved, and if desired, add brandy or vodka to extend shelf life. Transfer the prepared cordial to an airtight glass bottle and refrigerate for up to 3 months, or longer if alcohol is included.

How to Use

Take 1 to 2 tablespoons (15 to 30 ml) daily as a heart tonic or up to three times daily for additional cardiovascular support. Enjoy as is or dilute 2 tablespoons (30 ml) in ½ to ¾ cup (120 to 180 ml) warm water for a soothing drink.

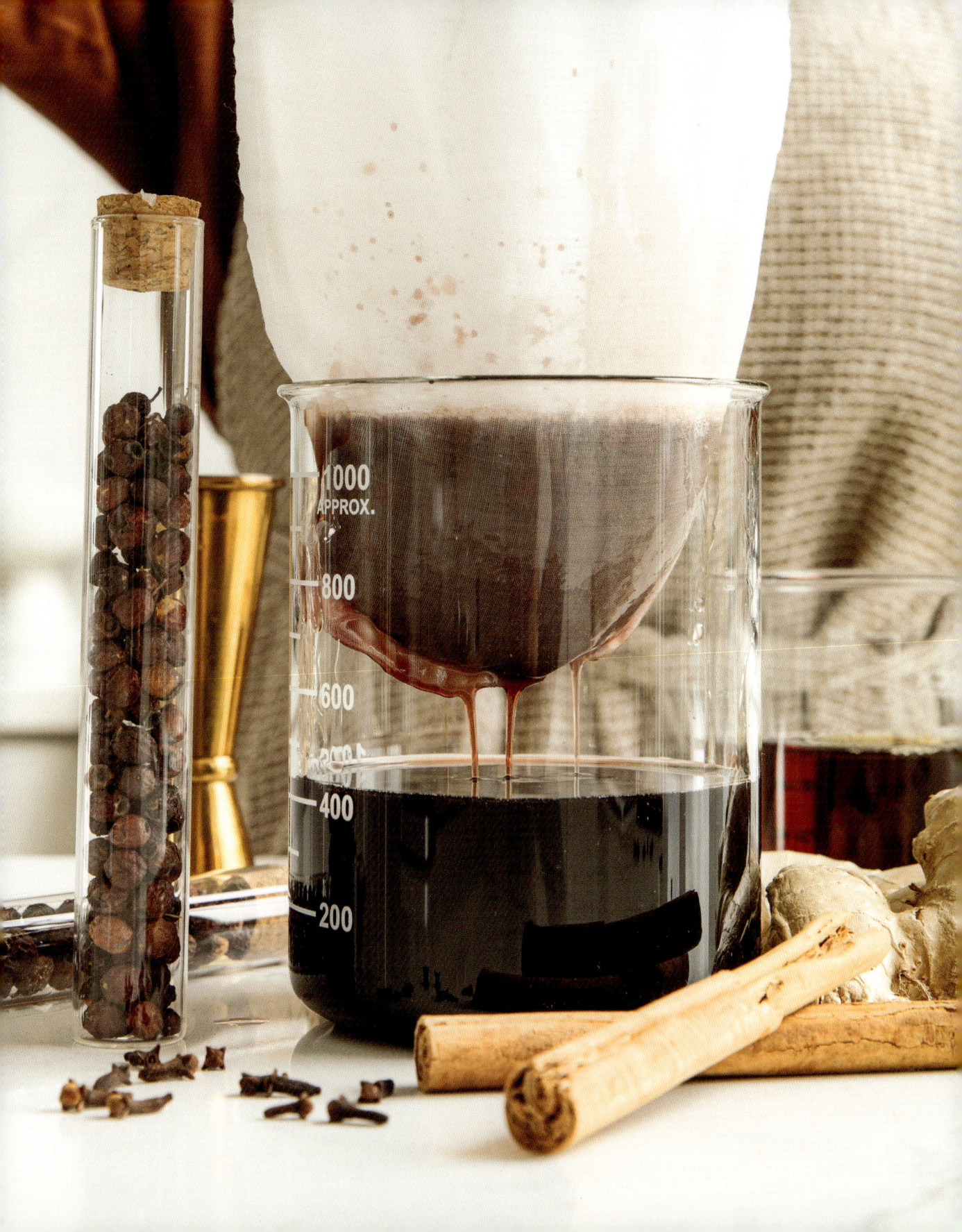

Chapter 4

Radiant Shield:
Herbs for Skin Health

Our skin, hair, and nails are more than just what we show the world—they're vital components of the integumentary system, a sophisticated network working to protect, sense, and adapt as we move through our environment. Our skin is our body's first line of defense, shielding us from pathogens and environmental threats while continuously repairing, renewing, and regenerating at the cellular level.

Key players in this system include keratinocytes, cells that produce keratin to keep skin resilient and waterproof, and melanocytes, cells that create melanin to protect against ultraviolet (UV) damage. In addition, langerhans cells act as immune sentries, identifying threats and triggering defenses. Deeper below the surface, fibroblasts synthesize collagen and elastin to maintain firmness and elasticity, while sebaceous glands keep skin hydrated and soft.

When stressors like pollutants, UV exposure, or internal imbalances disrupt this system, defenses can weaken, leading to dryness, irritation, or signs of aging. Here's where herbal allies shine. Calendula, with its gentle anti-inflammatory properties, soothes irritation and supports cellular healing. Blue tansy, often steam-distilled from wild Moroccan chamomile, is known for its calming nature—soothing reactive skin and helping to reduce redness, flare-ups, and uneven tone. Burdock aids detoxification and liver health, promoting clear skin from within. Aloe vera cools, hydrates, and repairs damaged tissues, while gotu kola stimulates fibroblasts to boost collagen production, keeping skin firm and supple.

This chapter includes recipes like Calendula-Infused Oil for Skin Healing to lock in moisture and support repair, and a Blue Tansy Cooling Gel Mask—a featherlight, aloe-based formula crafted to calm flushed, reactive skin and support barrier repair after sun, treatments, or stress. By nurturing these essential functions, herbs help your skin, hair, and nails stay resilient, radiant, and strong.

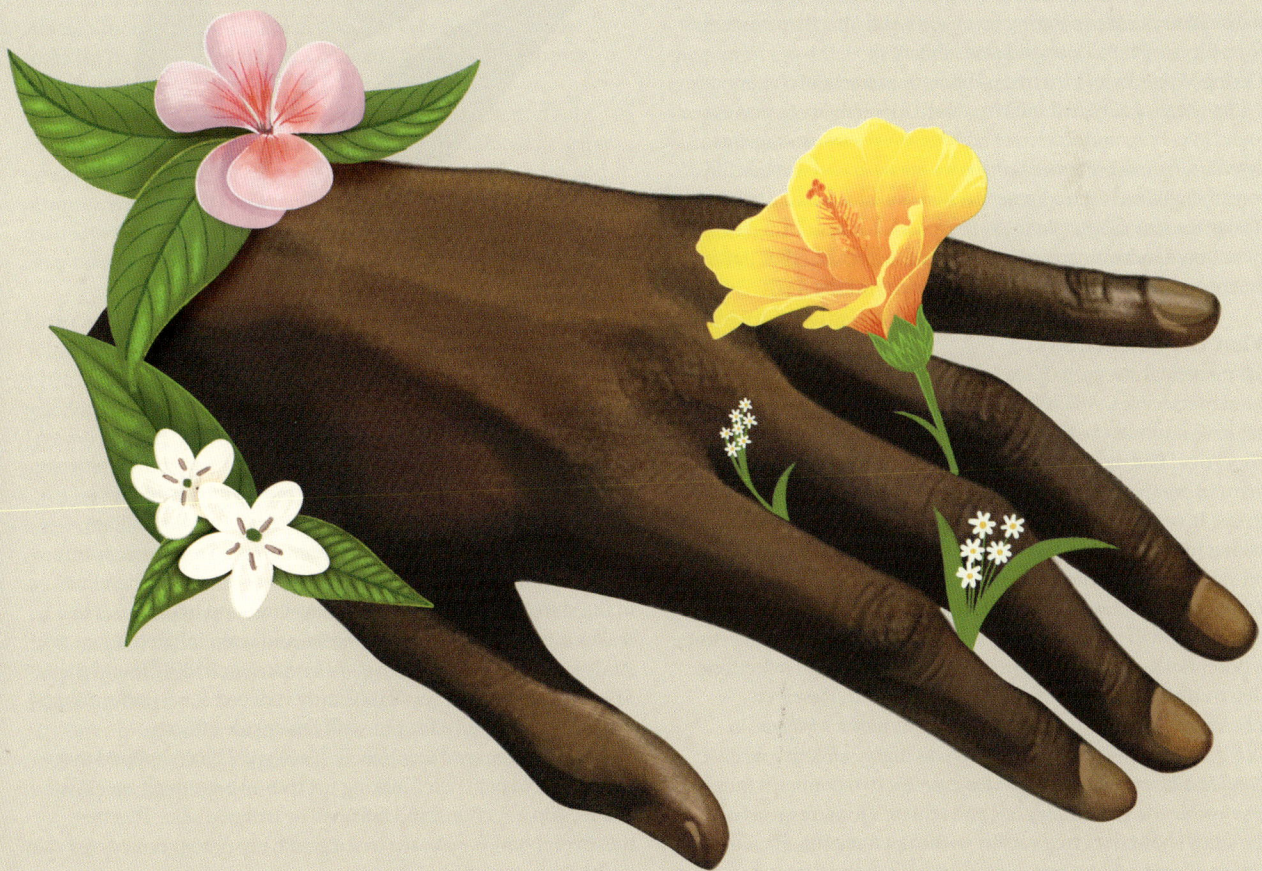

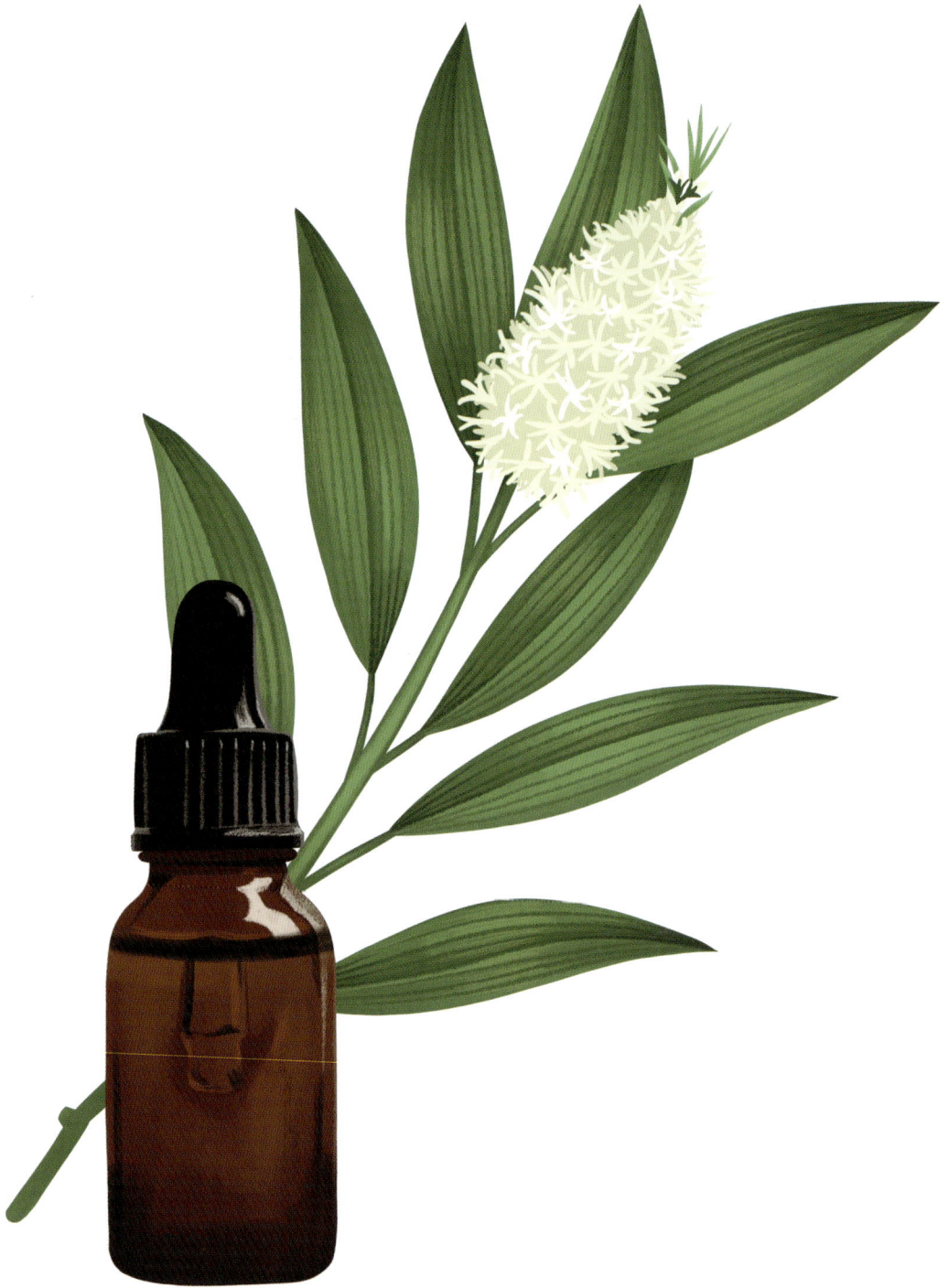

Tea Tree Oil Acne Spot Treatment

This simple yet effective tea tree spot treatment helps reduce breakouts while soothing inflammation and redness.

Yield: About 1½ teaspoons (7.5 ml)

1 teaspoon (5 ml) aloe vera gel (for hydration and soothing)

1 drop tea tree essential oil

½ teaspoon (2.5 ml) witch hazel (as a natural astringent)

Preparation

In a small bowl, mix the aloe vera gel, tea tree oil, and witch hazel until well combined. Transfer the mixture to a dark glass bottle and store it in a cool, dry place away from direct sunlight. Use within 6 months.

How to Use

Using a clean cotton swab, apply a small amount directly onto blemishes. Let it dry and leave it on overnight.

Apply once or twice daily to acne-prone areas, avoiding the eye area. If irritation occurs, reduce the frequency of application.

Fun Fact

In the 1920s, scientists found tea tree oil to be eleven times more effective than phenol, the standard antiseptic of the time. This discovery led to a surge in demand, and tea tree distilleries started popping up across Australia. Long before alcohol-based hand sanitizer was a thing, tea tree oil was already the MVP of germ-fighting!

Calendula *(Calendula officinalis)*
The Skin Soother

Calendula, with its vibrant golden-orange blossoms, is also known as "pot marigold." This healing herb has been used for centuries to soothe inflammation, promote wound healing, and protect the skin against infections.

In ancient Greece and Rome, calendula was commonly used in poultices and ointments to treat cuts, burns, and ulcers. Later, medieval European herbalists used it for skin irritations and infections and scattered calendula flowers in bathwater to promote glowing skin and enhance spiritual well-being. Meanwhile, in Ayurvedic and Traditional Chinese Medicine, calendula was used to clear heat, reduce swelling, and stimulate tissue repair.

Today calendula remains a staple in herbal skincare and is often used in preparations from gentle baby balms to intensive wound-care salves. It's prized not just for its effectiveness but also for its enduring connection to healing, beauty, and vitality.

What the Science Says

The flowers of calendula *(Calendula officinalis)* are full of skin-soothing and healing bioactive compounds. Some of the most powerful are **flavonoids**, antioxidants that help neutralize free radicals, reducing oxidative stress and protecting the skin from premature aging and cellular damage. Flavonoids, along with **triterpenoids**—a class of phytochemicals that help modulate inflammation and support tissue repair—help reduce inflammation, easing redness, swelling, and irritation. A 2024 study in *Pharmacological Research-Natural Products* confirmed that calendula was effective with these symptoms, making it a good remedy for eczema, dermatitis, and sunburn.

In addition, calendula contains **carotenoids**, fat-soluble pigments found in plants that act as antioxidants and are vital for skin and eye health. These include beta-carotene and lutein, which boost collagen production and stimulate fibroblast activity, thus speeding tissue repair. This makes this herb especially helpful for minor cuts, burns, and abrasions. A 2024 study in *European*

Journal of Medicinal Chemistry Reports revealed that patients who used calendula-based treatments had faster skin regeneration compared to those using conventional wound-care products. Carotenoids also improve skin elasticity and protect against environmental stressors like UV exposure and pollution.

In addition, research published in *Natural Product Research* in 2024 highlighted calendula's antibacterial and antifungal effects on skin infections such as staph bacteria and yeast overgrowth. These properties can also prevent infections from forming in wounds, which helps support healing without complications.

Calendula also contains **polysaccharides**—long chains of sugar molecules that help lock in moisture and support the skin's natural barrier—making it a go-to remedy for dry, sensitive, irritated, or damaged skin.

From soothing irritated skin to promoting faster healing and preventing infection, calendula remains an indispensable herb for skincare and natural healing.

Uses and Indications

You can use calendula for a wide variety of skin issues, healing, and overall skincare. It's a beneficial remedy to have on hand to treat cuts, scrapes, burns, and rashes, because its anti-inflammatory and regenerative properties help accelerate healing and its mild analgesic effects reduce discomfort. You can also use calendula to manage chronic skin conditions such as eczema and psoriasis, because it soothes irritation, reduces redness, and strengthens the skin barrier.

If you have acne or sensitive skin, calendula's gentle antimicrobial properties may help reduce breakouts and calm inflammation.

Interactions and Safety

Calendula is generally considered safe for topical and internal use. If you are allergic to plants in the Asteraceae family, such as chamomile, ragweed, or daisies, you may experience mild skin irritation when using calendula, so a patch test is recommended before widespread use.

Internally, calendula can be consumed as a tea or tincture for its anti-inflammatory and lymphatic-supporting properties. Consult a healthcare professional before using calendula internally if you're pregnant or breastfeeding, because its safety in these populations has not been extensively studied. Due to its mild relaxant effects, calendula may interact with certain medications, such as sedatives or blood pressure-lowering drugs. If you're taking these medications, check with your doctor first before adding calendula to your routine.

Growing and Harvesting

Calendula is a hardy, easy-to-grow plant that thrives in a variety of climates. It prefers well-drained soil and full sunlight, producing an abundance of bright, cheerful flowers throughout the growing season. The flowers are harvested when fully open, typically in the morning after the dew has dried, to ensure maximum potency.

To preserve calendula's medicinal properties, the flowers should be dried in a well-ventilated, shaded area and stored in an airtight container. Properly dried calendula retains its vibrant color and therapeutic compounds for several months, making it a valuable addition to home herbal apothecaries.

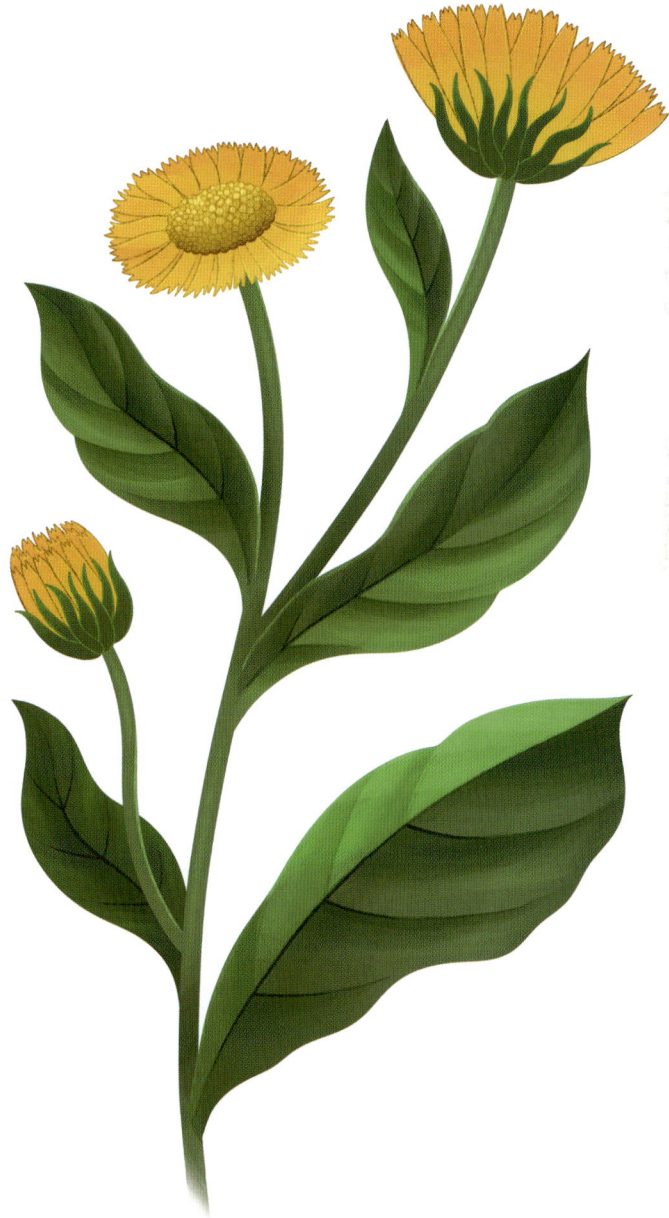

Calendula-Infused Oil for Skin Healing

Yield: About 1½ cups (360 ml)

This simple yet effective infused oil captures calendula's skin-soothing properties, making it a staple for treating minor cuts, burns, and irritations.

1 cup (120 g) dried calendula petals

1½ cups (360 ml) carrier oil (olive, sweet almond, or jojoba oil)

Preparation

Place the dried calendula petals in a clean glass jar and pour the carrier oil over them, ensuring the flowers are fully submerged. Seal the jar and place it in a warm, sunny spot for 4 to 6 weeks, shaking gently every few days to promote infusion. After the infusion period, strain the oil through a fine-mesh strainer or cheesecloth, discarding the spent flowers. Transfer the infused oil to a dark glass bottle and store it in a cool, dry place.

How to Use

Apply calendula oil directly to cuts, scrapes, burns, or irritated skin as needed. It can also be used as a massage oil for dry or inflamed skin, incorporated into a homemade salve, or blended with essential oils for an extra soothing effect.

Fun Fact

Calendula has held symbolic significance throughout history. It was used in religious rituals, added to culinary dishes for its bright color, and even used as a natural dye, giving a golden hue to fabrics and foods.

The Benefits of Growing Your Own Herbs

There is something undeniably grounding about growing the very herbs that you will later brew into tea or blend into tinctures. Even in a small urban space, a windowsill herb garden provides fresh, potent plants ready for harvest.

Herbs like peppermint thrive in containers, spreading rapidly and offering endless leaves for tea and digestion support. Calendula, with its bright golden blooms, is both medicinal and beautiful, infusing oils with skin-healing properties. Echinacea, revered for its immune-supporting compounds, adds resilience to any herb garden, while lemon balm, a calming nervous system tonic, grows vigorously in both pots and garden beds.

Cultivating herbs deepens the relationship between plants and person, making herbalism more than just something practiced—it becomes something lived. The act of watering, harvesting, and tending mirrors the care given to personal wellness.

Beyond convenience, homegrown herbs offer unmatched potency. Fresh leaves, snipped straight from the plant, contain higher concentrations of beneficial compounds compared to dried, store-bought varieties. The simple act of plucking a sprig of thyme or rosemary to add to a meal or medicine reinforces the connection between food, health, and nature.

When growing herbs for medicine, it's important to consider soil quality, sunlight exposure, and harvesting methods. Many medicinal herbs, such as nettle, dandelion, and burdock, thrive in wild spaces and can be foraged sustainably. However, growing them at home ensures access to pesticide-free, high-quality plants.

Drying and storing herbs properly extends their usefulness, ensuring a steady supply throughout the year. A simple drying rack, mason jars, and airtight containers can preserve herbal potency and create a year-round apothecary from a single growing season.

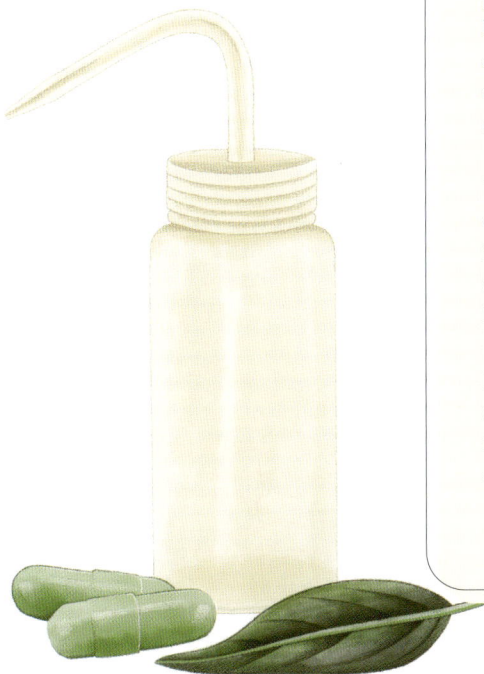

Aloe Vera *(Aloe barbadensis)*
The Natural Moisturizer

Aloe vera *(Aloe barbadensis)*, often referred to as the "plant of immortality," is prized for its healing properties. Ancient Egyptians documented its use for wounds, burns, and skin infections as early as 1550 BCE in the *Ebers Papyrus*. In Ayurvedic medicine, aloe was used for digestive health, wound healing, and balancing the body's internal heat. Traditional Chinese Medicine (TCM) also incorporates aloe for its cooling and detoxifying effects.

Greek and Roman physicians, including Dioscorides, praised aloe for its ability to cleanse wounds and support digestion. In medieval Europe, it was a key ingredient in herbal elixirs, valued for its ability to soothe inflammation and promote internal healing. Native American tribes also recognized aloe's benefits, using the gel to treat burns, insect bites, and skin irritations.

By the twentieth century, aloe vera became widely commercialized in skincare and health products, solidifying its reputation as one of the most versatile and widely used plants for hydration and skin repair. Today aloe remains a staple in both traditional and modern medicine, a testament to its enduring power as a healing botanical.

What the Science Says

The gel inside aloe vera leaves *(Aloe barbadensis miller)* contains over seventy-five bioactive compounds that give this herb its healing and hydrating properties. With 99 percent water content, aloe vera delivers deep hydration without clogging pores, making it a lightweight but effective moisturizer. This hydrating effect is further supported by **polysaccharides** like acemannan and glucomannan, which form a protective barrier over the skin, helping it retain moisture while reducing inflammation. Polysaccharides also stimulate immune function, enhance fibroblast activity, and boost collagen production, making aloe an excellent ally in skin repair and rejuvenation. A 2022 study published in *Arabian Journal of Chemistry* confirmed that aloe's polysaccharides improve skin hydration and elasticity, reinforcing its value as a natural moisturizer for dry and sensitive skin.

Aloe contains enzymes that reduce inflammation and help remove dead skin cells, speeding up skin renewal. The plant's anti-inflammatory effects come from its ability to inhibit certain specific enzymes that trigger redness, swelling, and pain. This makes aloe effective for sunburn relief, minor burns, and skin irritations. A 2021 study in the *Journal of Caring Sciences* found that aloe significantly accelerated burn healing, reducing pain, redness, and recovery time compared to conventional treatments. Researchers attributed these effects to aloe's ability to enhance collagen synthesis and promote tissue regeneration.

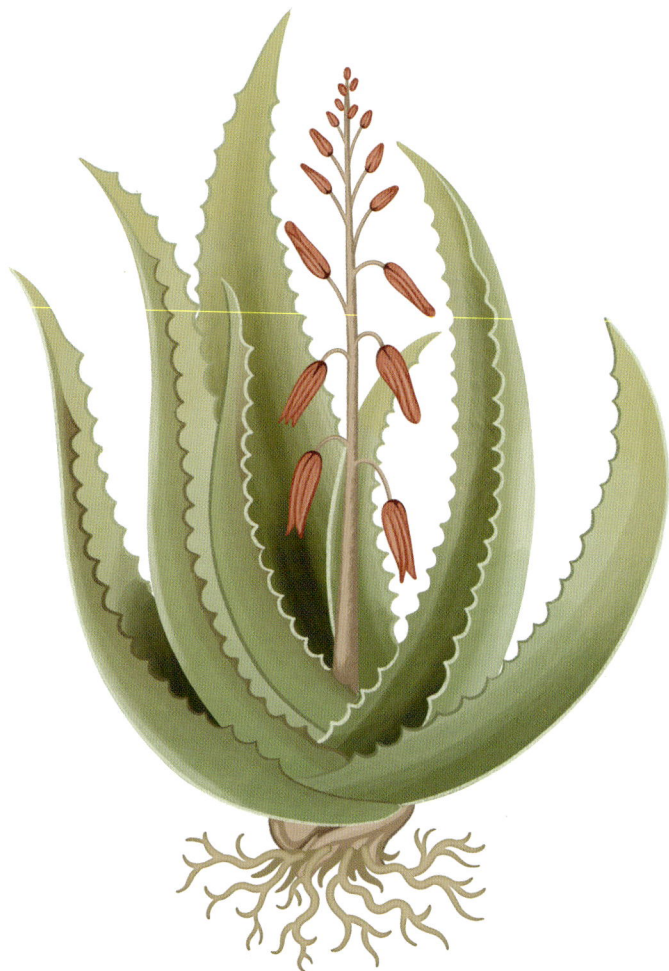

Another key compound in aloe vera are **anthraquinones**—naturally occurring aromatic compounds known for their laxative, antimicrobial, and anti-inflammatory properties. These include aloin and emodin, which provide mild antimicrobial and pain-relieving effects, making aloe suitable for minor skin infections. A 2017 study in *Nature* showed that aloe vera helped manage psoriasis and eczema, reducing scaling, redness, and itching when applied topically. The plant's antimicrobial compounds also help prevent infections in wounds, while its enzymatic activity supports skin exfoliation and tissue regeneration. Participants in randomized controlled trials reviewed in *Evidence-Based Complementary and Alternative Medicine* (2022) found that they had fewer acne breakouts and improved skin texture due to aloe's antimicrobial and anti-inflammatory properties.

Aloe vera is rich in vitamins A (beta-carotene), C, and E—potent antioxidants that help protect skin cells from oxidative stress and support cellular regeneration. In addition, B-complex vitamins assist in cellular energy production, aiding in tissue repair. Essential minerals such as calcium, magnesium, zinc, and selenium further contribute to wound healing and immune support, enhancing aloe's effectiveness for burns, cuts, and irritated skin.

Whether used to cool sunburns, accelerate wound healing, or improve hydration, aloe vera remains one of nature's most versatile and effective botanicals.

Uses and Indications

You can use aloe vera to treat burns, sunburns, and minor skin abrasions due to its cooling and regenerative properties. It's a staple in after-sun lotions, soothing gels, and first-aid treatments because of its ability to provide immediate relief and support faster healing.

If you have dry or sensitive skin, you can use aloe as a lightweight moisturizer that hydrates without clogging pores. You'll commonly find it in facial serums, masks, and creams as it enhances skin hydration and elasticity. Aloe's anti-inflammatory effects make it beneficial for managing conditions such as eczema, psoriasis, and dermatitis, as it helps reduce redness, itching, and irritation.

Aloe vera is also sometimes taken internally as a digestive aid, particularly in Ayurvedic and TCM traditions. You can use aloe juice to soothe the gastrointestinal tract, helping to alleviate acid reflux, gastritis, and inflammatory bowel conditions. That being said, some of the compounds in the plant can act as a strong laxative, so use with caution.

Interactions and Safety

Aloe vera is generally safe for topical use. But if you have sensitive skin, perform a patch test first, because you may experience mild irritation or allergic reactions.

Internally, aloe vera juice should be consumed cautiously, since excessive consumption can lead to abdominal cramping, diarrhea, and electrolyte imbalances. If you're pregnant or breastfeeding, avoid consuming aloe latex, as it may stimulate uterine contractions. Aloe may also interact with certain medications, including blood sugar–lowering drugs and diuretics, so those with diabetes or kidney conditions should consult a healthcare provider before using internally.

Growing and Harvesting

Aloe vera is a hardy, drought-tolerant succulent that thrives in warm, arid climates. It prefers well-drained soil and ample sunlight, making it an excellent addition to home gardens or indoor plant collections. The plant requires minimal maintenance, needing only occasional watering to prevent root rot.

To harvest aloe gel, select mature leaves from the outer edges of the plant. Cut the leaf close to the base, allow the yellow latex to drain (if internal use is not desired), and then slice the leaf lengthwise to extract the clear gel inside. Fresh aloe gel can be used immediately or stored in the refrigerator for up to a week for later use.

Aloe Vera Gel for Soothing Burns and Irritated Skin

This simple do-it-yourself aloe vera gel provides instant relief for burns, rashes, and skin irritation, offering hydration and protection with every application.

Yield: About 1½ cups (360 ml), depending on the size of the aloe leaf

1 to 2 large aloe vera leaves (enough to yield approximately 1½ cups [360 ml] of gel)

1 teaspoon (5 ml) vitamin E oil (optional, for extra hydration)

3 to 5 drops lavender essential oil (optional, for calming effects)

Preparation

Slice the aloe leaves lengthwise and use a spoon to scoop out the clear inner gel. Transfer the gel to a blender and blend until smooth. Measure out approximately 1½ cups (360 ml) of blended gel. Add the vitamin E oil and lavender essential oil, if using, and blend briefly to combine. Pour the gel into a clean, airtight container and store it in the refrigerator. Use within 1 to 2 weeks.

How to Use

Apply a thin layer of aloe gel to sunburns, minor cuts, or dry skin as needed. The cooling effect will help reduce discomfort and speed up healing.

Fun Fact

NASA has studied aloe vera's ability to purify the air, finding that it effectively removes toxins such as formaldehyde and benzene from indoor environments. This makes it not only a powerful skincare ingredient but also a beneficial addition to homes for improving air quality.

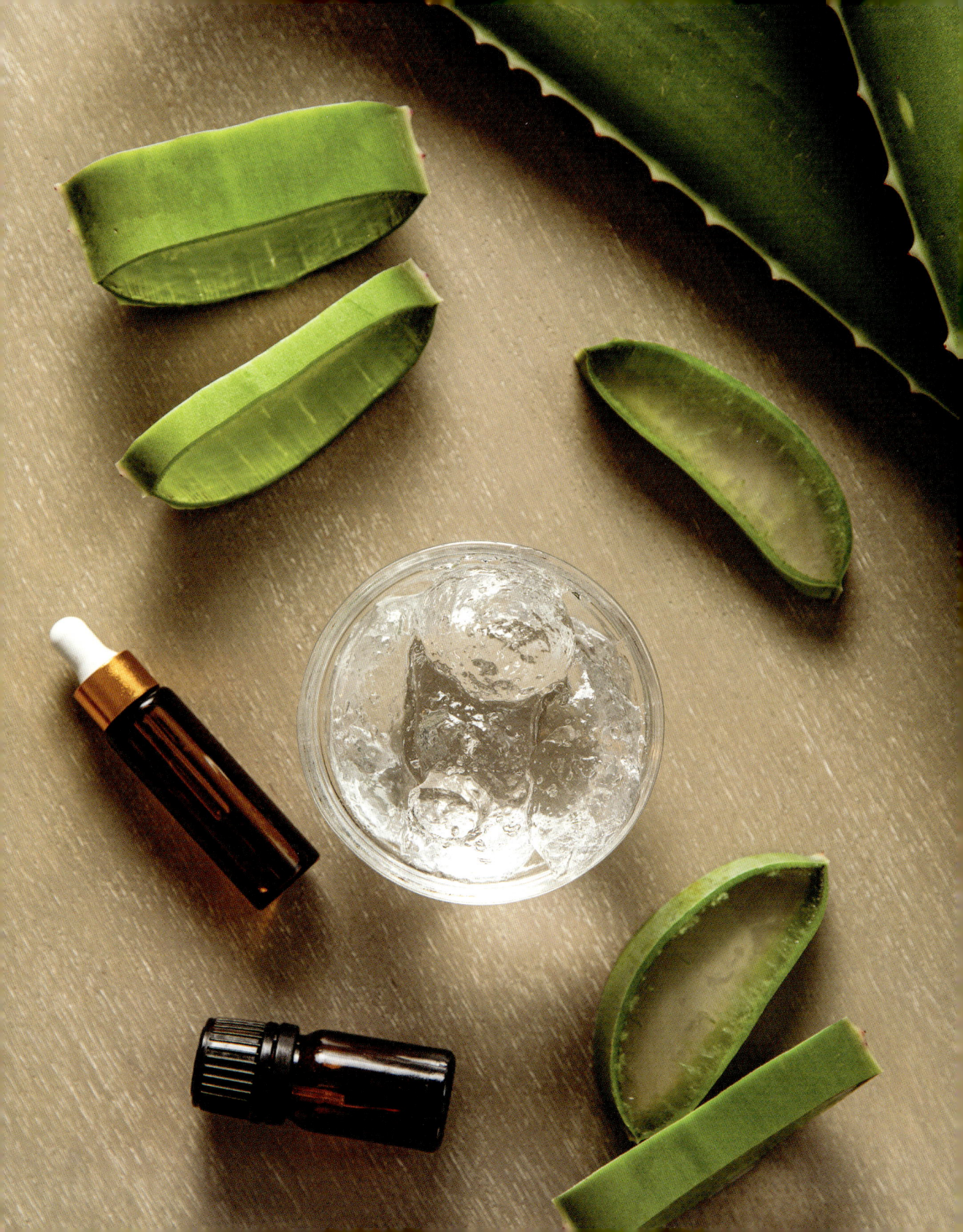

Blue Tansy (*Tanacetum annuum*)
The Skin Whisperer

Blue tansy, known for its vivid sapphire hue and calming aroma, has been prized in traditional Mediterranean and North African herbal medicine for centuries. Used historically in poultices and salves to ease inflammation, rashes, and insect bites, it remains a coveted skin soother in modern aromatherapy and botanical skincare. Despite its name, blue tansy bears no relation to the toxic common tansy (*Tanacetum vulgare*). Its vibrant blue essential oil comes from steam-distilled flowers and upper leaves—and its beauty is more than skin-deep.

In folk medicine, blue tansy was often used to "cool the skin" after sunburn or heat rash. Today it's the darling of clean skincare brands, featured in calming serums and oils formulated for sensitive, acne-prone, and inflamed skin.

What the Science Says

The vivid color of blue tansy (*Tanacetum annuum*) is due to chamazulene, a compound that forms during steam distillation when the natural precursor matricin is exposed to heat. Chamazulene belongs to a group of compounds called **sesquiterpenes**, which are known for their anti-inflammatory and antioxidant properties. These compounds work by suppressing the release of inflammatory agents that contribute to conditions such as acne, eczema, and irritated skin.

A 2022 study in *Molecules* analyzed the chemical composition of blue tansy and noted that chamazulene levels were directly associated with anti-inflammatory outcomes and soothing effects on the skin. In another study published in *Antibiotics* in 2023, blue tansy essential oil showed strong antioxidant activity, helping to neutralize harmful free radicals and reduce cellular stress in lab-based tests using skin cells. These findings suggest that blue tansy may help protect collagen and elastin from breakdown, making blue tansy a valuable ally for maintaining skin firmness and elasticity.

Further, blue tansy oil contains sabinene—a **monoterpene** with antimicrobial properties that help reduce the growth of acne-causing bacteria, as well as other naturally occurring compounds that enhance its skin-calming and barrier-repairing effects, making it especially useful for irritated or blemish-prone skin.

These combined effects help reduce swelling, redness, and histamine-driven reactions. Blue tansy is particularly helpful for calming irritated skin and restoring the skin's natural lipid barrier—key to managing sensitivity and chronic inflammation.

Uses and Indications

Blue tansy is a trusted remedy for reactive, inflamed, or sensitive skin. If you're dealing with acne, rosacea, or stress-triggered breakouts, blue tansy can help regulate the inflammatory response while protecting skin from further damage.

Diluted in a carrier oil such as jojoba, argan, or rosehip seed oil, blue tansy can be applied topically to reduce redness, support skin barrier recovery, and soothe irritation. Its gentle antimicrobial action also helps keep pores clear and balanced without overdrying, making it safe for daily use on acne-prone skin.

Blue tansy pairs well with other herbs like calendula and chamomile for a layered calming effect, especially in oil infusions or post-cleanse facial oils. You can also use it for facial steaming. A few drops added to hot water may help open pores and deliver its calming volatile compounds through inhalation and light topical contact.

Interactions and Safety

While blue tansy is generally safe for topical use, its essential oil is potent and should always be diluted to 1 to 2 percent before application. This equals about 6 to 12 drops per 1 ounce (28 ml) of carrier oil. Using it undiluted may cause sensitization in those with compromised skin barriers.

Blue tansy is a member of the Asteraceae family, so if you're allergic to plants such as chamomile, ragweed, or daisies, perform a patch test or consult a practitioner before using blue tansy. Do not use blue tansy internally, as adulterated forms may contain thujone, a potentially neurotoxic compound found in *Tanacetum vulgare*.

If you're pregnant or breastfeeding, avoid blue tansy unless under supervision. Always purchase essential oils from reputable suppliers who specify botanical origin (*Tanacetum annuum*) and proper gas chromatography-mass spectrometry (GC-MS) testing. Store the oil in an amber or cobalt bottle in a cool, dark place to maintain potency and protect chamazulene from degrading.

Growing and Harvesting

Blue tansy grows best in warm, dry climates with sandy, well-drained soil and full sun. Native to Morocco and parts of the Mediterranean, it grows to about 2 to 3 feet (60 to 91 cm) tall and produces yellow button-like flowers—not blue! The rich blue oil forms only during steam distillation, when heat converts matricin to chamazulene.

Harvest the flowers during full bloom, typically in late summer. The oil yield is low, and large quantities of the plant are needed to extract a few milliliters of essential oil. This contributes to blue tansy's relatively high cost and limited availability, making it a precious addition to botanical formulations.

Though rare in home gardens, blue tansy can be container-grown in sunny locations with care. Dried flowers may be used in infusions and compresses, but the essential oil is the most therapeutically potent form for skin health.

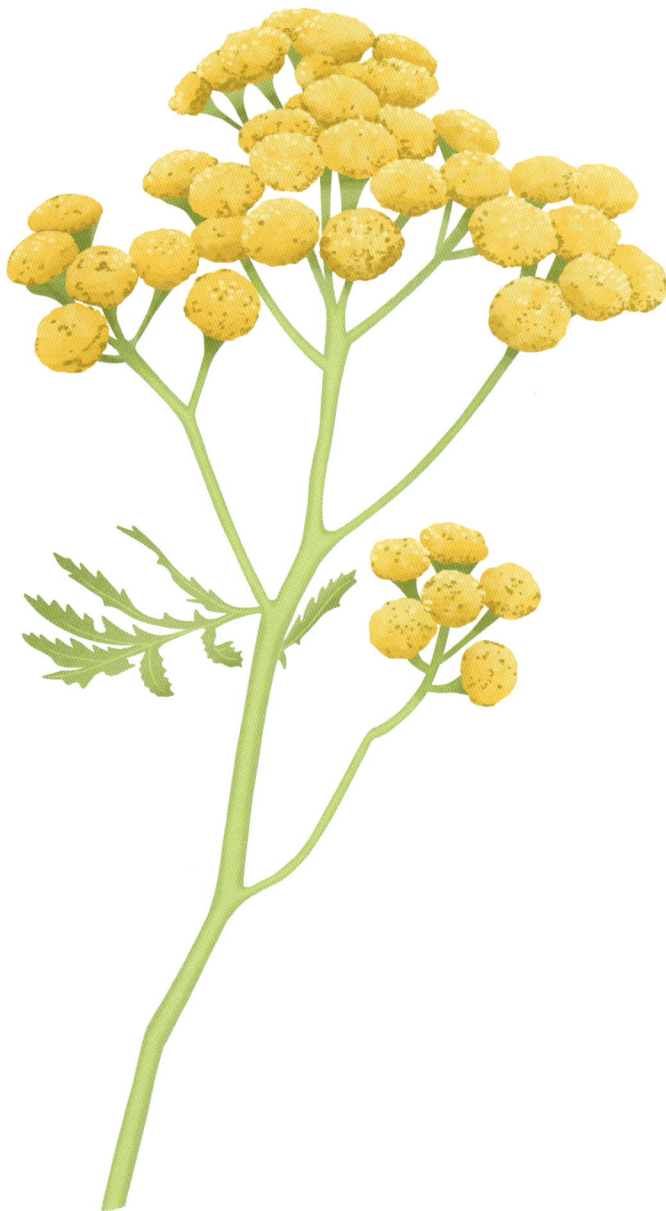

Blue Tansy Cooling Gel Mask

This featherlight aloe-based gel mask is designed to soothe redness, calm heat, and support barrier repair—perfect for post-sun, post-peel, or reactive skin days.

2 tablespoons (30 ml) aloe vera gel (pure, no alcohol)

2 teaspoons (10 ml) vegetable glycerin, divided

1 teaspoon (5 ml) calendula hydrosol (or rose water)

4 drops blue tansy essential oil (*Tanacetum annuum*)

1 drop lavender essential oil (optional, for extra calming)

¼ teaspoon (1 to 2 ml) leucidal liquid (or other natural preservative, optional but recommended for storage)

Preparation

In a non-metal bowl, combine the aloe vera gel, 1 teaspoon (5 ml) of the vegetable glycerin, and calendula hydrosol (or rose water). Stir gently until the texture is smooth and evenly blended. In a separate dish, add the essential oils to the remaining 1 teaspoon (5 ml) of glycerin, mixing a few drops at a time. This pre-mix helps disperse the oils more evenly throughout the formula, and reduces the risk of skin sensitivity. Once combined, pour this mixture into the gel base and stir gently. The final formula should take on a pale aqua or greenish-blue hue, depending on your aloe source. If you're using a preservative like leucidal liquid, incorporate it last and stir thoroughly to ensure an even distribution. Transfer the finished gel to a sterilized 2-ounce (60 ml) amber glass jar or airless pump container. Store in the refrigerator for an enhanced cooling effect and longer shelf life.

How to Use

After cleansing your face, apply a thin, even layer of the gel mask to clean skin, avoiding the eyes and lips. This mask does not dry down like clay—it remains dewy and breathable as it works. Leave it on for 10 to 15 minutes to allow the calming botanicals to penetrate and reduce inflammation. Gently rinse off with cool or lukewarm water and pat the skin dry with a clean towel. Follow with your usual serum or moisturizer. Use two or three times a week, or daily during periods of redness, breakouts, sunburn, post-exfoliation sensitivity, or reactive flare-ups.

The Ritual of Blue: Creating Space for Calm

Some herbs are medicinal. Others work on mood. Blue tansy quietly does both.

Long before it became the darling of high-end serums, blue tansy was cherished for what it offered beyond the skin. The oil carries a sweet, slightly fruity aroma that makes you feel like you are standing barefoot in a field after rain. There's something in it that settles the breath before you even realize you've exhaled.

While we often praise blue tansy for calming inflamed skin, its aromatic compounds also have a direct effect on the nervous system. Sabinene and chamazulene interact with the limbic brain, the area tied to emotion, memory, and stress response. In traditional aromatherapy, blue tansy is considered a cooling oil that helps ease tension—whether that shows up as heat in the skin or unease in the body.

Try this: Rub a single drop between your palms, then cup your hands over your nose and breathe deeply. Inhale slowly. Let the scent settle. That's an herbal intervention. Not flashy. Just present.

Working with blue tansy can also shift how we approach formulation. It is rare, costly, and low-yielding. This encourages care and intention. You will likely never use more than a few drops in a blend. That's part of its lesson. It reminds us that the strongest support doesn't always come from using more. It comes from using well.

Mini Ritual: Sensory Reset Oil

Blend 1 drop blue tansy, 2 drops Roman chamomile, and 1 drop lavender into 1 tablespoon (15 ml) of jojoba or calendula-infused oil. Gently massage a small amount onto your temples, jawline, or the center of the chest. Then pause. Inhale. Let your shoulders drop.

This is not a treatment. It's a reminder.

Some rituals are made for skin. Others are made for the moment between stress and softness. Let this one do both.

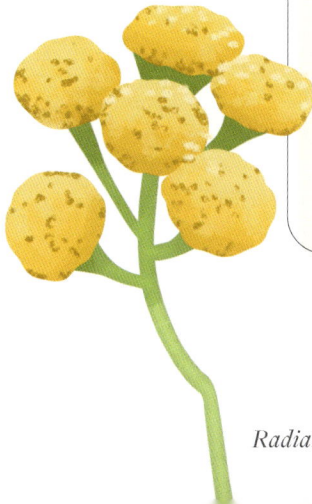

Chapter 5

Roots of Vitality: Herbs for the Reproductive System

The reproductive system is more than a collection of organs—it's the foundation of life, renewal, and vitality. For both men and women, this system plays a pivotal role in hormonal balance, energy levels, and overall well-being. Governed by the endocrine system, the reproductive system operates through a complex interplay of hormones like estrogen, progesterone, and testosterone, produced by cells in the ovaries, testes, and adrenal glands. These hormones influence fertility, mood, metabolism, and bone health.

Herbs have long been trusted to support reproductive health, offering natural ways to balance hormones, boost energy, and nourish this vital system. Maca, for instance, is renowned for enhancing stamina, libido, and hormone production. Chasteberry helps balance estrogen and progesterone, easing premenstrual syndrome (PMS) symptoms and regulating cycles. Red raspberry leaf, often used as a uterine tonic, strengthens and tones the uterine muscles, making it especially supportive during the menstrual cycle and in preparation for childbirth, while dong quai, a staple in Traditional Chinese Medicine, is known as "female ginseng" for its role in regulating cycles, easing cramps, and replenishing blood after menstruation.

This chapter introduces recipes like Black Cohosh Tincture for Menopause Relief and a soothing Chasteberry Cordial for Menstrual Irregularities, enhanced with warming spices for enjoyment. Supporting reproductive health with herbs nurtures not only physical balance but also the energy that fuels your life each day. Let's dive into the roots of vitality.

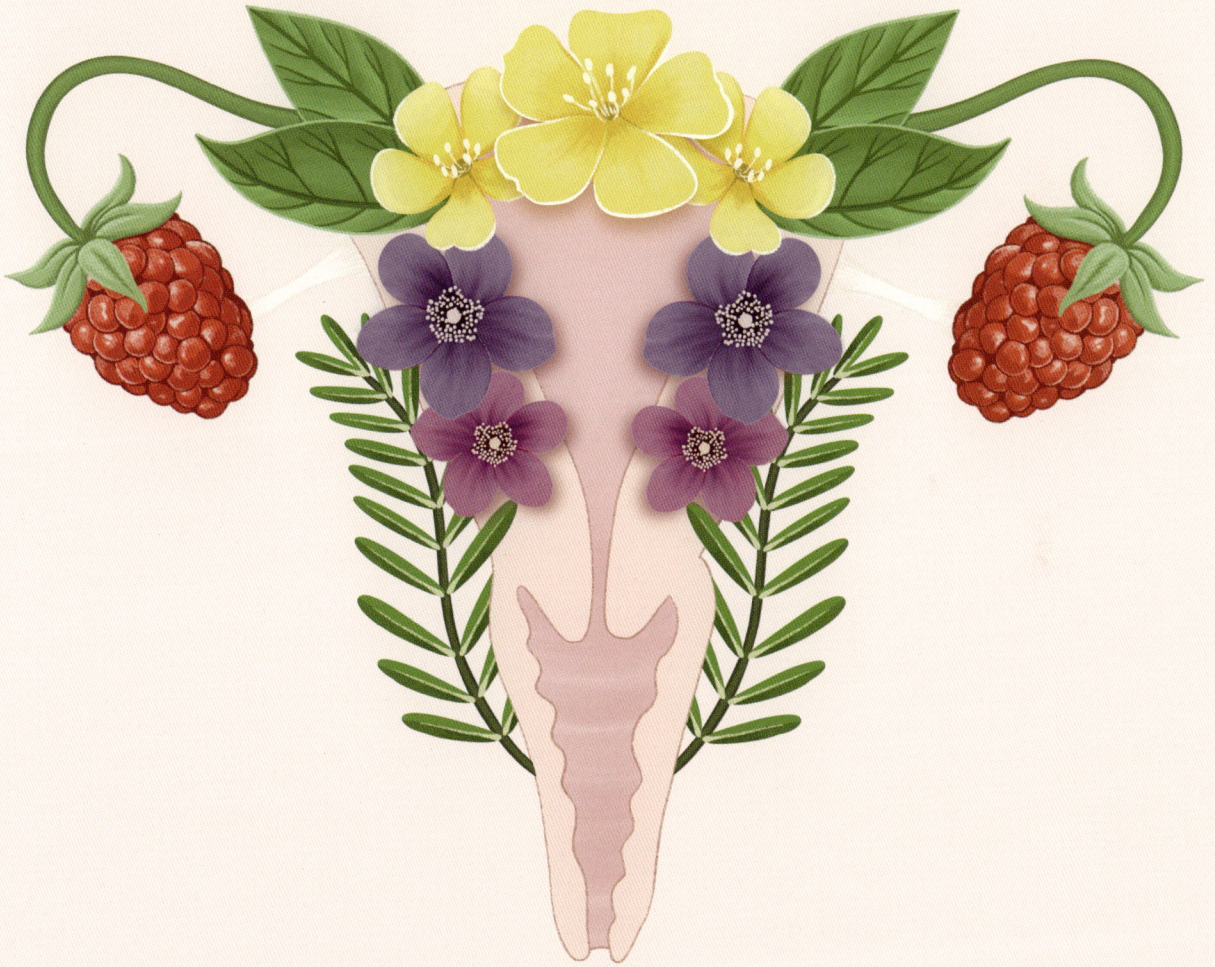

Red Raspberry Leaf *(Rubus idaeus)*
The Uterine Tonic

Red raspberry leaf has long been regarded as one of the most valuable herbs for uterine health, deeply woven into the traditions of midwifery and women's wellness. Used for centuries by Indigenous healers, European herbalists, and traditional midwives, red raspberry leaf was praised for its ability to strengthen the uterus, regulate menstrual cycles, and support pregnancy. Ancient records from Greece and Rome document its use as a fertility aid and a remedy for excessive menstrual bleeding. Native American tribes brewed the leaves into a tea to ease labor pains and facilitate a smoother birth process.

By the nineteenth century, red raspberry leaf had become a cornerstone of botanical medicine, frequently recommended by Eclectic physicians for menstrual irregularities and reproductive health. Midwives and herbalists also relied on it for postpartum recovery, as it was believed to help the uterus contract back to its normal size while replenishing essential nutrients lost during childbirth. Beyond pregnancy support, red raspberry leaf was commonly used to alleviate symptoms of premenstrual syndrome (PMS), such as cramping, bloating, and mood swings.

Modern herbalists continue to champion the use of red raspberry leaf, not only for its uterine-toning effects but also for its role in overall wellness.

What the Science Says

Red raspberry leaf *(Rubus idaeus)* is prized for its uterine-toning and reproductive-supporting properties. Its vibrant green leaves are rich in **tannins**, **flavonoids**, and **alkaloids**, all of which contribute to their therapeutic effects. The leaves are also packed with essential vitamins and minerals, including vitamins C, E, and B-complex, along with calcium, magnesium, potassium, and iron, all of which contribute to overall reproductive wellness.

One of the most notable compounds in red raspberry leaf is the alkaloid fragrine, which has been shown to strengthen the uterine muscles, supporting more efficient contractions during labor and helping to regulate menstrual flow. Unlike synthetic uterotonics, which force contractions, red raspberry leaf provides a gentler effect, working in harmony with the body's natural rhythms. This toning action helps regulate menstrual cycles, ease cramping, and prepare the uterus for labor, without inducing premature contractions. A 2016 study in the *Journal of Herbal Medicine* highlighted red raspberry leaf's ability to ease menstrual cramping and regulate menstrual cycles, reinforcing its uterine-toning properties.

As far as other compounds go, flavonoids like quercetin and kaempferol provide potent antioxidant protection, reducing oxidative stress and inflammation, which helps ease hormonal imbalances and menstrual discomfort. Tannins offer astringent properties, which help tighten and tone tissues, making it particularly beneficial for uterine health. These tannins help balance menstrual bleeding, reducing excessive flow while supporting overall cycle regularity. This makes red raspberry leaf particularly useful for heavy periods.

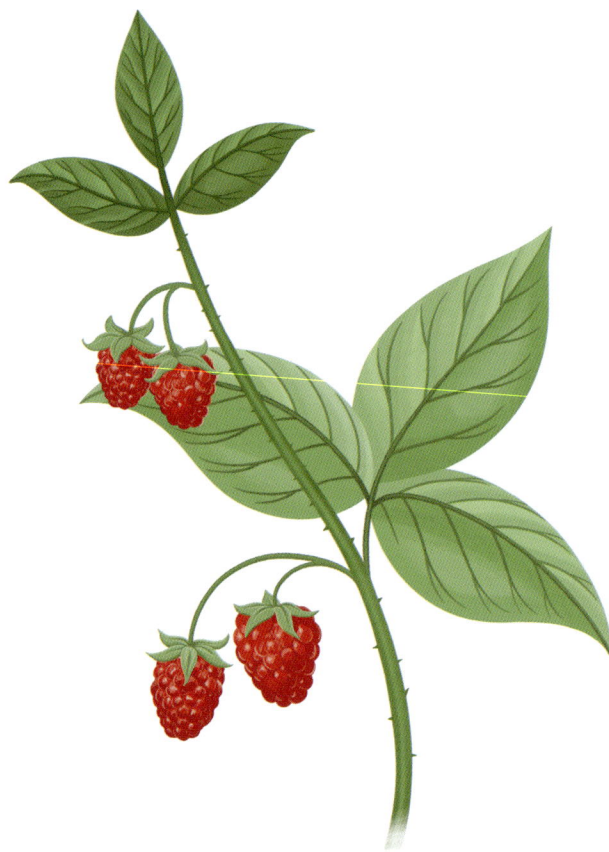

During pregnancy, red raspberry leaf is often used in the third trimester to strengthen the uterus in preparation for labor. A 2001 study in *Midwifery* found that women who consumed red raspberry leaf during pregnancy experienced a shorter second stage of labor and were less likely to require forceps-assisted delivery. While clinical research remains limited, midwives and herbal practitioners have long recommended red raspberry leaf for its uterine-toning properties and its traditional use in supporting recovery after childbirth.

By nourishing the uterus and reducing inflammation, red raspberry leaf provides comprehensive reproductive support at various life stages.

Uses and Indications

Red raspberry leaf is most commonly used as a supportive herb for women's reproductive health. You can use it to support menstrual regulation, fertility, pregnancy, postpartum recovery, and menopause.

Red Raspberry Leaf Nourishing Herbal Tea

A nourishing herbal tea made from red raspberry leaf provides gentle yet powerful support for reproductive health. You can prepare this tea each day to help regulate menstrual cycles, ease cramps, and support uterine tone.

Yield: 1 cup (240 ml)

1 tablespoon (8 g) dried
red raspberry leaf

1 teaspoon (2 g) dried nettle leaf
(optional, for additional mineral support)

1 cup (240 ml) hot water

Honey or lemon (optional)

Preparation

Place the dried red raspberry leaf and nettle, if using, in a tea strainer or teapot. Pour the hot water over the herbs and let steep for 10 to 15 minutes. Strain and enjoy warm. Add honey or lemon if desired for flavor.

How to Use

Drink 1 to 3 cups daily to support reproductive health. During pregnancy, consult with a midwife or healthcare provider before use. The cooling effect will help reduce discomfort and speed up healing.

For people who menstruate, red raspberry leaf can help balance heavy or irregular cycles, reduce cramping, and alleviate symptoms of PMS. If you are in menopause, its mineral-rich composition helps support hormonal balance and overall well-being.

Red raspberry leaf can be used for fertility support, as it nourishes and strengthens the reproductive system, creating a healthier environment for conception. During pregnancy, it can be used in the third trimester to strengthen the uterus and prepare for labor. Many midwives recommend it as part of a holistic approach to prenatal care. Beyond pregnancy, you can use red raspberry leaf postpartum to support uterine recovery, aiding in the return of the uterus to its pre-pregnancy state.

Interactions and Safety

Red raspberry leaf is considered safe for most individuals when used appropriately. However, while traditionally used in pregnancy, it is generally recommended only in the second and third trimesters, as its uterine-toning effects may not be suitable for early pregnancy. If you have a history of preterm labor or uterine complications, consult a healthcare provider before use.

If you're taking blood-thinning medications, use caution, as red raspberry leaf contains natural astringents that could potentially interact with anticoagulants. If you have a kidney disorder, monitor your intake of this herb to avoid excess mineral accumulation due to the mineral content of red raspberry leaf. Mild side effects such as nausea or digestive discomfort are rare but possible, particularly with high doses.

Growing and Harvesting

Red raspberry plants thrive in temperate climates and are commonly found growing in the wild or cultivated in gardens. They prefer well-drained soil and full sunlight, producing lush green leaves and sweet red berries. While the fruit is widely enjoyed, it is the leaves that hold medicinal value.

The best time to harvest red raspberry leaves is in late spring or early summer before the plant flowers. The leaves should be dried in a shaded, well-ventilated area to preserve their medicinal compounds. Once dried, they can be stored in an airtight container for several months, retaining their potency for teas and infusions.

Black Cohosh (*Actaea racemosa*)
The Menopause Ally

Black cohosh has long been valued as a vital herb for women's health, particularly for easing the transition through menopause. Indigenous tribes of North America, including the Cherokee and Iroquois, traditionally used the root to relieve menstrual cramps, support childbirth, and calm nervous tension. Early European settlers quickly adopted it into their medical practices, and by the nineteenth century, black cohosh was a staple in Eclectic medicine, used to address menstrual irregularities, arthritis, and even respiratory conditions.

Interest in black cohosh surged again in the twentieth century as scientists explored its potential as a natural alternative to hormone replacement therapy. It remains one of the most well-researched botanical options for addressing menopausal discomfort and is widely available in various forms, including capsules, tinctures, and teas.

What the Science Says
Black cohosh (*Actaea racemosa*) derives its medicinal strength from its thick, knotted root, which contains a wide array of bioactive compounds that support hormonal balance, mood regulation, and inflammation relief. Among the most important constituents are **triterpene glycosides**, such as actein and cimigenol, which interact with serotonin receptors in the brain. These compounds work to regulate mood and body temperature, which can reduce menopausal symptoms such as hot flashes and night sweats.

Black cohosh also contains **phenolic acids**, including caffeic and **ferulic acids**, which provide antioxidant and anti-inflammatory effects. This helps ease muscle tension and joint pain, making it a useful remedy for stiff joints, tension headaches, and menstrual cramping. Its **flavonoids** help calm the nervous system, while **alkaloids** and **volatile oils** enhance its muscle-relaxing effects.

Black cohosh was once believed to act as a phyto (plant-based) estrogen, but unlike synthetic estrogen treatments, it doesn't contain hormones. It's now believed to work by interacting with estrogen receptors that help the body adapt to hormonal fluctuations, making it a safe alternative to hormone replacement therapy with fewer significant side effects. A study published in *Annals of Internal Medicine* in 2002 showed that black cohosh was as effective as low-dose hormone replacement therapy in alleviating vasomotor symptoms (hot flashes and sweating), without the associated risks of blood clots or hormone-sensitive cancers.

Black cohosh appears to work primarily in the hypothalamus, the brain's temperature-regulating center. This may explain this herb's ability to reduce hot flashes and night sweats. Scientific research supports the herb's effectiveness in managing menopausal symptoms like these. A 2010 systematic review in *Menopause* found that black cohosh extract significantly reduced the frequency and intensity of hot flashes compared to a placebo. Three years later, a study in *Chinese Medicine* confirmed its ability to improve sleep quality and reduce night sweats.

Black cohosh influences dopamine and noradrenaline pathways, which help stabilize mood. Since menopause often causes anxiety, irritability, and mild depression, black cohosh's ability to modulate neurotransmitters is especially beneficial for emotional balance during hormonal transitions. All in all, black cohosh remains a widely trusted option for women seeking natural support through menopause and for menstruation symptoms.

Uses and Indications
You can use black cohosh to manage your menopause-related symptoms, including hot flashes, night sweats, mood swings, and sleep disturbances. It's also helpful if you are experiencing perimenopausal (the period before menopause) symptoms such as irregular periods and hormonal mood shifts.

Before menopause, you can also use black cohosh to relieve premenstrual syndrome (PMS) and menstrual cramps. Its muscle-relaxing properties can help ease uterine spasms, while its mild sedative effects promote relaxation. It can also be used for tension headaches, joint pain, and inflammatory conditions.

Interactions and Safety
Although black cohosh is generally well-tolerated by most people, some precautions are advised. The herb is not recommended if you have a liver disorder, as rare cases of liver toxicity have been reported. Furthermore, women with a history of estrogen-sensitive conditions, such as breast cancer, should consult their healthcare provider before using black cohosh, though current research suggests it does not stimulate estrogen-dependent tumor growth.

You're unlikely to experience any side effects from black cohosh, but mild gastrointestinal discomfort, headaches, or dizziness are possible. Long-term safety studies are limited, so seek professional guidance before using the herb for extended periods. If you are pregnant or breastfeeding, avoid black cohosh due to its effects on uterine contractions.

Growing and Harvesting

Black cohosh is a shade-loving perennial native to the woodlands of eastern North America. It thrives in moist, well-drained soil with dappled sunlight, often growing beneath a canopy of trees. In late summer, the plant produces tall, spiky clusters of white flowers that attract pollinators, though it is the knotted, dark brown root that holds medicinal value.

Roots are typically harvested in late autumn after the plant has died back, allowing for the highest concentration of active compounds. After harvesting, the roots are cleaned, dried, and stored in airtight containers to preserve their potency. Due to increasing demand and overharvesting in the wild, ethical sourcing and sustainable cultivation are critical for preserving black cohosh populations.

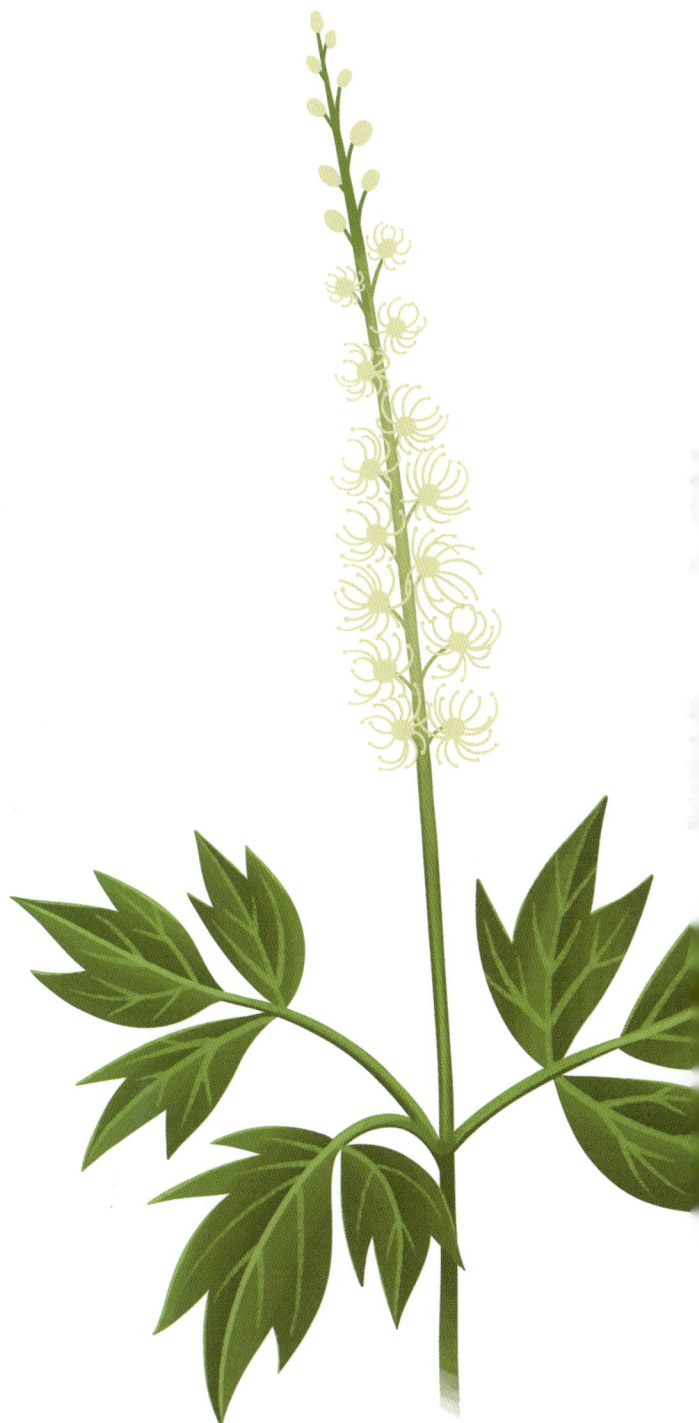

Black Cohosh Tincture for Menopause Relief

Yield: 1 cup (240 ml)

A tincture is one of the most effective ways to extract black cohosh's medicinal properties, ensuring a concentrated and long-lasting remedy for menopausal support.

2 tablespoons (12 g) dried black cohosh root

1 cup (240 ml) vodka or brandy (at least 40% alcohol)

Preparation

Place the dried black cohosh root in a clean, airtight glass jar. Pour the vodka or brandy over the herb, ensuring the root is fully submerged. Seal the jar tightly and shake it gently. Store in a cool, dark place for 4 to 6 weeks, shaking the jar every few days to encourage extraction. After the steeping period, strain the mixture through a fine-mesh strainer or cheesecloth into a clean bowl. Transfer the liquid tincture to a dark glass dropper bottle for storage.

How to Use

Take 30 to 40 drops (1 to 1½ droppers full) in water or tea up to twice daily to help manage menopausal symptoms. Consistency is key, and effects may take a few weeks to become noticeable.

Fun Fact

Black cohosh's nickname, "bugbane," comes from its historical use as an insect repellent. The plant was traditionally burned or crushed to ward off mosquitoes and other pests, making it useful beyond herbal medicine.

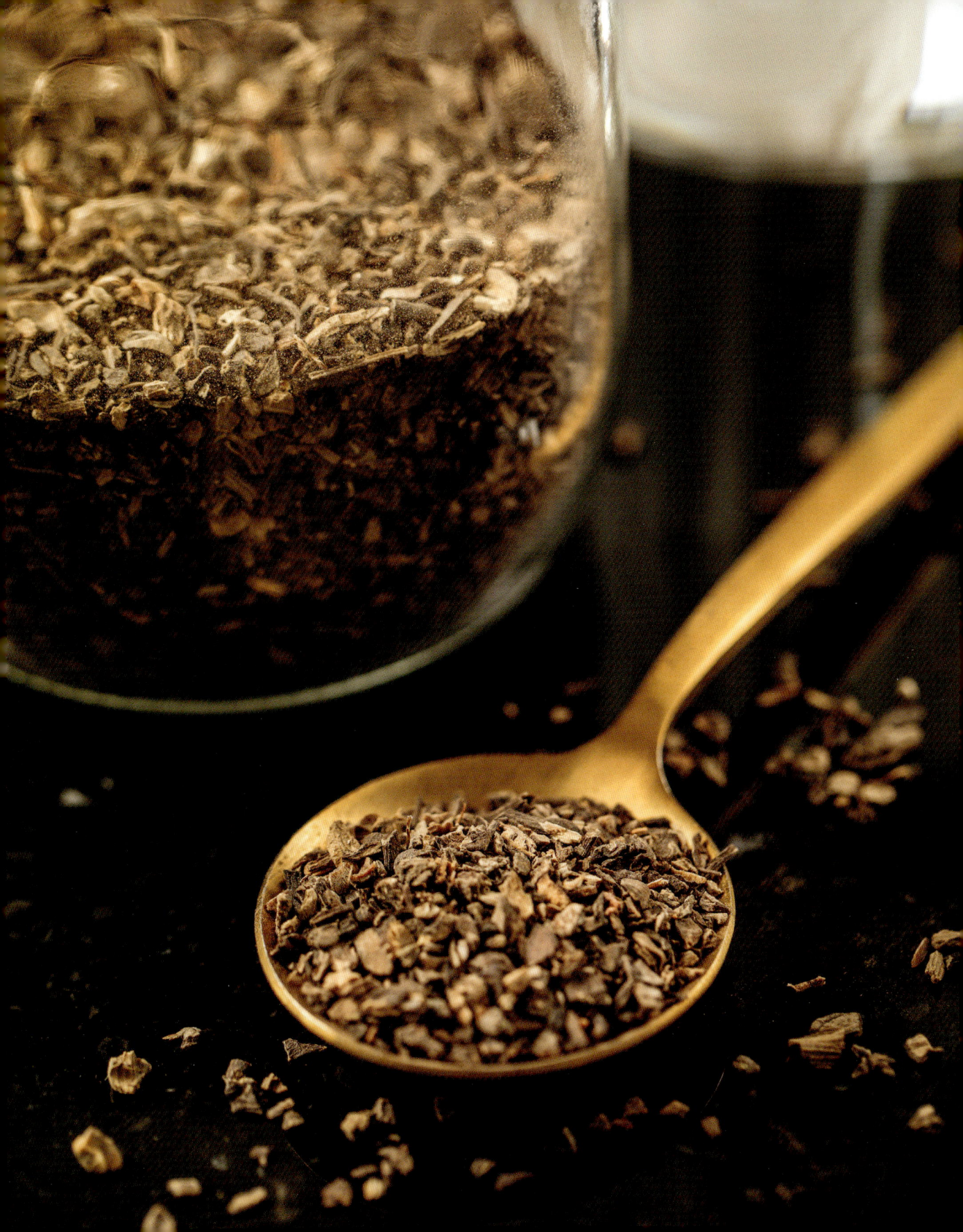

Chasteberry (*Vitex agnus-castus*)
The Hormone Balancer

Chasteberry, a small, berry-producing shrub native to the Mediterranean, has long been valued for its hormonal-balancing properties. Traditionally used in Greek, Roman, and European folk medicine, this herb supports menstrual health, fertility, and menopausal transitions. In European folk medicine, chasteberry was used to alleviate symptoms of premenstrual syndrome (PMS), including bloating, breast tenderness, and mood swings. Ayurvedic and Traditional Chinese Medicine practitioners also used it to stabilize menstrual cycles and ease discomfort related to hormonal fluctuations. By the nineteenth century, Eclectic physicians in the United States frequently prescribed chasteberry for irregular menstruation, absent periods, and menopausal symptoms.

Chasteberry remains a staple in herbal medicine and is often found in teas, tinctures, and supplements tailored for women's health.

What the Science Says

The medicinal effects of chasteberry (*Vitex agnus-castus*) stem from its ability to influence the pituitary gland, which plays a central role in regulating reproductive hormones. Unlike synthetic hormone therapies, chasteberry does not contain hormones but instead helps balance the body's natural production of estrogen and progesterone. This makes it an ideal option for those seeking gentle, plant-based hormonal support.

One of chasteberry's key mechanisms is its ability to lower prolactin levels, a hormone that, when elevated, can disrupt ovulation and menstrual regularity, which can be beneficial for individuals experiencing irregular cycles, luteal phase deficiency, or fertility challenges. A 2024 clinical review in the *Archives of Gynecology and Obstetrics* demonstrated chasteberry's ability to balance prolactin levels and, in turn, regulate menstrual cycles and balance hormone levels. A randomized controlled trial published in *Molecules* in 2021 further supported this, showing that chasteberry helped normalize irregular menstrual cycles and also improved fertility outcomes in women with luteal phase defects.

Chasteberry is particularly well-known for its ability to reduce PMS symptoms such as bloating, breast tenderness, mood swings, and headaches. It can also help with dopamine regulation, which leads to improved mood stability, making it especially beneficial for individuals experiencing hormonal anxiety, irritability, or mild depressive symptoms.

A 2001 study in the *British Medical Journal* found that women taking chasteberry extract experienced a significant reduction in PMS symptoms, including mood disturbances and breast tenderness. Some studies have also suggested that chasteberry may help reduce hormonal acne, particularly breakouts associated with fluctuating estrogen and progesterone levels. Researchers are also continuing to explore its potential benefits for menopause, as some evidence suggests chasteberry may help with symptoms like night sweats and irritability.

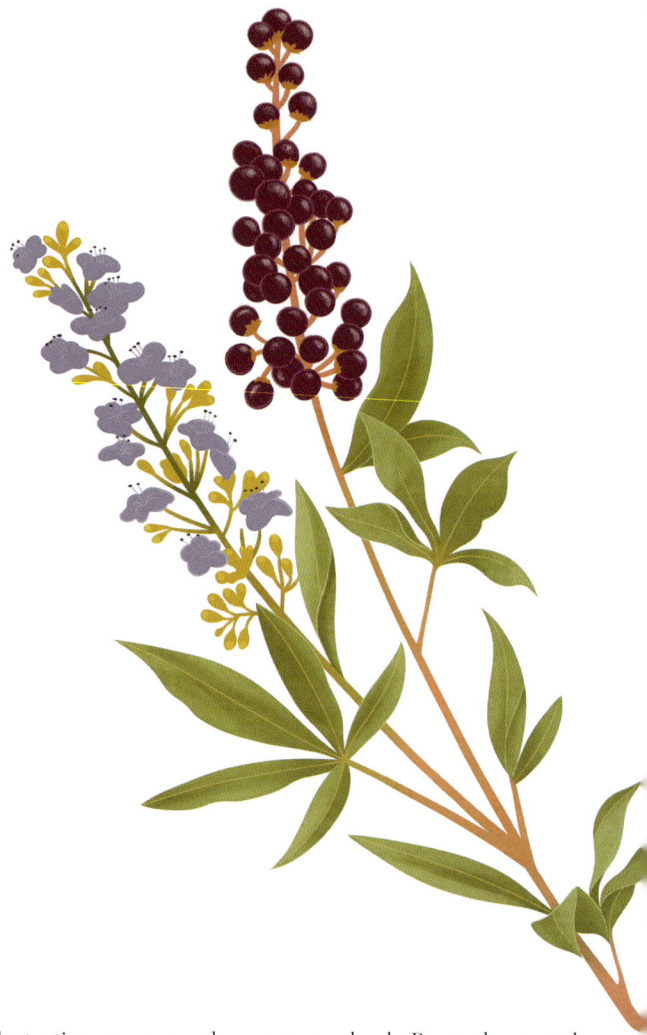

Uses and Indications

Use chasteberry to support hormonal balance, particularly if you're experiencing irregular cycles, luteal phase deficiency, or hormone-related acne. It is especially beneficial for reducing common PMS symptoms such as bloating, breast tenderness, mood swings, and headaches.

If you are menopausal, you can use chasteberry to help ease hot flashes, night sweats, and mood fluctuations. Some herbalists also recommend it for those discontinuing hormonal birth control to aid in restoring the body's natural cycle. Chasteberry is also widely used for polycystic ovary syndrome (PCOS), as it helps regulate cycles and may support ovulation in those with hormonal imbalances.

Beyond reproductive health, you can use chasteberry to support mental well-being, particularly in cases of hormone-related anxiety or mild depression.

Recipe

Chasteberry Cordial for Menstrual Irregularities

This warming, hormone-balancing cordial combines chasteberry's regulatory effects with supportive herbs to help ease menstrual irregularities, reduce PMS symptoms, and promote overall cycle balance.

> *Yield: 1½ cups (360 ml)*

2 tablespoons (12 g) dried chasteberries

1 tablespoon (8 g) dried red raspberry leaf (optional)

1 teaspoon (1.6 g) dried cinnamon chips (for warming circulation and hormone balance)

1 teaspoon (2 g) dried ginger root

1 cup (240 ml) brandy or vodka (for preservation)

½ cup (120 ml) raw honey or maple syrup/

Preparation

In a clean glass jar, lightly crush the dried chasteberries to release their medicinal compounds. Add the raspberry leaf, if using, cinnamon, and ginger. Pour in the brandy or vodka, ensuring all ingredients are fully submerged. Seal the jar and store it in a cool, dark place for 4 to 6 weeks, shaking occasionally. After the infusion period, strain the mixture through a fine-mesh strainer or cheesecloth, pressing the herbs to extract as much liquid as possible. Stir in the raw honey or maple syrup until fully dissolved. Transfer the cordial to a sterilized glass bottle and store it in a cool, dark place or refrigerate for up to a year.

How to Use

Take 1 to 2 teaspoons (5 to 10 ml) daily to support hormonal balance and ease menstrual discomfort. This cordial can be taken on its own or added to warm water, herbal tea, or even sparkling water for a delicious and supportive drink.

Interactions and Safety

Chasteberry is generally well-tolerated, but it should be used with caution if you're taking hormone-based medications, including hormonal birth control, hormone replacement therapy, or medications for conditions like endometriosis. Because it influences dopamine receptors, it may also interact with medications for Parkinson's disease or psychiatric conditions.

You may experience mild side effects such as nausea, dizziness, or digestive discomfort, particularly when starting chasteberry for the first time. If you have a hormone-sensitive condition, such as breast cancer, it's important to consult a healthcare provider before use. Due to its effects on hormone levels, chasteberry is not typically recommended during pregnancy, though some midwives use it postpartum to help restore hormonal balance.

Growing and Harvesting

Chasteberry thrives in warm, Mediterranean-like climates with well-drained soil and full sunlight. This hardy deciduous shrub can grow up to 15 feet (4.5 m) tall, producing fragrant lilac-colored flowers in the summer, followed by small, dark berries in the fall.

The berries, which contain the highest concentration of medicinal compounds, are typically harvested in late summer or early autumn when fully ripe. Once collected, they should be dried in a well-ventilated area away from direct sunlight to preserve their potency. Dried chasteberries can be stored in airtight containers for several months for use in teas, tinctures, and herbal preparations.

Dong Quai *(Angelica sinensis)*
The Female Tonic

Dong quai *(Angelica sinensis)*, often referred to as the "female ginseng," has been a cornerstone of Traditional Chinese Medicine (TCM) for thousands of years, revered for its ability to balance hormones, nourish the blood, and support reproductive health. Dong quai was first recorded in ancient Chinese medical texts during the Han dynasty, when it was prescribed for menstrual irregularities, postpartum recovery, and overall vitality. It was traditionally classified as a warming and harmonizing herb, frequently included in formulas designed to support women's health.

Across Asia, dong quai has been deeply embedded in holistic healing traditions, often used to regulate *qi* (vital energy) and promote smooth blood circulation. In TCM, it is especially valued for nourishing *xue* (blood), which is essential for a healthy reproductive system, pregnancy, and overall vitality. As knowledge of herbal medicine spread beyond East Asia, dong quai gained recognition in Western herbalism, where it became popular for easing symptoms of premenstrual syndrome (PMS), supporting menopause, and addressing hormonal imbalances. By the nineteenth century, it was included in Western botanical texts as a tonic for women's reproductive health, often recommended by herbalists and Eclectic physicians.

Today dong quai remains one of the most widely used herbs in women's health, often used for menstrual regulation, hormonal balance, postpartum recovery, and overall well-being.

What the Science Says
Dong quai *(Angelica sinensis)* is one of the most widely used herbs for women's reproductive health, with a long-standing reputation for balancing hormones, promoting circulation, and easing menstrual discomfort. Unlike synthetic hormones, dong quai is phytoestrogenic, meaning it may help regulate estrogen activity in a way that supports hormonal equilibrium rather than artificially increasing hormone levels. This type of regulation is beneficial because it allows the body to maintain its own hormonal rhythm, making it a gentler option for those seeking support during times of hormonal fluctuation. A 2020 review in a book chapter, *Fundamental Principles of Herbal Medicine,* highlighted dong quai's regulatory effect on estrogen receptors, suggesting that it helps stabilize hormonal fluctuations without acting as a direct estrogen replacement.

The root of dong quai contains bioactive compounds such as **ferulic acid**, **coumarins**, and ligustilide, which work together to reduce inflammation, improve blood flow, and relax smooth muscles, making it particularly beneficial for menstrual irregularities, PMS symptoms, and menopausal discomfort. Its ability to enhance circulation to the pelvic region supports healthy uterine function, while its antispasmodic properties help relieve menstrual cramps and muscle tension. A study in *Phytomedicine* (2016) demonstrated dong quai's ability to improve blood circulation and reduce menstrual discomfort through its effects on vascular dilation and muscle relaxation. In addition to all of this, dong quai's antioxidant profile protects cells from oxidative stress, a key factor in aging and hormonal imbalances.

Dong quai is often recommended for menopausal symptoms, with some research suggesting it may help reduce hot flashes, night sweats, and mood swings. A 2019 study in the *Journal of Evidence-Based Integrative Medicine* found that dong quai significantly improved menopause-related symptoms, particularly hot flashes and sleep disturbances, reinforcing its use as a natural support for hormonal transitions. Traditionally, it has also been used for postpartum recovery, helping to restore vitality and replenish blood after childbirth.

With its unique combination of circulatory, hormonal, and anti-inflammatory benefits, dong quai remains a cornerstone herb for those seeking natural hormonal balance and reproductive health support.

Uses and Indications
Use dong quai to support menstrual health—especially if you're dealing with irregular cycles, menstrual cramps, heavy bleeding, or the absence of menstruation (amenorrhea). It's particularly helpful for promoting healthy blood flow, easing PMS symptoms, and supporting overall hormonal balance. Dong quai also supports uterine function, making it a go-to ally for cycle regulation and menstrual comfort.

You can also use dong quai to alleviate menopausal symptoms such as hot flashes, night sweats, and mood swings. Its ability to regulate estrogen levels makes the transition through menopause smoother while promoting overall vitality and emotional well-being.

Beyond reproductive health, you can use dong quai as a general blood tonic, which helps combat anemia, enhance circulation, and support cardiovascular health. You'll find dong quai is a common ingredient in many herbal blends that increase energy levels, support liver detoxification, and improve overall well-being. Some herbalists also recommend dong quai for those recovering from illness or surgery due to its nourishing and revitalizing properties.

Interactions and Safety

Dong quai is usually well-tolerated, but it does have a mild blood-thinning effect, so if you're taking anticoagulant medications such as warfarin or aspirin, it's a good idea to consult your healthcare provider before use. If you experience heavy menstrual bleeding, you should also use caution when taking dong quai, as it may increase blood flow.

Avoid dong quai if you're pregnant, particularly in early pregnancy, because it may stimulate uterine contractions. If you have a hormone-sensitive condition, such as estrogen-positive breast cancer, fibroids, or endometriosis, seek professional guidance before use.

Mild side effects like digestive discomfort, light sensitivity, or dizziness are rare but possible. To minimize any adverse reactions, it's best to start with a low dose. Always follow the package directions or consult a qualified herbal practitioner for personalized guidance.

Growing and Harvesting

Dong quai is a perennial herb native to China, Korea, and Japan and thrives in cool, moist environments with well-drained, nutrient-rich soil. It prefers partial shade and can withstand cooler temperatures, making it a hardy plant once established.

The root, which has the most medicinal value, is typically harvested in the autumn when its bioactive compounds are at their peak. After harvesting, the roots are cleaned, sliced, and dried for medicinal use. Traditional processing methods, such as steaming or slow drying, are often employed to enhance its therapeutic properties. Proper storage in airtight containers helps preserve potency for use in teas, tinctures, and herbal formulations.

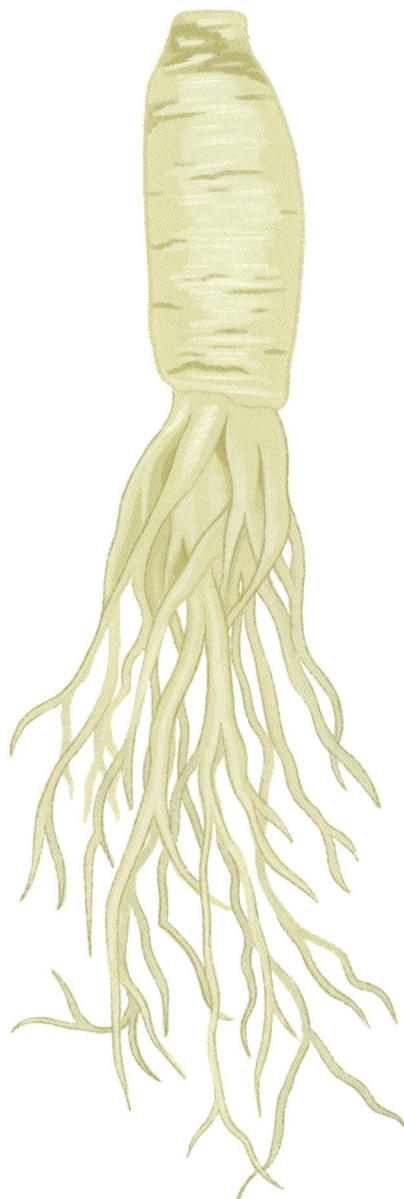

Dong Quai Nourishing Herbal Tonic

This warming blend is traditionally used to promote menstrual regularity, ease discomfort, and revitalize the body. Gentle yet effective, it can be incorporated into a daily routine to maintain overall reproductive and systemic wellness.

Yield: 2 cups (480 ml)

2 tablespoons (12 g) dried dong quai root (for blood nourishment and hormonal balance)

1 teaspoon (2 g) dried ginger root (for circulation and warming effects)

1 teaspoon (2.7 g) dried cinnamon bark (for additional circulatory and digestive support)

2 cups (480 ml) water

1 tablespoon (15 ml) raw honey (optional, for sweetness)

Preparation

In a small saucepan, combine the dried dong quai, ginger, cinnamon, and water. Bring to a simmer over low heat and let steep for 20 to 30 minutes. Strain the liquid into a cup and add honey, if desired.

How to Use

Drink 1 cup (240 ml) daily for general reproductive support or up to 2 cups (480 ml) during menstruation to ease cramping and regulate flow.

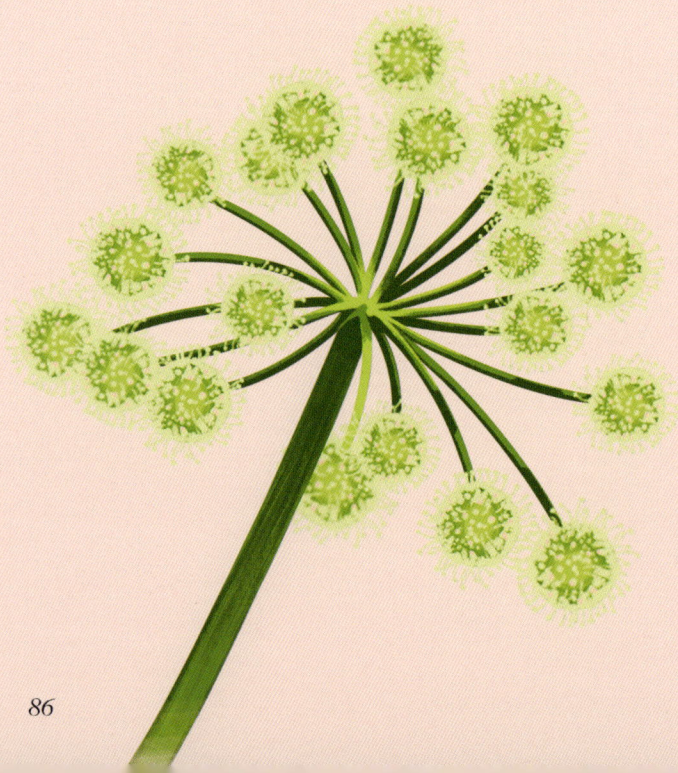

Maca *(Lepidium meyenii)*
The Fertility Booster

Maca, a hardy root vegetable native to the high-altitude regions of the Peruvian Andes, has long been celebrated for its revitalizing effects on energy, stamina, and fertility. For over two thousand years, the Indigenous Quechua people have cultivated and consumed maca, often drying and grinding the root into flour or boiling it into a nourishing tonic. It is considered sacred food—both sustenance and medicine.

Legend has it that Andean warriors ate maca before battle to enhance strength and endurance, while women relied on it to promote fertility, vitality, and resilience during pregnancy. Maca was also used ceremonially, offered to the gods as a symbol of life force and agricultural abundance. Its cultivation was so highly valued that at times it was used as currency or tribute in trade with neighboring communities.

Today maca's legacy as a revered Andean botanical continues, with its traditional uses providing the foundation for its modern popularity as a root of resilience and reproductive support.

What the Science Says

Maca *(Lepidium meyenii)* has long been valued for its ability to enhance fertility, support hormonal balance, and improve energy levels. Unlike direct hormonal stimulants, maca works by nourishing the endocrine system, helping the body self-regulate hormone production rather than introducing external hormones.

The bioactive compounds in maca play a key role in its hormone-balancing effects. Among the most significant are macamides, unique **alkaloids** found exclusively in maca, that support endocrine function by influencing the hypothalamus and pituitary gland, the body's hormonal command center. By supporting the hypothalamic-pituitary-adrenal (HPA) axis—the central network that controls how your body responds to stress, manages energy, and produces hormones—maca helps the brain communicate more effectively with the adrenal and reproductive glands. This in turn promotes healthy levels of estrogen, progesterone, and testosterone, making maca beneficial for both men and women.

Scientific research has provided strong support for maca's effects on sexual health for men and hormonal balance for women. For example, a 2001 clinical trial in the *Asian Journal of Andrology* found that maca supplementation significantly improved sperm concentration and motility in men experiencing infertility, reinforcing its role in male reproductive health. In addition, a 2022 study in *Phytomedicine* demonstrated that maca reduced menopausal symptoms, including hot flashes and mood fluctuations, by helping to stabilize estrogen levels without acting as a **phytoestrogen**.

Earlier research in *BMC Complementary and Alternative Medicine* (2010) highlighted maca's ability to enhance sexual function and libido in both men and women, confirming its traditional reputation as a reproductive tonic. These findings align with maca's long-standing use in Indigenous medicine as a natural remedy for fertility, to stabilize hormone levels, and for overall vitality.

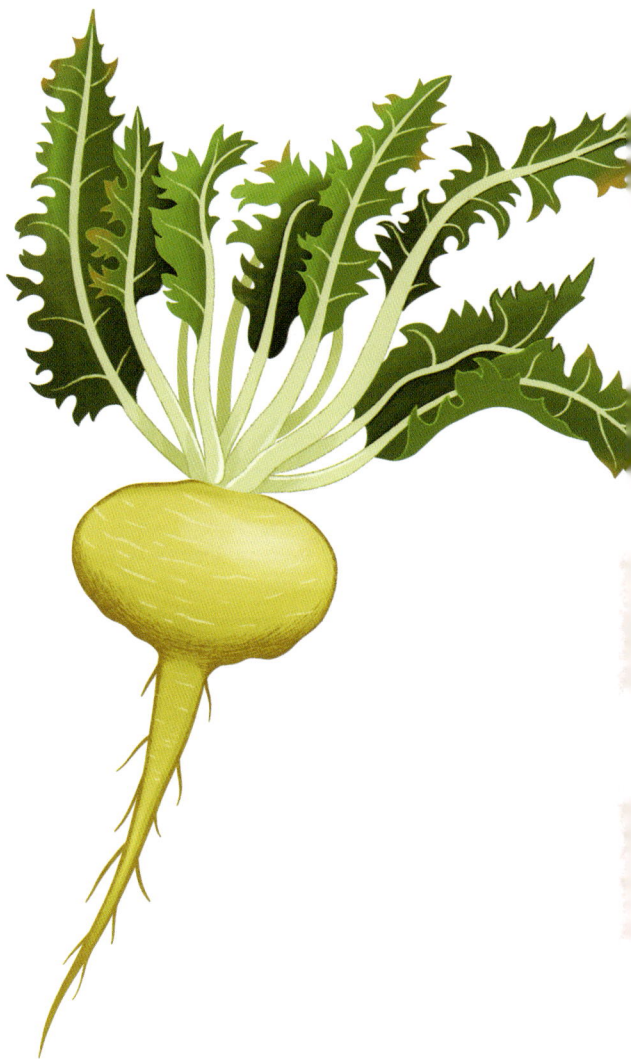

Another important group of compounds found in maca are glucosinolates, sulfur-containing compounds that support hormonal detoxification. These compounds aid the liver in metabolizing excess hormones, helping to prevent estrogen dominance and maintain optimal endocrine function. Additionally, maca contains **flavonoids** with antioxidant and anti-inflammatory properties that help protect reproductive tissues from oxidative stress, a factor that can negatively impact fertility and hormone function. The root is also a rich source of essential minerals, including calcium, magnesium, zinc, and iron, all of which contribute to reproductive health and energy production.

Maca's adaptogenic properties help reduce stress-related hormonal imbalances by regulating cortisol levels, which is key because chronic stress can interfere with menstrual cycles, ovulation, and testosterone production. By keeping cortisol in balance, maca supports the body's natural ability to adapt to stress, promoting more stable hormone levels. Research also suggests that maca may enhance dopamine and serotonin activity—neurotransmitters that influence mood, libido, and overall well-being.

Uses and Indications

Maca is commonly used to support reproductive health in both men and women.

For women, it can be used to help regulate menstrual cycles, reduce premenstrual syndrome (PMS) symptoms, and improve overall fertility. Maca is particularly beneficial if you're experiencing irregular periods, polycystic ovary syndrome (PCOS), or perimenopausal symptoms.

For men, maca is often used to enhance sperm quality, boost testosterone levels, and improve libido. Unlike synthetic testosterone boosters, maca supports natural hormone production without causing hormonal imbalances or dependency.

Beyond reproductive health, you can use maca to enhance energy, endurance, and mental clarity. Its adaptogenic nature makes it an excellent choice if you're experiencing fatigue, burnout, or high levels of stress. Because it supports adrenal function, it can also be a useful ally if you're recovering from chronic stress, adrenal fatigue, or HPA axis dysregulation.

Interactions and Safety

Maca is generally well-tolerated and safe but there are a few caveats you need to be aware of. Due to its hormone-modulating effects, if you have a hormone-sensitive condition, such as estrogen-positive breast cancer, endometriosis, or uterine fibroids, please consult a healthcare provider before using maca.

If you have a thyroid disorder, use maca with caution, as excessive intake may interfere with thyroid hormone balance. While rare, mild side effects such as digestive discomfort or headaches may occur, particularly when taking large doses.

If you're pregnant or breastfeeding, consult a healthcare professional before incorporating maca into your routine, as research on its safety in these populations is limited.

Growing and Harvesting

Maca thrives in the harsh, high-altitude conditions of the Peruvian Andes, growing in rocky, nutrient-rich soil at elevations above 12,000 feet (3.7 km). This extreme environment—marked by intense ultraviolet radiation, drastic temperature swings, and low oxygen levels—gives maca its potent adaptogenic qualities. Because of these unique growing conditions, maca isn't an ideal plant for home gardens or typical climates. Instead, it's best used in its powdered or encapsulated form, where its resilience is preserved and concentrated.

Hormone Balance Tincture

This hormone-balancing tincture combines maca with other adaptogenic and hormone-supportive herbs to promote endocrine health, improve fertility, and enhance overall vitality.

2 tablespoons (14 g) dried maca root powder

1 tablespoon (6.6 g) dried ashwagandha root (for adrenal support)

1 teaspoon (2 g) dried shatavari root (for reproductive health)

1 cup (240 ml) vodka or brandy (at least 40% alcohol)

Preparation

Combine all the dried herbs in a clean glass jar and pour the alcohol over them, ensuring the herbs are fully submerged. Seal the jar tightly and store it in a cool, dark place for 4 to 6 weeks, shaking it gently every few days. After the tincture has steeped, strain it through cheesecloth or a fine strainer, pressing the herbs to extract as much liquid as possible. Transfer the tincture to a dark glass dropper bottle for storage.

How to Use

Take 1 to 2 droppers full (1 to 2 ml) daily to support hormonal balance and reproductive health. This tincture can be taken on its own or added to water or tea.

Fun Fact

Maca's ability to grow in extreme conditions has earned it the nickname "Peruvian ginseng," even though it is not botanically related to ginseng. It's a staple food for Andean communities, where it is often consumed as a porridge or blended into traditional drinks.

Tribulus (*Tribulus terrestris*)
The Strength and Vitality Herb

Tribulus, often referred to as "puncture vine" due to its sharp, spiky fruit, has a long-standing reputation as a tonic for strength, endurance, and reproductive health. This herb has been revered in Ayurvedic, Traditional Chinese Medicine (TCM), and Mediterranean herbal traditions for centuries. In Ayurveda, Tribulus has been used to support kidney function, enhance male virility, and balance hormones in both men and women. In TCM, Tribulus is valued for its ability to dispel wind, soothe liver stagnation, and improve circulation. The ancient Greeks and Romans consumed Tribulus as a natural performance enhancer, believing it to boost physical stamina and overall vitality.

In modern herbalism, Tribulus is best known for its role in supporting testosterone levels, improving libido, and enhancing athletic performance. While widely marketed as a supplement for bodybuilders and athletes, Tribulus offers much broader benefits, including cardiovascular support, hormone balance, and adaptogenic properties that help the body respond to stress. It is considered a safe and effective herb for those looking to improve strength, vitality, and overall well-being.

What the Science Says

Tribulus (*Tribulus terrestris*) is widely used in traditional medicine for its hormonal, cardiovascular, and adaptogenic benefits. Its medicinal properties are found in its fruit, leaves, and roots, which contain a diverse array of bioactive compounds.

Tribulus supports reproductive health through its key bioactive compounds: **steroidal saponins**, especially protodioscin. These plant-based compounds stimulate the hypothalamic-pituitary-gonadal (HPG) axis, helping the body naturally increase testosterone and dehydroepiandrosterone (DHEA) levels without the risks associated with synthetic hormones. This makes Tribulus a valuable herb for supporting male fertility, libido, and muscle strength, as well as balancing estrogen and androgen levels in women.

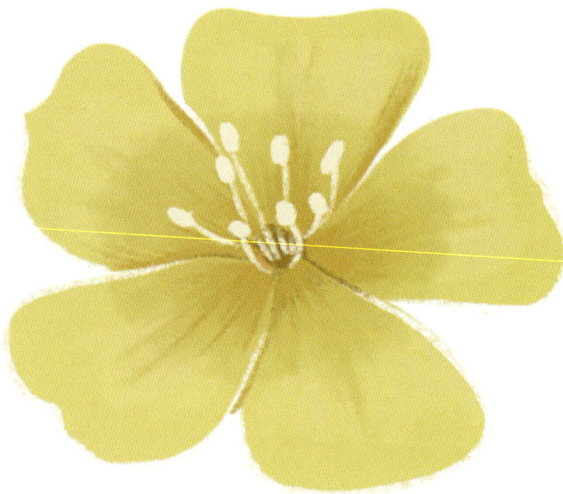

A 2018 study in the *Journal of Dietary Supplements* found that Tribulus supplementation improved sperm concentration, motility, and testosterone levels in men experiencing infertility. A 2021 *Phytomedicine* review further supported its role in male reproductive function and hormonal modulation. In women, a 2014 *BMC Complementary and Alternative Medicine* study linked Tribulus to improved hormonal balance and symptom relief in those with polycystic ovary syndrome (PCOS).

Tribulus also contains **lignans**, plant-based **polyphenols** that can bind to estrogen receptors and either mimic or modulate estrogen activity depending on the body's hormonal environment. This regulatory effect supports hormonal balance in both men and women. Additionally, **coumarins**—aromatic compounds with natural blood-thinning and vasodilatory properties—help enhance circulation and relax blood vessels. This contributes to Tribulus's cardiovascular benefits and makes it especially valuable for promoting endurance, physical performance, and erectile function in men.

Tribulus also contains **flavonoids** that provide antioxidant and anti-inflammatory benefits, protecting cells from oxidative stress and supporting healthy circulation. In addition, Tribulus's **alkaloids** contribute to its adaptogenic properties, helping the body regulate stress responses and maintain balanced energy metabolism—especially during periods of physical or emotional strain.

With its synergistic combination of hormone-balancing, circulation-enhancing, and adaptogenic properties, Tribulus remains a trusted herb for those looking to optimize reproductive health, boost physical resilience, and support overall well-being.

Uses and Indications

Tribulus is widely used as natural support for reproductive health, physical performance, and overall vitality. Men can take it to enhance testosterone production, improve libido, and support muscle growth. It also supports prostate health, improves sperm quality, and enhances cardiovascular function.

For women, Tribulus can help balance estrogen and progesterone levels, making it beneficial if you're experiencing menstrual irregularities, PCOS, or menopause-related hormone imbalances. Because of its mild diuretic properties, it can also be used to promote urinary tract health and reduce water retention.

Athletes and individuals looking to improve endurance and recovery can use Tribulus as a natural performance enhancer. Tribulus can improve oxygen delivery to muscles, reduce fatigue, and enhance post-workout recovery. It can also be used to combat stress and fatigue, making it a useful adaptogen for those experiencing burnout, adrenal fatigue, or chronic exhaustion.

Interactions and Safety

Tribulus is generally well-tolerated by most people when used in appropriate doses, but there are some precautions to consider. You may experience mild digestive discomfort or headaches, particularly if you take high doses. Because Tribulus can influence hormone levels, consult a healthcare provider before use if you have a hormone-sensitive condition, such as estrogen-positive breast cancer or a prostate disorder. Due to its potential effects on blood sugar and blood pressure, Tribulus should be used with caution if you're taking antihypertensive or antidiabetic medications. The same goes if you have a kidney disorder, as its diuretic properties may impact fluid balance. If you're pregnant or breastfeeding, avoid Tribulus, as its effects on pregnancy and lactation have not been thoroughly studied.

Growing and Harvesting

Tribulus is a hardy, drought-resistant plant that thrives in arid and semi-arid regions across Asia, the Mediterranean, and parts of North and South America. It grows well in sandy or rocky soils and is often found in disturbed areas, such as roadsides and fields.

The medicinal parts of the plant, including the fruit, leaves, and roots, are typically harvested in late summer or early fall. The fruit is dried and ground into powder for use in extracts and supplements, while the roots and leaves are sometimes used in traditional decoctions or tinctures. Proper storage in airtight containers preserves its potency and ensures its long-term efficacy.

Fun Fact

Tribulus has also been used in Ayurvedic medicine for centuries as a spiritual herb believed to promote inner strength, confidence, and resilience. In traditional practices, it was often given to warriors before battle to enhance endurance and courage.

Tribulus Strength-Boosting Cordial

This invigorating herbal cordial combines Tribulus with warming spices to create a delicious and energizing tonic that supports strength, stamina, and reproductive health.

Yield: 4 cups (960 ml)

¼ cup (12 g) dried Tribulus fruit

1 cinnamon stick

1 teaspoon (2 g) dried ginger root

1 teaspoon (3 g) raw cacao nibs

2 cups (480 ml) water

1 cup (240 ml) raw honey

1 cup (240 ml) brandy or vodka (optional, for preservation)

Preparation

In a medium saucepan, combine the dried Tribulus fruit, cinnamon stick, ginger root, cacao nibs, and water. Simmer gently over low heat for 30 minutes, stirring occasionally to ensure even extraction of the medicinal compounds.

Remove the mixture from the heat and allow it to cool slightly. Strain the liquid through a fine strainer or cheesecloth into a clean bowl, pressing the solids to extract as much liquid as possible.

Stir in the raw honey until fully dissolved, and if desired, add brandy or vodka to extend the cordial's shelf life. Transfer to an airtight glass bottle and refrigerate for up to 3 months, or longer if alcohol is included.

How to Use

Take 1 to 2 tablespoons (15 to 30 ml) daily as a vitality tonic or up to three times daily for additional stamina and strength support. This cordial can be taken alone or diluted in warm water.

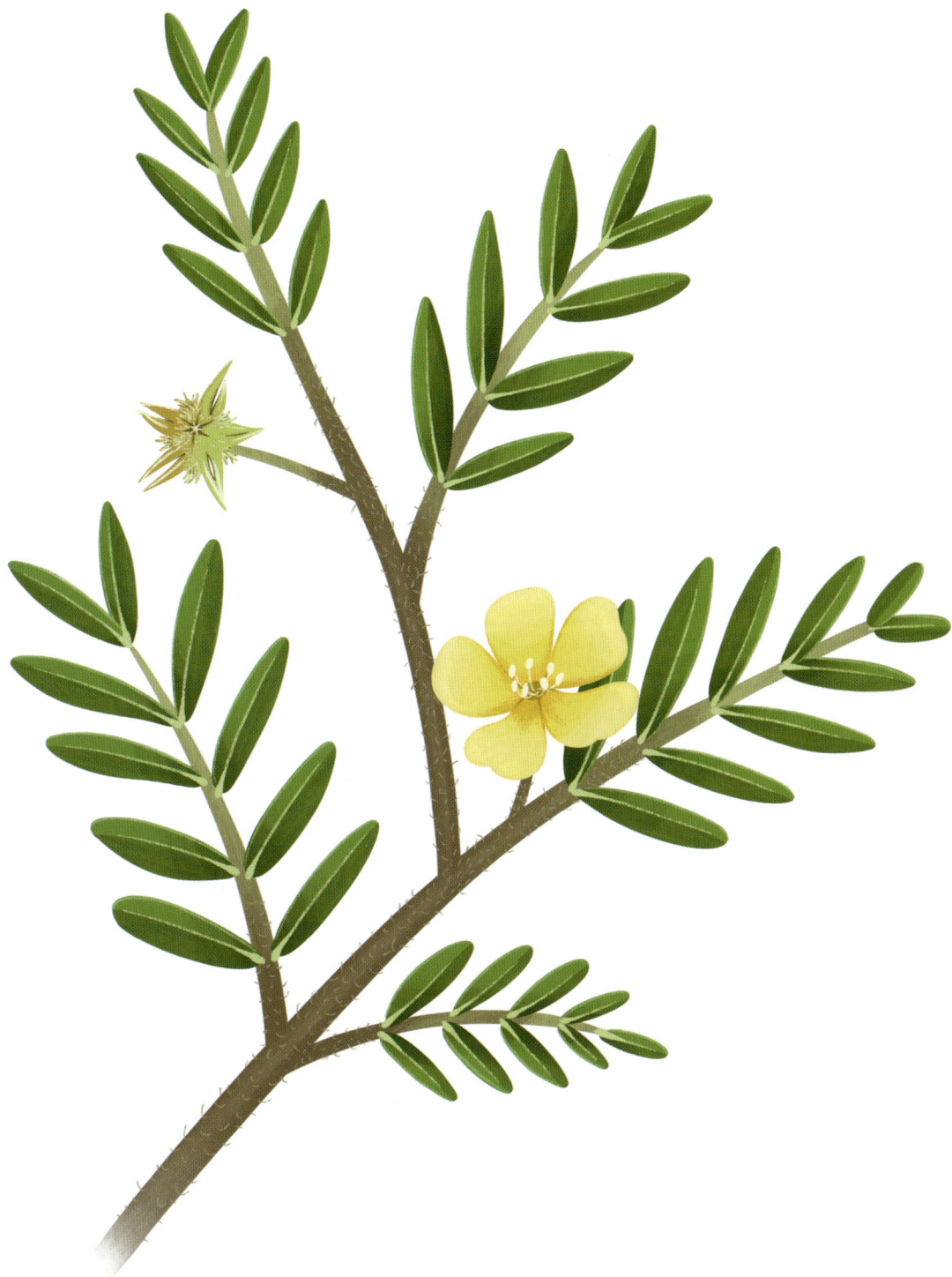

Chapter 6

Mind Matters: Herbs for Mental Health, Cognition, and Mood

Welcome to the realm of the mind, where herbal allies nurture resilience, focus, and much more. Our mental wellness hinges on the intricate workings of the brain, where neurons communicate via electrical and chemical signals to regulate our mood, memory, and stress response. Neurotransmitters like serotonin and dopamine orchestrate this balance, guiding everything from how we feel to how we connect with others. But when stress disrupts this delicate system, elevated cortisol levels can overwhelm brain processes, leaving us feeling overwhelmed, unfocused, or emotionally drained.

The nervous system is the body's command center, constantly processing information and helping us respond to the world around us. It relies on a healthy network of brain cells to stay sharp and balanced. These cells not only send signals but also clean up waste and deliver nutrients the brain needs to function at its best. If something interferes with this system, such as stress, inflammation, or poor nutrition, it can affect our ability to focus, feel calm, or maintain a stable mood.

Herbs can restore harmony, helping to balance stress hormones, enhance neurotransmitter activity, and improve blood flow to the brain. Ashwagandha, an adaptogen, calms the hypothalamic-pituitary-adrenal (HPA) axis, regulating cortisol and supporting nerve health. Rhodiola bolsters neurotransmitter function, improving endurance and reducing fatigue. Reishi mushroom, a calming and immune-supportive herb, fortifies the nervous system. Gotu kola, a revered brain tonic, improves memory and nurtures neuronal pathways, while ginkgo enhances blood circulation to the brain, boosting cognitive function.

This chapter includes recipes like a soothing Ashwagandha Extract for Stress Relief and a refreshing Gotu Kola Tea for Mental Clarity. With these herbal allies at hand, you can steady your mind, restore balance, and support restful sleep. Let's explore the path to clarity, calm, and focus.

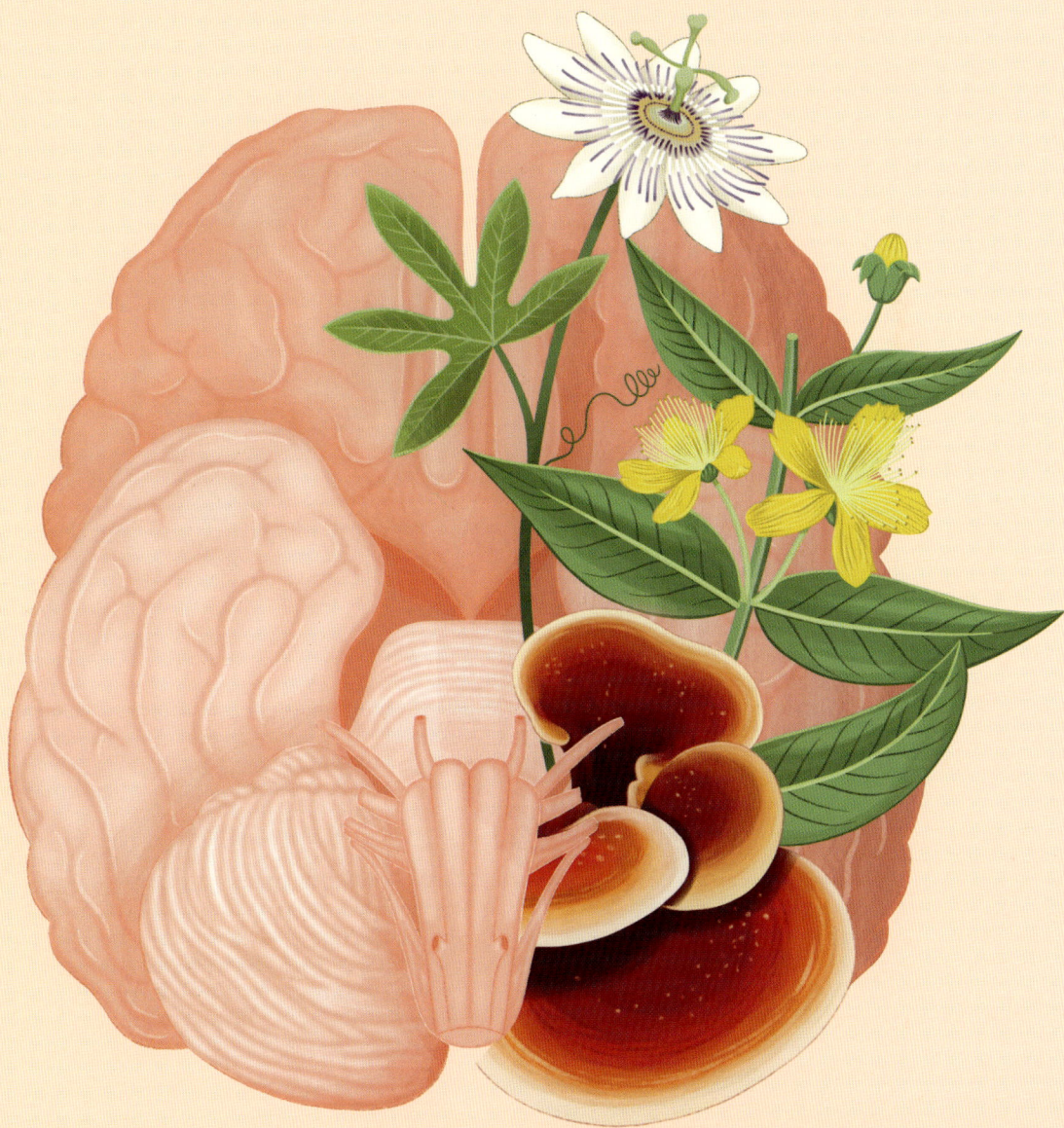

Ashwagandha *(Withania somnifera)*
The Resilient Relaxer

Ashwagandha has been a foundational herb in Ayurvedic medicine for over three thousand years, prized for its adaptogenic properties and ability to promote strength, endurance, and mental clarity. In Sanskrit, its name translates to "smell of a horse," a nod to both its distinct aroma and its reputation for imparting vitality and resilience. Traditionally, ashwagandha was used to support warriors and scholars alike, helping to sharpen focus, restore energy, and enhance physical stamina. It has long been classified as a *rasayana*, or rejuvenator, meaning it is used to promote longevity and overall well-being.

Today ashwagandha remains one of the most widely studied adaptogens, used to balance stress hormones, support cognitive function, and improve sleep quality. Its popularity continues to grow as research confirms its broad-spectrum benefits for physical, mental, and emotional health.

What the Science Says

The medicinal potency of Ashwagandha *(Withania somnifera)* lies in its roots and leaves, both of which are rich in bioactive compounds that provide adaptogenic, neuroprotective, and hormone-balancing effects. The most well-researched of these are withanolides—naturally occurring **steroidal lactones** known for their ability to modulate stress responses and reduce inflammation. These compounds help regulate the stress hormone cortisol, which is released when we feel tense, under threat, or otherwise triggered into fight-or-flight mode. Withanolides also support immune resilience, nervous system stability, and overall homeostasis.

The primary mechanism of action of ashwagandha is its ability to modulate the hypothalamic-pituitary-adrenal (HPA) axis, the system that governs the body's response to stress. By helping regulate cortisol production—the body's main stress hormone—ashwagandha supports a more balanced stress response. It also enhances gamma-aminobutyric acid (GABA) signaling, which means it boosts the activity of gamma-aminobutyric acid, a calming neurotransmitter that reduces neuron excitability. This helps quiet an overactive nervous system, promoting relaxation, improving sleep quality, and stabilizing mood. Ashwagandha also interacts with dopamine and serotonin receptors, further supporting emotional resilience, reducing anxiety, and enhancing mental focus.

Ashwagandha's benefits for cognitive function have been confirmed through modern research. A 2017 study in the *Journal of Dietary Supplements* found that ashwagandha extract significantly improved memory, attention, and information processing speed in adults experiencing cognitive decline. This supports its historical reputation for sharpening focus and enhancing mental clarity.

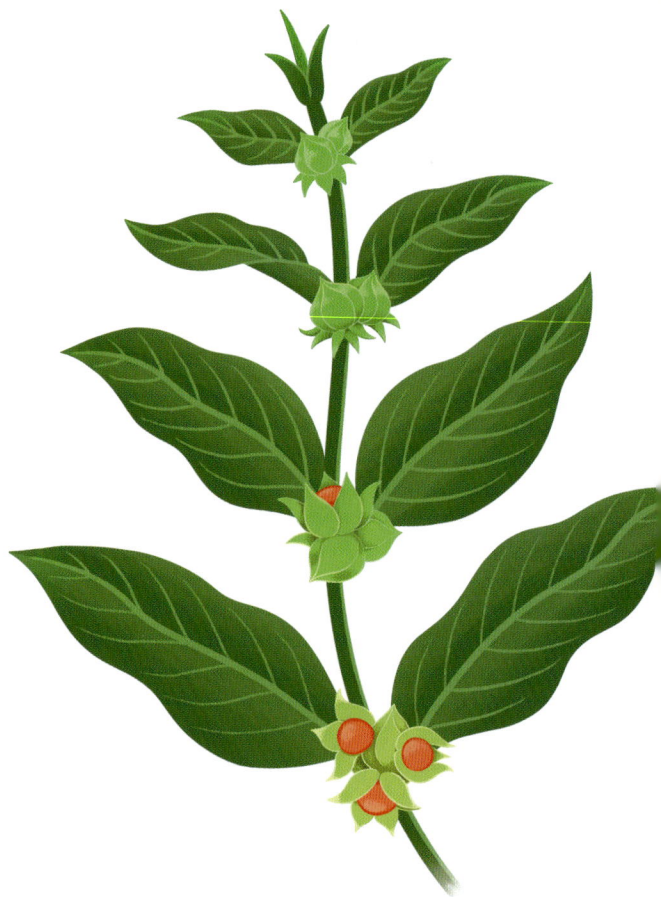

Research suggests that ashwagandha may also benefit thyroid health. A 2018 study published in the *Journal of Alternative and Complementary Medicine* showed that ashwagandha supplementation helped support endocrine balance by regulating thyroid hormone levels in participants with subclinical hypothyroidism.

One of the traditional uses for ashwagandha has long been as a rejuvenator after strenuous physical activity, and the herb has also been studied extensively in this capacity. A 2015 study published in the *Journal of the International Society of Sports Nutrition* found that ashwagandha supplementation significantly improved muscle strength, endurance, and recovery in resistance-trained men.

Altogether, ashwagandha's ability to reduce stress and promote emotional well-being, improve physical endurance, and boost cognitive function makes it one of the most versatile adaptogens in herbal medicine.

Ashwagandha Extract for Stress Relief

Try this simple recipe to experience ashwagandha's adaptogenic benefits.

Yield: 2 cups (480 ml)

½ cup (53 g) dried ashwagandha root

2 cups (480 ml) brandy or vodka

Preparation

Place the dried ashwagandha root into a clean glass jar with a tight-fitting lid. Pour the alcohol over the root, ensuring it is fully submerged. Seal the jar and store it in a cool, dark place for 2 to 4 weeks, shaking it every few days to encourage extraction. After the steeping period, strain the extract using a fine-mesh strainer or cheesecloth. Transfer the liquid to a dark glass bottle for storage.

How to Use

Take 1 to 2 droppers (about 1 to 2 ml) in water or tea as needed to promote relaxation, reduce stress, and support nervous system balance. For best results, use consistently over time.

Uses and Indications

Use ashwagandha to support stress management, boost energy levels, and enhance cognitive function. You can also add this herb to your wellness routine to aid in adrenal support, sleep improvement, and hormonal balance. Its adaptogenic properties make it particularly valuable if you're experiencing chronic stress, burnout, or nervous system exhaustion.

Interactions and Safety

Ashwagandha is generally considered safe, but some individuals should use caution. If you're pregnant, avoid ashwagandha as it may stimulate uterine contractions. If you have hyperthyroidism, consult your healthcare provider before taking ashwagandha, which may increase thyroid hormone levels. If you're taking sedatives or anti-anxiety medications, ashwagandha may enhance these effects, so be mindful of potential interactions. Always be sure to select high-quality, standardized extracts to ensure the product has optimal potency and meets safety standards.

Growing and Harvesting

Ashwagandha thrives in warm, dry climates with sandy, well-drained soil and full sun exposure. Native to India and parts of Africa, it grows best in regions with long summers and minimal rainfall. Though it can be grown in temperate zones, it requires an extended growing season or greenhouse cultivation to reach full maturity.

The plant is typically harvested in late fall when its leaves begin to yellow, signaling that the roots have developed their full medicinal potency. The roots are carefully dug up, washed, and dried in a well-ventilated area away from direct sunlight to preserve their bioactive compounds. Once dried, they can be stored whole or ground into powder for long-term use.

Ashwagandha's hardy nature reflects its adaptogenic properties; it thrives under stress and helps us do the same by building resilience and restoring balance.

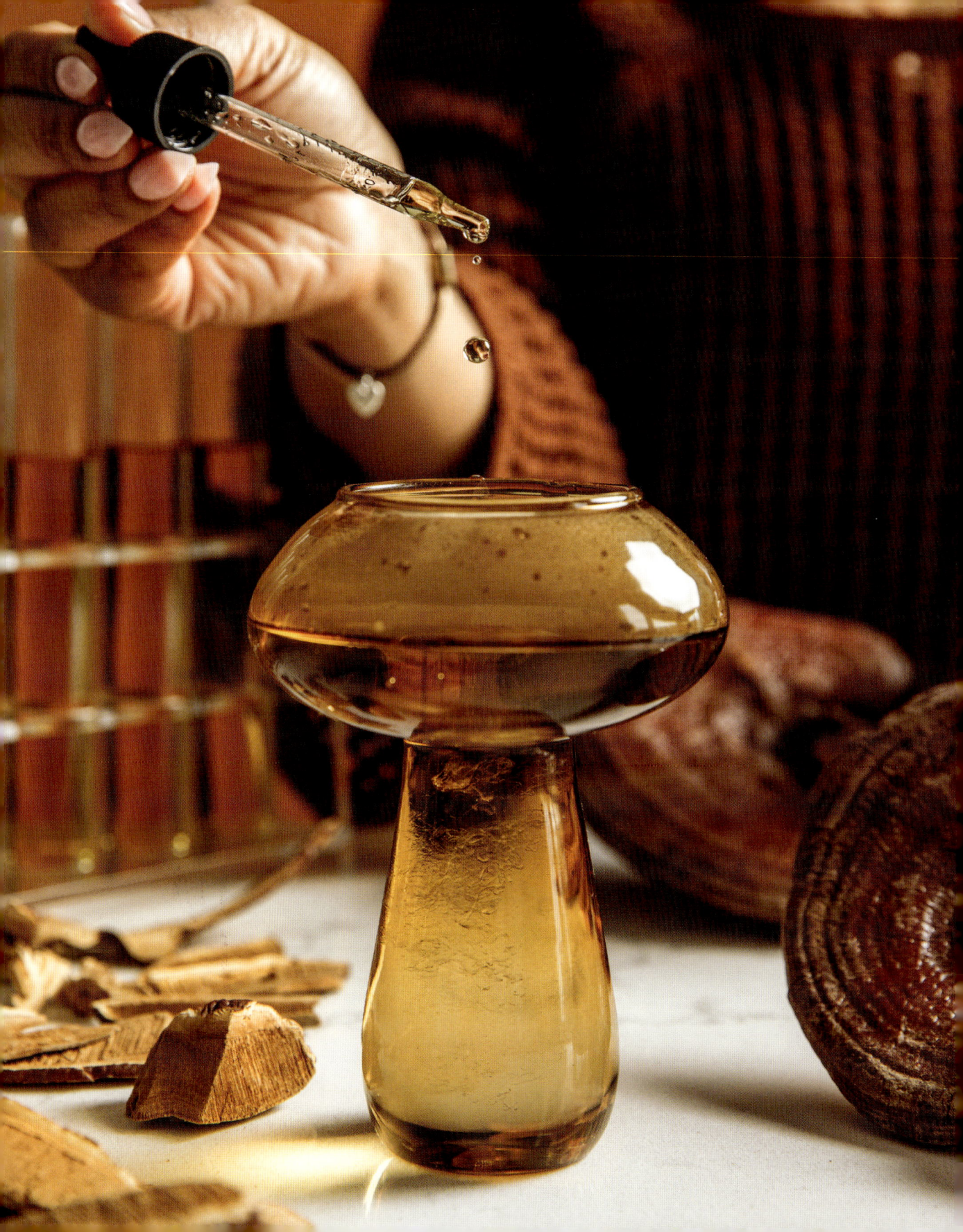

Reishi Mushroom (*Ganoderma lucidum*)
The Calming Adaptogen

Reishi mushroom, often called the "mushroom of immortality," has been a staple in Traditional Chinese Medicine (TCM) and Japanese Kampo medicine for over two thousand years. In ancient China, it was reserved for emperors and high-ranking officials, as it was believed to promote longevity, inner peace, and resilience against disease. Reishi was historically used to nourish the Shen, or spirit, in TCM, making it a valuable herb for calming the mind, reducing stress, and supporting emotional balance.

Reishi's reach extended beyond Asia to Western herbalism practitioners when research confirmed its immune-supporting, stress-reducing, and anti-inflammatory properties. Today it is a commonly sought-after natural adaptogen, helping people cope with chronic stress, anxiety, and sleep disturbances, while enhancing overall well-being.

What the Science Says

Reishi's therapeutic properties stem from its rich composition of bioactive compounds, primarily **triterpenes**, **polysaccharides**, and **ganoderic acids**, which provide anti-inflammatory, adaptogenic, and neuroprotective effects. Research has confirmed the latter; a 2017 study in *Neural Regeneration Research* suggested that reishi extract may support cognitive function and protect against neurodegenerative diseases, reinforcing its role in long-term brain health.

One of reishi's primary mechanisms of action is its ability to modulate the hypothalamic-pituitary-adrenal (HPA) axis, the system that governs the body's stress response. By balancing cortisol levels, reishi helps the body adapt to stress more efficiently, preventing the excessive release of stress hormones that contribute to anxiety, fatigue, and sleep disturbances.

A 2011 study in *Phytotherapy Research* found that reishi extract significantly reduced fatigue and improved well-being in individuals experiencing chronic stress. Another study in *Food Reviews International* (2025) demonstrated that reishi polysaccharides enhanced sleep quality by increasing non-REM sleep, supporting its traditional use for promoting deep relaxation and restfulness.

Reishi also acts as a nervous system regulator, with triterpenes playing a role in calming overactive neural pathways. These compounds have been shown to interact with GABA receptors, similar to mild sedatives but without the risk of dependence. This makes reishi particularly beneficial for reducing stress and anxiety, promoting a balanced mood, and enhancing sleep and emotional resilience.

With its ability to reduce stress, promote relaxation, enhance sleep, and support emotional stability, reishi stands as one of the most revered adaptogenic herbs in modern and traditional medicine alike.

Uses and Indications

Reishi is often used to reduce stress, support emotional resilience, promote restful sleep, and enhance overall well-being. Its adaptogenic effects make it particularly beneficial if you're dealing with chronic stress, burnout, or difficulty winding down after a long day.

Safety and Interactions

Reishi is generally well-tolerated, though it does produce mild anticoagulant effects, which means it may interact with any blood-thinning medications. If you're pregnant, breastfeeding, or taking prescription medications, consult a healthcare provider before use.

Growing and Harvesting

Reishi mushrooms thrive in warm, humid environments and are typically found growing on decaying hardwood trees, such as oak, maple, and hemlock. In the wild, they prefer shaded forested areas with ample moisture. While it is naturally rare, modern cultivation has made reishi more accessible, allowing it to be grown on hardwood logs or supplemented sawdust blocks in controlled environments.

Cultivating reishi requires patience, as it takes several months to fully mature. Spores or mycelium are introduced into prepared logs or substrate where the fungus slowly develops. The characteristic kidney-shaped fruiting bodies with their glossy red surface begin forming after an extended growth period. When mature, reishi can be harvested by carefully cutting the mushrooms at the base.

Once harvested, reishi must be dried thoroughly to preserve the medicinal compounds. This is typically done by slicing the mushrooms and air-drying them in a well-ventilated space, away from direct sunlight. Once fully dried, reishi can be stored in airtight containers for long-term use in decoctions, tinctures, and powdered extracts.

Reishi Mushroom Extract for Relaxation

This deeply calming extract captures the full spectrum of reishi's adaptogenic and nervous system–supportive compounds, making it ideal for reducing stress and promoting relaxation.

Yield: 4 cups (960 ml)

½ cup (28 g) dried reishi mushroom slices

2 cups (480 ml) filtered water

2 cups (480 ml) 40% alcohol (such as vodka or brandy)

Preparation

Add the reishi mushroom slices and water to a small saucepan. Bring to a gentle simmer, cover, and let it simmer for 45 to 60 minutes to extract the beneficial compounds. Strain the liquid, pressing out as much extract as possible from the mushrooms, and allow it to cool completely. Combine the strained reishi decoction with alcohol in a glass jar, shaking well to mix. Store the jar in a cool, dark place for 4 to 6 weeks, shaking it every few days to encourage extraction. After the steeping period, strain the liquid and transfer it to a clean bottle for long-term storage.

How to Use

Take 1 to 2 dropperfuls (about 30 to 60 drops) daily, either directly under the tongue or diluted in a small amount of water or tea. Reishi is best taken in the evening to support relaxation and restful sleep.

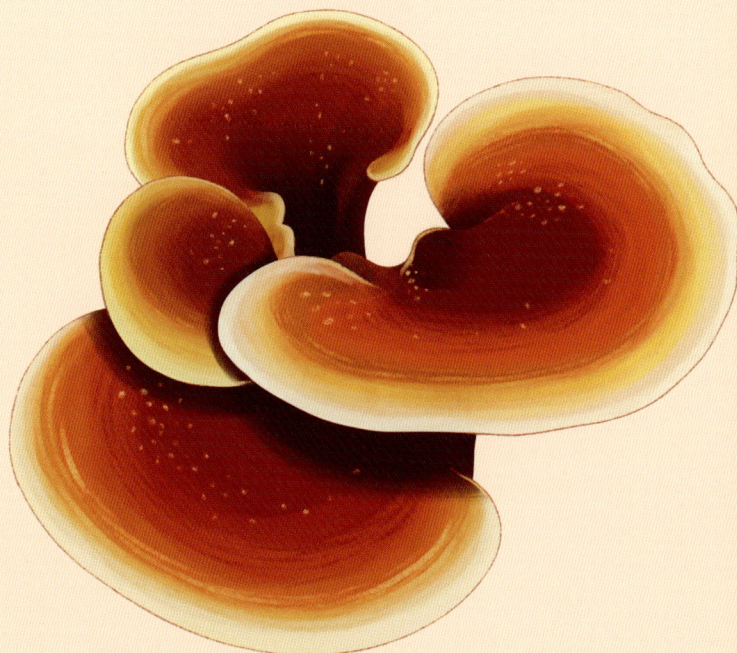

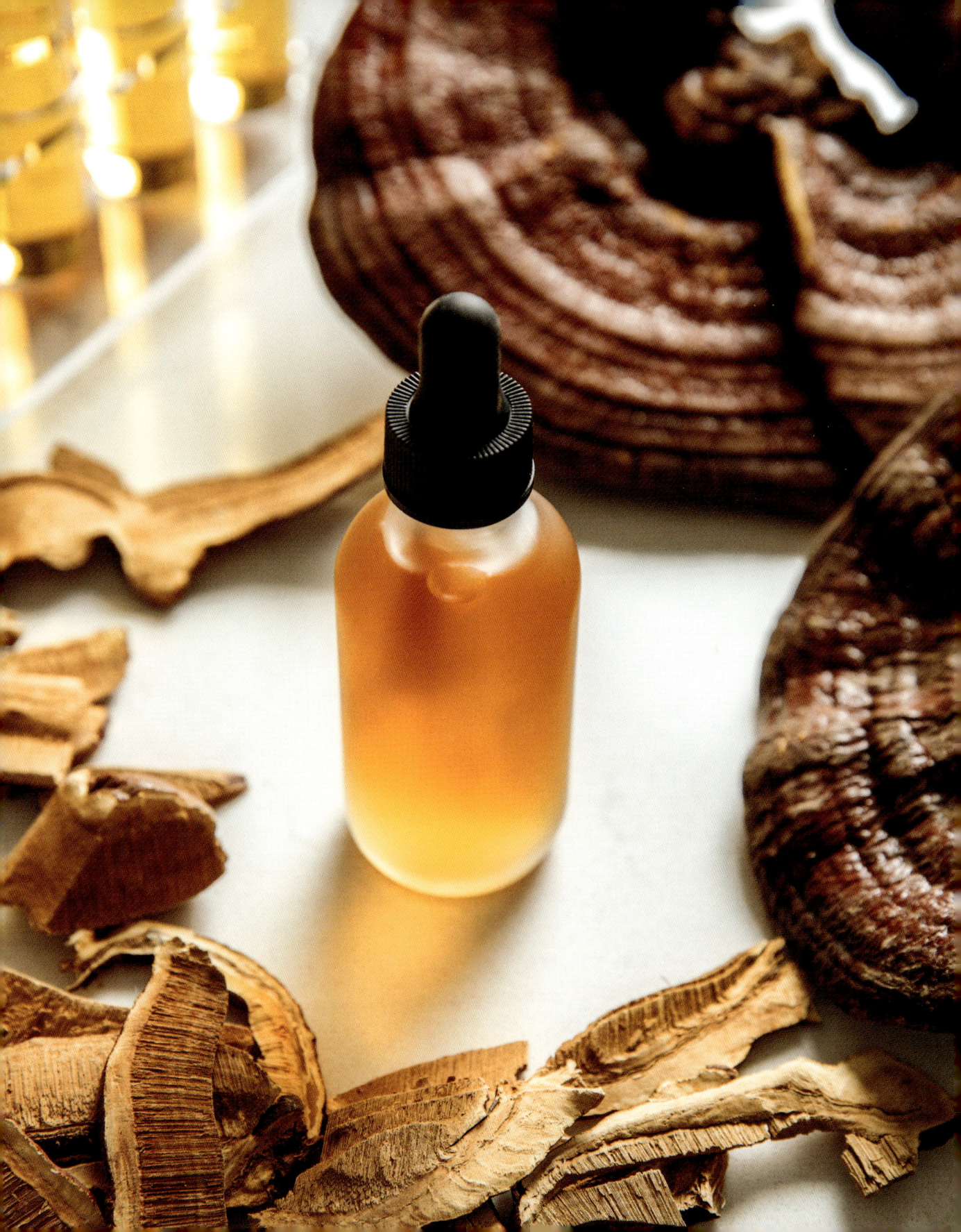

Skullcap *(Scutellaria lateriflora)*
The Nervous System Nurturer

Skullcap has long been revered in North American herbal traditions for its ability to soothe the nervous system and promote relaxation. Used by Indigenous tribes and early European settlers, it was often included in remedies for stress, nervous exhaustion, and tension headaches. The herb gained further recognition in the nineteenth century, when Eclectic physicians prescribed it as a "nerve tonic" for people experiencing chronic stress, anxiety, and insomnia.

Unlike stronger sedatives, skullcap was prized for its ability to promote calm without dulling mental clarity, making it a go-to remedy for those experiencing nervous tension without needing excessive sedation. Today it remains a gentle but effective herbal ally for emotional balance and nervous system support.

What the Science Says
Skullcap contains a rich profile of bioactive compounds that contribute to its calming and neuroprotective effects. The aerial parts of the plant are abundant in **flavonoids** such as baicalin, baicalein, and wogonin, which have been shown to regulate neurotransmitter activity and reduce oxidative stress in the brain. A study in *Nutritional Perspectives: Journal of the Council on Nutrition* (2024) supported this, showing that skullcap's flavonoids shielded brain cells from damage due to oxidative stress.

Like passionflower, one of skullcap's most valuable properties is its ability to increase gamma-aminobutyric acid (GABA) levels in the brain. GABA is the primary inhibitory neurotransmitter, responsible for reducing excessive neural excitability and promoting relaxation. Research suggests that low GABA levels are linked to anxiety, restlessness, and stress-related conditions, making skullcap a valuable herb for supporting emotional stability. Research published in *Phytomedicine* in 2003 showed that skullcap compounds interact with GABA receptors—much like pharmaceutical anxiolytics, which are medications used to reduce anxiety—but without the risk of dependency. Another study published in *British Journal of Wellbeing* (2010) found that skullcap extract enhanced mood and reduced anxiety in healthy individuals without causing sedation. These findings suggest that skullcap may be particularly beneficial for individuals dealing with chronic stress, nervous tension, or mood fluctuations.

Beyond its calming effects, skullcap has anti-inflammatory and antioxidant properties that support overall cognitive health and nervous system resilience. With its ability to modulate neurotransmitters, reduce oxidative stress, and promote a balanced nervous system, skullcap remains a go-to herb for emotional and mental well-being.

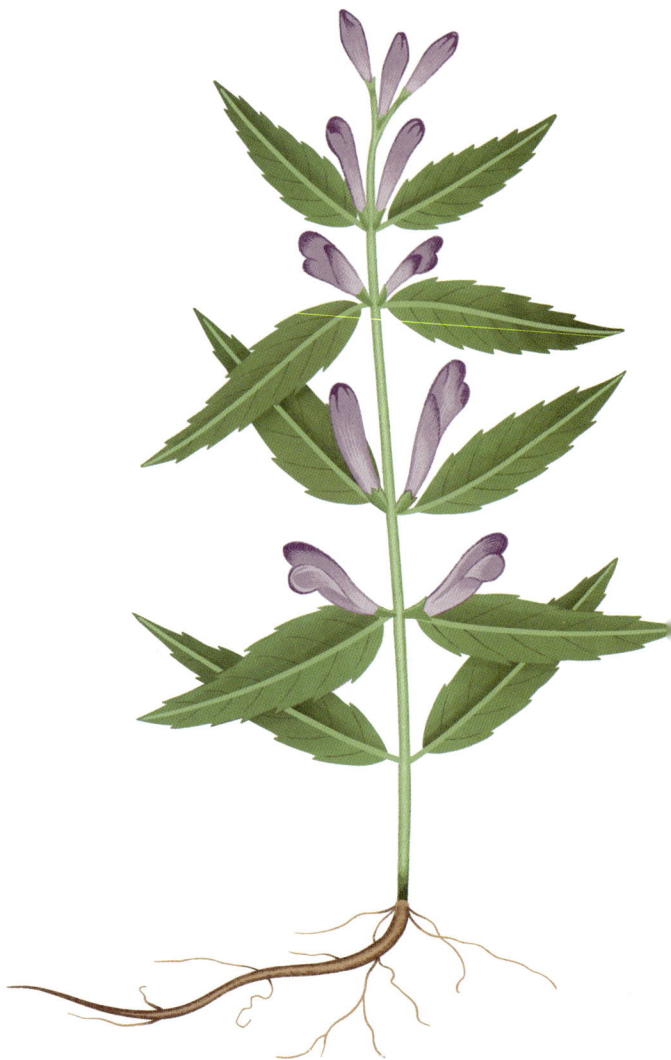

Uses and Indications
Use skullcap to reduce stress, ease nervous tension, and promote emotional balance. It is ideal for daytime use in managing anxiety or stress-related symptoms as, unlike stronger sedatives, it provides calming support without excessive drowsiness. You can also use skullcap to reduce muscle tension, tension headaches, and sleep disturbances.

Safety and Interactions
Skullcap is generally safe when used in moderation, but if you're taking sedative or anti-anxiety medication, be aware that it may enhance the effects. If you're pregnant, breastfeeding, or taking prescription medications, consult a healthcare provider before use.

Recipe

Skullcap Calming Infusion

This soothing herbal tea is a gentle way to calm the mind and body, making it a perfect evening ritual after a long or stressful day.

Yield: 1 cup (240 ml)

1 teaspoon (1.5 g) dried skullcap leaves

½ teaspoon (0.75 g) chamomile flowers (optional, for enhanced relaxation)

¼ teaspoon (0.25 g) lavender buds (optional, for a soothing aroma)

1 cup (240 ml) boiling water

Raw honey or maple syrup (optional, for sweetness)

Preparation

Place the dried skullcap leaves, chamomile, if using, and lavender, if using, in a tea infuser or directly into a mug. Pour the hot water over the herbs and let steep for 10 to 15 minutes. Strain, if necessary, then sweeten with honey or maple syrup if desired.

How to Use

Drink 1 cup (240 ml) in the evening to unwind after a stressful day or as needed to promote a relaxed state without excessive drowsiness.

Growing and Harvesting

Skullcap thrives in moist, well-drained soil with partial to full sunlight. It is commonly found growing along riverbanks and in meadows, making it well-suited for herb gardens with ample water access. While it prefers temperate climates, skullcap can also be cultivated in pots, allowing for controlled growing conditions.

The aerial parts of the plant, including the leaves and flowers, are harvested when the plant is in full bloom, typically in late summer. For best potency, it is recommended to harvest in the early morning when the plant's essential oils are most concentrated. The harvested material should be dried in a shaded, well-ventilated area to preserve its active compounds. Once dried, skullcap can be stored in airtight containers away from heat and moisture to maintain its therapeutic benefits.

With its ability to thrive in various environments and its relatively low-maintenance requirements, skullcap is an excellent addition to any herbal garden, providing a steady supply of calming, nervous system–supportive medicine.

Fun Fact

Skullcap gets its name from its flowers, which resemble a miniature medieval helmet.

Gotu Kola *(Centella asiatica)*
The Mind-Sharpening Herb

Gotu kola has been treasured in Ayurvedic and Traditional Chinese Medicine (TCM) for thousands of years due its ability to enhance memory, mental clarity, and cognitive function. In Ayurvedic tradition, it is considered a *medhya rasayana*, a rejuvenating herb that specifically benefits the mind and nervous system. Gotu kola has even been used by yogis and monks to promote spiritual enlightenment and meditation, earning its reputation as "the herb of enlightenment."

In TCM, gotu kola is valued for its ability to improve circulation, nourish the blood, and strengthen mental faculties. In Southeast Asia, it has been traditionally used as a cooling herb to promote longevity and skin health. Today gotu kola continues to be recognized as a natural brain tonic that supports both cognitive and nervous system health.

What the Science Says

The cognitive-enhancing effects of gotu kola *(Centella asiatica)* stem from its aerial parts, which are rich in **triterpenoids**—a class of plant-based compounds known for their anti-inflammatory, antioxidant, and tissue-repairing properties. These compounds have been extensively studied for their role in brain function, circulation, and neuroprotection.

One of gotu kola's key benefits is its ability to increase blood flow to the brain, helping deliver more oxygen and nutrients where they're needed most. This boost in circulation has been linked to better memory, sharper focus, and overall brain performance. Research suggests that compounds in gotu kola may also increase levels of brain-derived neurotrophic factor (BDNF)—a protein that supports the growth of new brain cells and helps the brain form and strengthen connections, both of which are essential for learning and memory.

Gotu kola is also a potent antioxidant and anti-inflammatory herb, protecting the brain from oxidative stress—a major contributor to cognitive decline and neurodegenerative conditions. Research published in *Evidence-Based Complementary and Alternative Medicine* (2012) found that gotu kola extract improved cognitive function in individuals experiencing mild cognitive impairment, suggesting its potential role in preventing age-related memory loss. Additionally, a study in *Phytotherapy Research* (2014) demonstrated that gotu kola enhanced working memory and reduced anxiety-related behaviors in animal models, further supporting its use as a nootropic (cognitive enhancer).

Gotu kola is also known to help reduce mental fatigue and stress. By modulating neurotransmitters such as dopamine and serotonin, gotu kola helps balance mood and improve mental clarity.

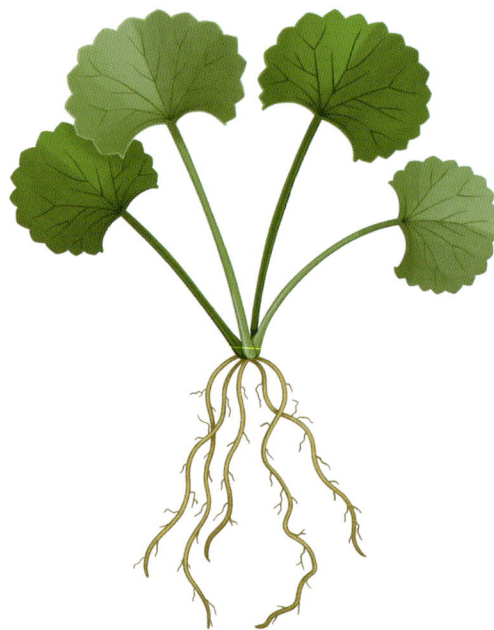

This makes it particularly beneficial for treating "brain fog," nervous exhaustion, or difficulty concentrating due to stress.

Due to its impact on blood circulation, gotu kola has also been studied for its role in supporting vascular health and reducing symptoms of chronic venous insufficiency (CVI). Research in *Phytotherapy: A Quick Reference to Herbal Medicine* (2003) found that gotu kola extracts strengthened blood vessels and improved microcirculation, suggesting additional benefits for cardiovascular and skin health.

With its ability to enhance blood flow, stimulate neurogenesis, protect against oxidative damage, and support mental focus, gotu kola continues to be one of the most trusted herbs for cognitive health and longevity.

Uses and Indications

Gotu kola is primarily used to enhance cognitive function, sharpen focus, and improve memory retention. It is highly beneficial if you're struggling with mental fatigue, stress-induced brain fog, or mild anxiety. An excellent herb for promoting relaxation while maintaining mental alertness, gotu kola is a good choice for those who require sustained concentration without sedation.

Interactions and Safety

Most people can take gotu kola without any problems because it's generally well-tolerated when used in moderate amounts. However, in high doses, it may cause mild digestive discomfort or drowsiness. If you're taking sedatives, anti-anxiety medications, or blood thinners, consult a healthcare provider before use, as gotu kola may enhance the effects of these medications. Pregnant or breastfeeding individuals should also seek professional advice before incorporating gotu kola into their routine.

Gotu Kola Tea for Mental Clarity

A warm cup of gotu kola tea is a gentle and effective way to support focus, memory, and mental clarity.

Yield: 1 cup (240 ml)

1 to 2 teaspoons (4 to 8 g) dried gotu kola leaves

1 cup (240 ml) boiling water

Raw honey or lemon (optional, for flavor enhancement)

Preparation

Place the dried gotu kola leaves into a tea infuser or directly into a mug. Pour the hot water over the leaves and let steep for 5 to 10 minutes. Strain, if necessary, and enjoy warm. Sweeten with honey or lemon if desired.

How to Use

Drink up to 2 cups (480 ml) daily to support mental clarity, cognitive function, and focus. For best results, consume consistently over time.

Growing and Harvesting

Native to South and Southeast Asia, gotu kola thrives in warm, tropical climates and is commonly found in marshy wetlands, along riverbanks, and in damp, shaded environments. It prefers rich, moist soil and can grow as a ground cover, spreading quickly through creeping stems.

Gotu kola can be grown at home in pots or garden beds with consistently damp soil. It grows well in partial shade but can tolerate full sun as long as the soil remains moist. Regular watering is crucial to keep the plant from drying out.

Harvesting is best done once the plant has established a healthy spread of leaves, typically a few months after planting. The leaves, which contain the highest concentration of bioactive compounds, can be harvested continuously throughout the growing season. Simply snip the leaves and tender stems, allowing the plant to regrow. Fresh leaves can be used immediately in teas, tinctures, or culinary preparations, while dried leaves should be stored in an airtight container away from direct light to preserve their potency.

When properly maintained, gotu kola is a resilient and prolific plant, making it an excellent addition to any herbal garden. Its ability to regrow after harvesting ensures a steady supply for those who incorporate it regularly into their wellness routine.

Fun Fact

According to legend, gotu kola was a favorite herb of elephants—animals often associated with long life and exceptional memory. This has contributed to its reputation as a brain-boosting herb that promotes longevity and mental sharpness.

Passionflower *(Passiflora incarnata)*
The Calming Herb

Passionflower, native to the woodlands of North America, has been cherished for centuries for its calming and sedative effects. Indigenous tribes, including the Cherokee and Algonquin peoples, traditionally used passionflower tea and infusions to ease anxiety, promote sleep, and soothe nervous tension. Spanish explorers who encountered passionflower were captivated by its strikingly intricate blooms and named it "flor de la pasión" because they saw religious symbolism in its floral structure.

By the eighteenth and nineteenth centuries, passionflower had made its way into European herbal medicine, where it became a widely used natural remedy for insomnia, nerves, and restlessness and to balance mood. Today passionflower remains a trusted botanical ally for reducing stress, promoting relaxation, and improving sleep quality.

What the Science Says

Passionflower exerts its calming effects through a unique combination of bioactive compounds, particularly **flavonoids** such as apigenin, chrysin, and vitexin. These compounds have been shown to increase gamma-aminobutyric acid (GABA) levels in the brain. GABA is the brain's main inhibitory neurotransmitter, responsible for slowing down overactive neural activity and promoting a sense of calm. Low GABA levels have been linked to anxiety, stress, and sleep disturbances. Raising GABA levels helps reduce nervous system excitability and induce a state of relaxation, making passionflower a natural option for balancing the nervous system.

A study published in *Phytomedicine* (2011) found that passionflower extract significantly reduced symptoms of generalized anxiety disorder (GAD), with effects comparable to prescription anti-anxiety medications but without the risk of dependency. Another study in *Sleep Science* (2017) demonstrated that passionflower improved sleep quality, particularly in individuals who experienced mild sleep disturbances.

Additionally, research published in *Anesthesia & Analgesia* in 2008 found that passionflower could ease presurgical anxiety, making it a promising alternative to pharmaceutical sedatives in certain cases. These studies highlight passionflower's potential as a natural, non-habit-forming option for stress relief, relaxation, and sleep support.

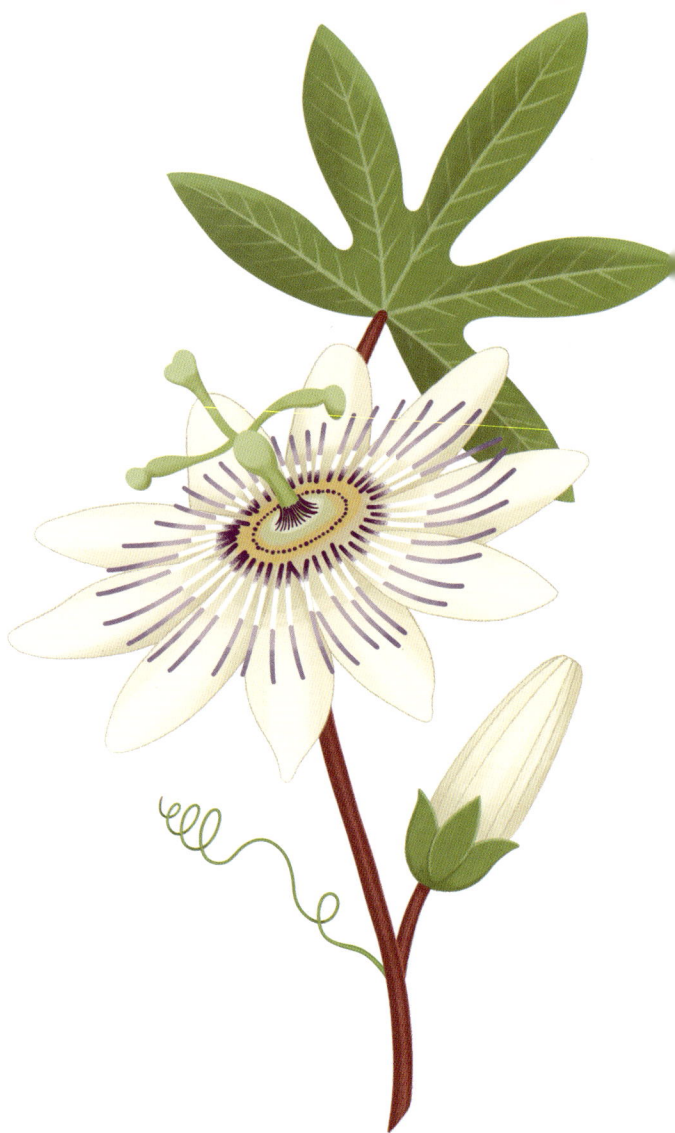

Beyond anxiety and sleep, passionflower's antioxidant and anti-inflammatory properties help protect the brain from oxidative stress, which can contribute to mental fatigue and cognitive decline. The flavonoid content in passionflower has also been linked to improved mood stability, making it useful for individuals dealing with stress-related mood fluctuations or tension headaches.

With its ability to enhance GABA activity, ease stress-related tension, and promote deep, restorative sleep, passionflower remains one of the most widely used and respected calming herbs in herbal medicine.

Uses and Indications

Passionflower can be used to ease anxiety, promote relaxation, and improve sleep quality. It can be especially beneficial if you experience restlessness, have racing thoughts, or struggle to wind down at night. You can also use passionflower to support mood stability and reduce nervous tension in response to stress.

Safety and Interactions

When used in moderate amounts, passionflower is generally safe. However, because of its sedative effects, it should be used with caution if you're taking sleep aids, anti-anxiety medications, or other central nervous system depressants. Consult with a healthcare provider before using passionflower if you're pregnant or breastfeeding.

Growing and Harvesting

Passionflower thrives in warm, temperate climates, flourishing in well-drained soil with plenty of sunlight. It grows as a climbing vine, requiring a trellis or fence for support. While it prefers warm conditions, it can be grown in containers and brought indoors in colder climates.

The leaves, flowers, and stems are harvested in late summer when the plant is in full bloom. They can be used fresh or dried in teas, tinctures, and extracts. To preserve potency, dry the plant in a shaded, well-ventilated area and store it in airtight containers away from light and moisture.

For those growing passionflower for its fruit, patience is needed, as it may take over a year to produce. The ripe fruit, which appears in late summer to early fall, is mildly sweet and edible. Passionflower is both a medicinal and an ornamental addition to any herbal garden.

Fun Fact

The passionflower vine is a favorite plant for pollinators, attracting bees and butterflies with its intricate flowers and nectar-rich blooms. Historically, Native American tribes used passionflower not just as medicine but also as a food source, eating its mildly sweet fruit as a natural treat.

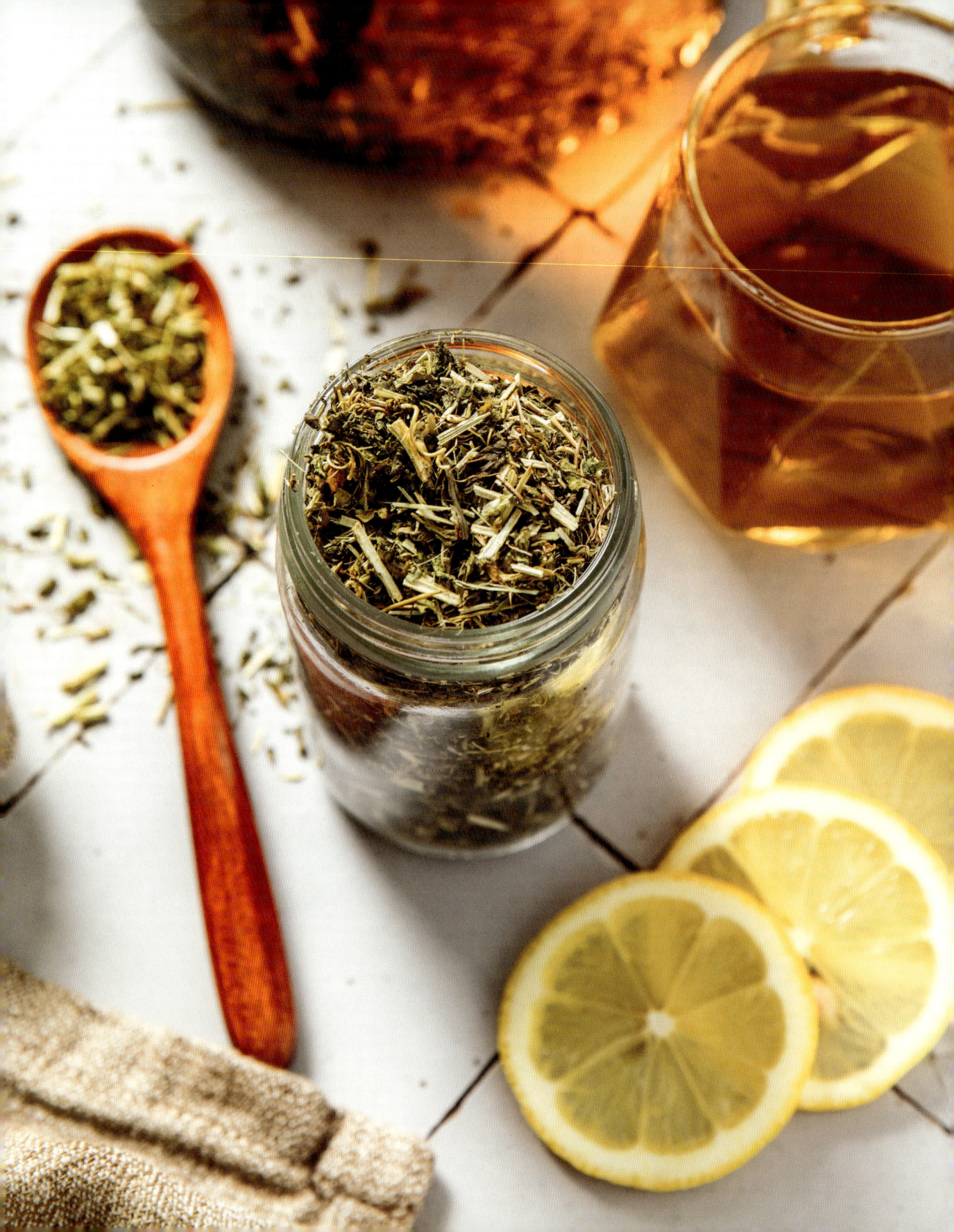

Passionflower Tea for Calming Anxiety

This gentle herbal tea provides a natural way to ease stress and promote relaxation, making it an excellent addition to a bedtime routine or a genuine and much needed moment of self-care during a stressful day.

Yield: 1 cup (240 ml)

1 to 2 teaspoons (2 to 4 g) dried passionflower

1 cup (240 ml) boiling water

Raw honey or lemon (optional, for flavor and added relaxation benefits)

Preparation

Place the dried passionflower into a tea infuser or directly intoa mug. Pour the hot water over the herb and let steep for 10 minutes. Strain, if necessary, and enjoy warm. Sweeten with honey or lemon if desired.

How to Use

Drink 1 cup (240 ml) in the evening to unwind before bed or sip during the day to ease nervous tension and promote relaxation.

St. John's Wort *(Hypericum perforatum)*
The Mood Harmonizer

A cherished staple of European folk medicine, St. John's wort earned its name because it typically blooms in late June around the feast day of St. John the Baptist. Its golden-yellow flowers were traditionally gathered to ward off negative energies, but its more practical use for centuries has been as a natural remedy for lifting spirits and easing emotional distress. In ancient Greece, physicians such as Dioscorides and Galen relied on its ability to ease melancholy and nervous tension in their patients. Later, in the Middle Ages, St. John' wort was widely used across Europe to dispel dark moods and promote inner balance.

Historically, St. John's wort had a role beyond mental well-being. The bright red oil extracted from its flowers was used often as a healing salve, applied to wounds and burns and used to soothe nerve pain. Today it remains one of the most extensively studied herbs for its role in treating mild to moderate depression and improving overall emotional resilience, making it a popular natural alternative to prescription medicines.

What the Science Says
The aerial parts of St. John's wort *(Hypericum perforatum)* are packed with bioactive compounds, including hypericin and hyperforin, which help balance neurotransmitters such as serotonin, dopamine, and norepinephrine—key chemicals responsible for regulating mood. Hyperforin, in particular, is believed to inhibit the reuptake of these neurotransmitters—meaning it prevents brain cells from reabsorbing chemicals like serotonin, dopamine, and norepinephrine too quickly. This action, similar to how some conventional antidepressants work, allows these mood-regulating neurotransmitters to stay active in the brain longer, promoting a greater sense of emotional balance and well-being.

In addition to its mood-enhancing effects, St. John's wort contains **flavonoids**, **tannins**, and **phenolic acids**, all of which contribute to its antioxidant, anti-inflammatory, and neuroprotective properties. Together, these phyto (plant-based) compounds help protect the nervous system from oxidative stress, which can exacerbate symptoms of depression and anxiety.

Several clinical studies have demonstrated St. John's wort's effectiveness in treating mild to moderate depression. A 2008 meta-analysis published in the *Cochrane Database of Systematic Reviews* found that St. John's wort extracts were just as effective as standard antidepressants in improving mood, with fewer reported side effects. Another study published in 2016 in *BMC Medicine* reinforced these findings, showing that St. John's wort worked comparably to drugs like fluoxetine (Prozac), making it a viable natural option for mood support.

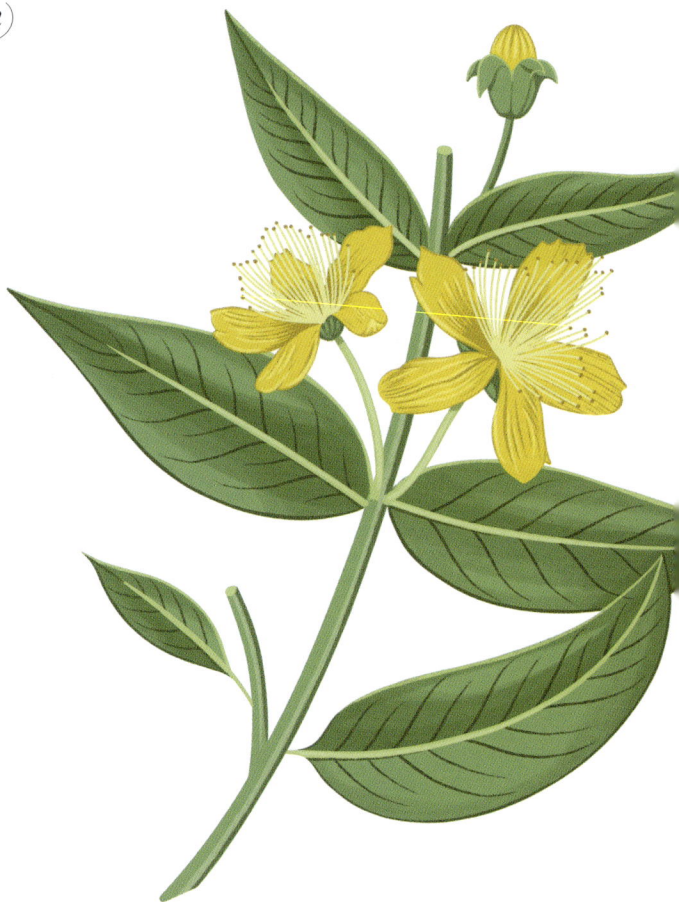

While St. John's wort is widely used for depression, it also shows promise in managing seasonal affective disorder (SAD), premenstrual mood disturbances, and stress-related fatigue. Additionally, some research suggests St. John's wort may help improve sleep quality in those struggling with low mood, though it should be taken earlier in the day due to its potential to interfere with melatonin production.

With its ability to enhance neurotransmitter activity, protect the nervous system, and support long-term emotional well-being, St. John's wort continues to be a trusted herbal ally for those seeking a natural approach to mental wellness and balance.

Uses and Indications

Take St. John's wort to ease mild to moderate depression and/ or help alleviate low mood, irritability, and fatigue. It may also be helpful if you struggle with seasonal affective disorder (SAD), stress management, or emotional resilience. Finally, it can be taken to promote mental clarity and reduce nervous tension, particularly during times of emotional transition or hormonal fluctuations.

Interactions and Safety

While generally well-tolerated, St. John's wort interacts with many medications, including antidepressants, birth control, blood thinners, and immunosuppressants. Consult your healthcare provider before using St. John's wort if you are on any prescription medications. Photosensitivity is another potential side effect, so those taking it regularly should limit excessive sun exposure or use sunscreen.

Growing and Harvesting

St. John's wort thrives in temperate climates with well-drained soil and full sun exposure. It is a hardy perennial that can grow in the wild along roadsides, meadows, and rocky slopes, but it also adapts well to home gardens. The plant prefers slightly sandy or loamy soil and requires minimal maintenance once established.

The best time to harvest St. John's wort is in mid- to late summer when its bright yellow flowers are in full bloom. Harvesting is done by snipping the top few inches of the flowering stems, as these contain the highest concentrations of hypericin and hyperforin, the key mood-supporting compounds. The flowers and leaves can be used fresh or dried for teas, tinctures, and infused oils.

To dry St. John's wort, bundle the stems together and hang them upside down in a cool, dark, and well-ventilated space. Once fully dried, the flowers and leaves can be stored in an airtight container away from direct sunlight to preserve their potency. Properly dried St. John's wort retains its medicinal qualities for up to a year, making it a valuable addition to any herbal apothecary.

Fun Fact

During medieval times, St. John's wort was hung above doorways to ward off evil spirits and negative energy. It was believed that placing the plant under one's pillow could prevent nightmares and promote joyful dreams, further reinforcing its long-standing reputation as a mood-lifting herb.

St. John's Wort Mood-Boosting Tea

This gentle herbal tea combines the mood-balancing effects of St. John's wort with the calming properties of lemon balm and the uplifting aroma of orange peel.

Yield: 1 cup (240 ml)

1 teaspoon (1.5 g) dried St. John's wort flowers

½ teaspoon (0.33 g) dried lemon balm leaves (optional, for additional calming effects)

¼ teaspoon (0.75 g) dried orange peel (optional, for a refreshing citrus note)

1 cup (240 ml) boiling water

Raw honey or agave syrup (optional)

Preparation

Place the St. John's wort flowers, lemon balm, if using, and orange peel, if using, into a tea infuser or directly into a mug. Pour the hot water over the herbs and let steep for 5 to 10 minutes. Strain, if necessary, then sweeten with honey or agave syrup if desired. Enjoy warm as a gentle, mood-balancing remedy.

How to Use

Drink 1 to 2 cups (240 to 480 ml) daily, preferably earlier in the day, as St. John's wort may interfere with sleep cycles if taken too late.

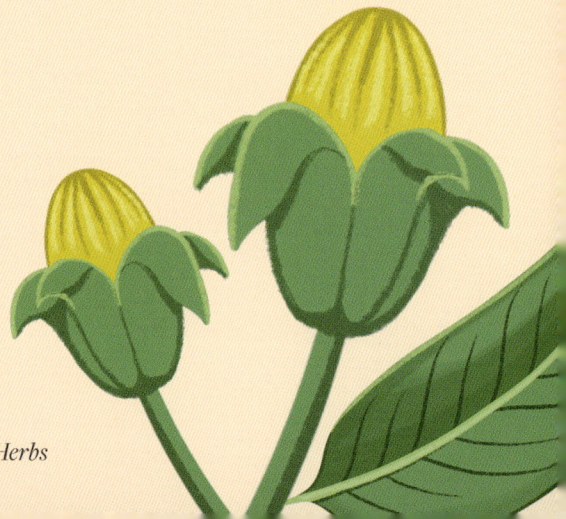

Seasonal Herbal Practices: Aligning Remedies with Nature

Just as our daily routines shift with the seasons, so too should our approach to herbalism. Aligning herbal practices with nature allows us to work in harmony with the body's natural rhythms and seasonal changes. Each season brings its own set of challenges, from spring allergies to winter colds, and herbs provide the perfect way to support the body during these transitions.

Spring is a time of renewal and cleansing, making it the perfect season for detoxifying herbs that support the liver and kidneys. Nettle, dandelion, and burdock root help clear out stagnation, promote circulation, and provide a fresh start for the body after the sluggishness of winter. These herbs can be enjoyed in mineral-rich infusions, fresh salads, or light teas that nourish and cleanse.

As temperatures rise in summer, the focus shifts to cooling, hydrating, and protecting the body from heat-related stress. Herbs like peppermint, hibiscus, and lemon balm help regulate body temperature, prevent dehydration, and soothe inflammation. Infusing these herbs into refreshing iced teas or incorporating them into infused waters can make hydration more enjoyable while keeping the body cool and balanced.

Fall signals a return to structure—busier schedules, cooler weather, and more time spent indoors—all of which can challenge the immune system. As temperatures drop, this is the season to lean on immune-supportive herbs like elderberry, astragalus, and echinacea. Syrups, tinctures, and warming decoctions help strengthen the body's defenses and provide daily support against seasonal illnesses.

Winter calls for deep nourishment, warmth, and resilience. The cold and dry conditions of the season can make the body more susceptible to stiffness, fatigue, and lowered immunity. Warming spices like ginger, cinnamon, and cloves stimulate circulation, support digestion, and provide comfort. Adaptogenic herbs like ashwagandha and reishi help the body withstand stress and maintain energy levels. Sipping on spiced herbal broths and infused tonics ensures the body stays resilient through the colder months.

By rotating herbs in sync with nature's cycles, herbalism becomes more intuitive, ensuring that the body receives exactly what it needs at the right time.

Chapter 7

Good Bones: Herbs for the Skeletal and Muscular System

The skeletal and muscular systems are the core structures that support our ability to move. At the cellular level, these systems are in constant motion—osteoblasts and osteoclasts work together to renew and reshape bones, adapting to our body's demands, while muscle fibers contract and relax in response to motor neuron signals. These movements rely on a precise balance of calcium, magnesium, and proteins like actin and myosin, which power every motion we make.

Bones and muscles endure daily wear and tear, requiring consistent care to maintain strength and flexibility. Nutrients like calcium and magnesium are critical for bone density and muscle function, while collagen fibers in connective tissues provide resilience to joints. Inflammation from stress or overuse, if unchecked, can lead to stiffness, joint pain, and soreness, further highlighting the need for a proactive approach to skeletal and muscular health.

Herbs offer natural, effective ways to support these systems. Turmeric's anti-inflammatory compounds ease muscle soreness and improve joint mobility by regulating inflammatory pathways. Horsetail, rich in silica, strengthens bones, joints, and connective tissues while also benefiting hair, nails, and skin. Nettle provides a wealth of minerals to reduce cramps and support muscle recovery, and Boswellia soothes joints, reducing pain and swelling.

Recipes in this chapter include a warming Golden Milk for Joint and Muscle Health and a mineral-rich Nettle Extract for Bone and Muscle Health. Together, these herbs help keep your body strong, flexible, and resilient—empowering every step, lift, and stretch.

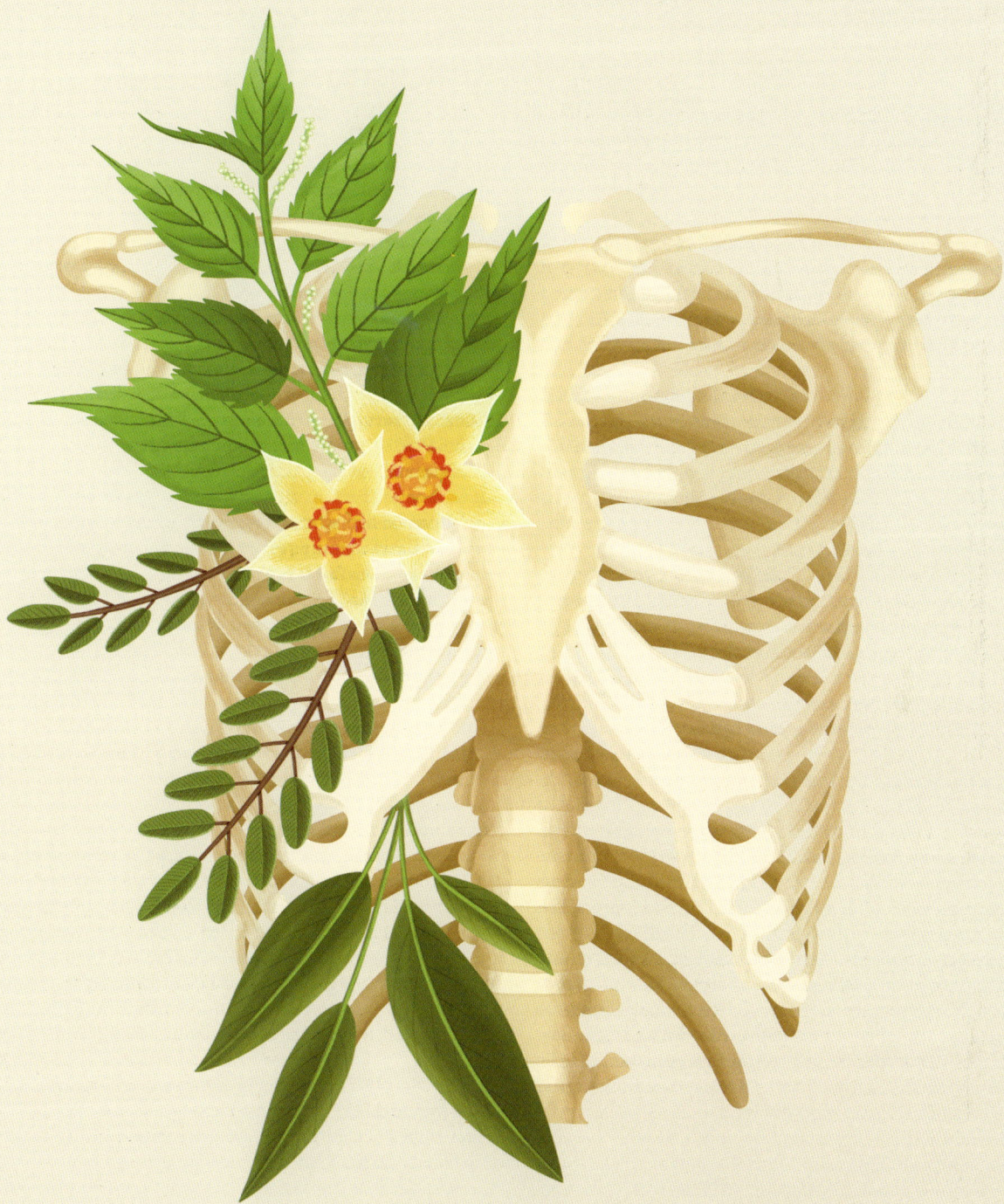

Horsetail *(Equisetum arvense)*
The Bone Builder

Horsetail, an ancient plant that has existed for over 300 million years, is one of the oldest surviving plant species on Earth. This prehistoric herb was highly valued in Greek, Roman, and Traditional Chinese Medicine for its ability to strengthen bones, joints, and connective tissues. Ancient physicians, including Dioscorides and Galen, recommended horsetail for wound healing, bone fractures, and urinary health, and herbalists across Europe and Asia used it to fortify hair, nails, and skin.

In traditional Western herbalism, horsetail was often prepared as a tea or poultice because its high silica content made it a natural bone-building tonic. Thanks to this, horsetail became a trusted remedy for osteoporosis, arthritis, and connective tissue repair. Today this herb remains a popular natural therapy that helps strengthen and regenerate bones, reduce joint pain, and improve mobility.

What the Science Says

Horsetail *(Equisetum arvense)* is exceptionally rich in silica, a key mineral for collagen production, bone density, and connective tissue resilience. Silicon, the bioavailable form of silica, enhances calcium absorption, helping to strengthen bones, joints, and cartilage while supporting hair, skin, and nail health.

One of horsetail's primary mechanisms of action is its role in bone mineralization. A 2004 study published in the *Journal of Bone and Mineral Research* found that horsetail extract increased bone density and calcium retention in postmenopausal women, supporting its use in osteoporosis prevention and bone repair. Another study in *Expert Opinion on Biological Therapy* (2021) demonstrated that horsetail's silica content promotes osteoblast (bone-building cell) activity, which is essential for bone regeneration and fracture healing.

Horsetail also exhibits anti-inflammatory and diuretic properties, which contribute to joint mobility and detoxification. A 2020 study in *Traditional and Integrative Medicine* revealed that horsetail extract reduced joint stiffness and improved flexibility in participants with osteoarthritis, likely due to its ability to reduce inflammation and improve connective tissue strength.

Beyond skeletal benefits, horsetail is widely recognized for its impact on hair, skin, and nails. Its silica and **flavonoids** help maintain elasticity and hydration, making it a valuable beauty-enhancing herb as well. *International Journal of Molecular Sciences* (2023) found that horsetail extract reduced signs of aging, confirming its role in collagen support and tissue regeneration.

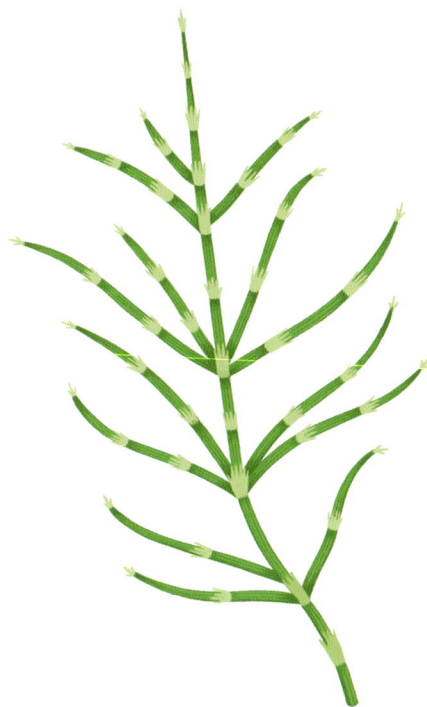

By enhancing calcium absorption, strengthening bones and joints, and supporting connective tissues, horsetail is an excellent herb to have in your medicine chest to promote skeletal resilience, flexibility, and long-term structural health.

Uses and Indications

Horsetail is commonly used to support bone density, enhance joint flexibility, strengthen connective tissues, and promote healthy hair, skin, and nails. It is particularly beneficial for those recovering from fractures, managing osteoporosis, or seeking mineral-rich support for overall structural integrity.

Safety and Interactions

Horsetail is generally safe for short-term use, but long-term use may lead to thiamine (vitamin B_1) deficiency due to its content of thiaminase—an enzyme that breaks down thiamine in the body, making it harder to absorb and utilize. Over time, this can reduce B_1 levels, especially if dietary intake is low.

Use horsetail cautiously if you have kidney disease, as its natural diuretic properties may place added strain on these organs. If you're pregnant or breastfeeding, consult a healthcare provider before use.

Growing and Harvesting

Horsetail thrives in damp environments, often growing in wetlands, riverbanks, and moist meadows. It prefers acidic, nutrient-poor soils and spreads quickly through underground

Horsetail Mineral-Boosting Tea

This mineral-rich tea is an excellent daily tonic for bone health, joint flexibility, and connective tissue support.

1 teaspoon (0.75 g) dried horsetail herb

½ teaspoon (1 g) dried nettle leaves (optional, for added minerals)

¼ teaspoon oat straw (0.5 g) (optional, for calcium support)

1 cup (240 ml) boiling water

A splash of lemon juice (optional, to enhance mineral absorption)

Raw honey or agave syrup to taste (optional)

Preparation

Add the horsetail and nettles and oat straw, if using, to a tea infuser or directly into a mug. Pour the hot water over the herbs and let steep for 10 to 15 minutes to fully extract its bone-nourishing minerals. Strain, if necessary, and add a splash of lemon juice to aid in mineral absorption. Sweeten with honey or agave syrup if desired.

How to Use

Enjoy warm as a daily infusion to fortify bones, support joint mobility, and replenish essential minerals. For best results and safety, use daily for no more than 2 to 3 weeks at a time, followed by a 1- to 2-week break. Rotate with other mineral-rich herbs as needed.

rhizomes, making it a resilient and self-sustaining plant. Due to its deep-reaching root system, horsetail efficiently absorbs minerals from the soil, contributing to its high silica content.

For cultivation, horsetail can be grown in containers or designated garden areas where its vigorous spreading won't interfere with other plants. It requires partial to full sunlight and consistent moisture to thrive. While it does not produce flowers or seeds in the traditional sense, horsetail propagates through spores or root division, making it relatively easy to establish in the right conditions.

Harvesting is best done from late spring to early summer when the plant's mineral content is at its peak. The aerial stems are clipped and either used fresh or dried for long-term storage. Drying should be done in a shaded, well-ventilated area to preserve its medicinal properties. Once dried, horsetail can be stored in airtight containers and used in teas, extracts, or powdered formulations to support bone, joint, and connective tissue health.

Fun Fact

Horsetail is a living fossil, dating back hundreds of millions of years to the time of the dinosaurs. Ancient horsetail plants grew as tall as modern trees, dominating prehistoric landscapes long before flowering plants evolved.

Turmeric (*Curcuma longa*)
The Inflammation Fighter

Turmeric has been a staple in Ayurvedic, Chinese, and Southeast Asian medicine for over four thousand years, prized for its ability to reduce inflammation, ease pain, and promote overall well-being. Ancient texts such as the *Charaka Samhita* and *Sushruta Samhita*—foundational Ayurvedic medical treatises—describe the use of turmeric as a remedy for joint discomfort, digestive issues, and skin conditions. Traditional healers incorporated turmeric into pastes, decoctions, and medicated oils for both internal and external healing.

In Ayurveda, turmeric was classified as a warming herb that balances excess "kapha" and "vata," making it ideal for addressing stiffness, swelling, and poor circulation. Traditional Chinese Medicine (TCM) practitioners used turmeric to invigorate blood flow and clear stagnation, particularly for conditions involving joint and muscle pain.

As global trade routes expanded, turmeric's reputation spread to the Middle East and Europe, where it was valued not just for its medicinal benefits but also as a culinary herb and textile dye. Today modern science continues to validate turmeric's long-standing use, confirming its potent anti-inflammatory, antioxidant, and pain-relieving properties.

What the Science Says

Turmeric's medicinal power lies in curcumin, its primary bioactive **polyphenol**, which has been extensively studied for its anti-inflammatory, antioxidant, and pain-relieving effects. One of curcumin's key actions is its ability to block NF-κB, a protein complex that turns on genes linked to inflammation. When overactivated, NF-κB can lead to pain, swelling, and tissue damage—especially in conditions like arthritis and muscle strain. A 2016 study in the *Journal of Medicinal Food* found that curcumin supplementation significantly reduced joint pain and stiffness in osteoarthritis patients, with effects comparable to nonsteroidal anti-inflammatory drugs (NSAIDs) but without the usual gastrointestinal side effects.

Curcumin's antioxidant properties also make it an essential herb for muscle recovery and protection. By neutralizing free radicals that contribute to oxidative stress and tissue damage, it helps preserve muscle function and accelerates post-exercise recovery. Research in the *Journal of the International Society of Sports Nutrition* (2014) demonstrated that curcumin supplementation reduced muscle soreness and inflammation in athletes following intense exercise.

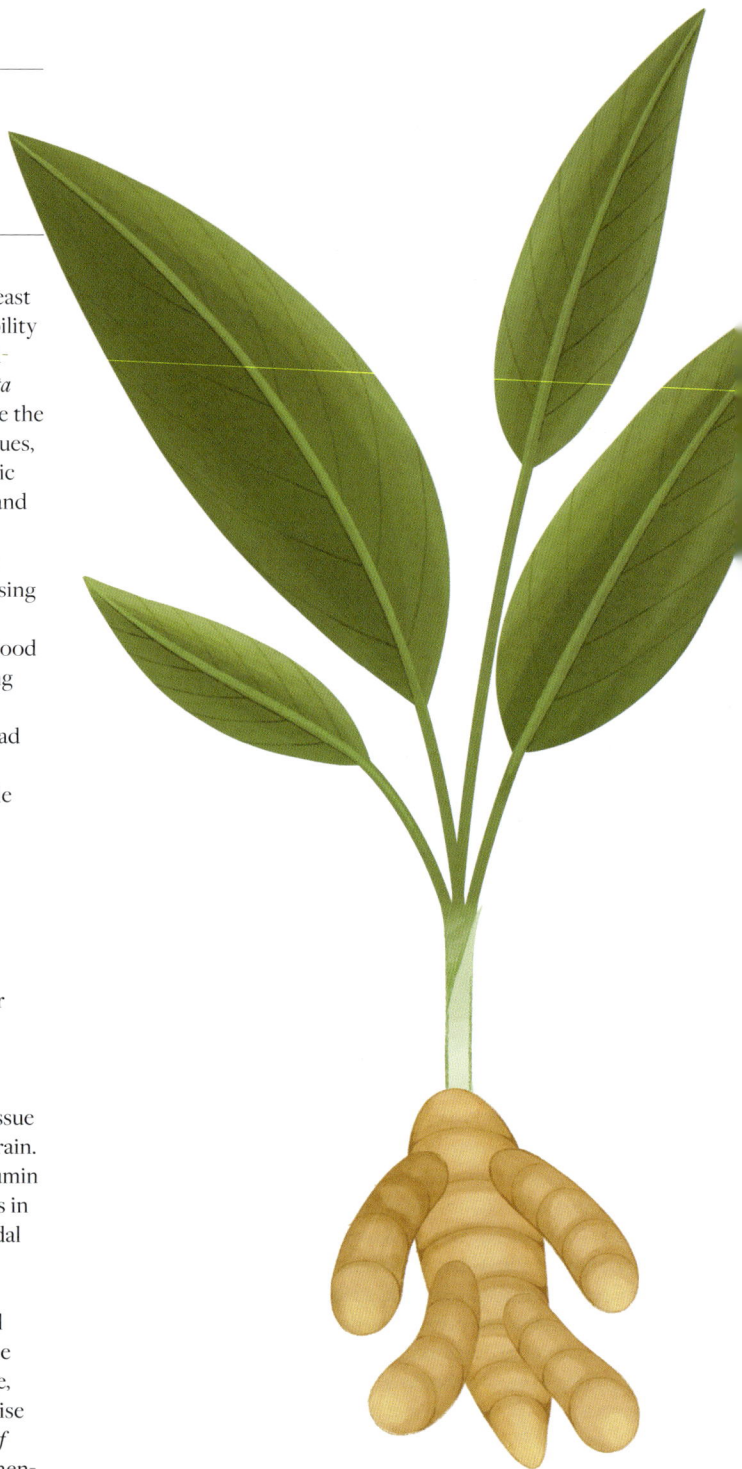

Curcumin is poorly absorbed on its own, but its ability to reduce inflammation is so powerful that it has been studied extensively to find a way to boost its bioavailability. Studies show that combining curcumin with black pepper (piperine) increases its absorption by up to 2,000 percent, enhancing its therapeutic effects. Tumeric is also more easily absorbed when it is paired with healthy fats such as coconut oil, olive oil, or ghee, and warming spices like ginger and cinnamon, which also offer complementary anti-inflammatory benefits.

By blocking inflammatory pathways, protecting tissues from oxidative stress, and supporting muscle and joint function, turmeric is one of the most well-researched and effective natural remedies for pain relief and mobility.

Uses and Indications

Turmeric is commonly used to help reduce joint pain, improve mobility, ease muscle soreness, and support post-workout recovery. It can be particularly beneficial for managing arthritis or other chronic pain conditions, or simply for maintaining flexibility and comfort in daily movement.

Safety and Interactions

Turmeric is considered safe when consumed in moderate amounts, but high doses may cause digestive upset, especially if you have a sensitive stomach. Since turmeric thins the blood, consult your healthcare provider before using turmeric if you're taking anticoagulants or blood-thinning medications. Avoid turmeric if you have gallbladder disease, because it stimulates bile production, which may worsen symptoms.

Growing and Harvesting

Turmeric thrives in warm, humid climates and is traditionally cultivated in regions such as India, Southeast Asia, and Central America. This tropical plant, a member of the ginger family, requires well-draining, loamy soil and consistent moisture to flourish. It grows best in partial shade but can tolerate full sun in milder climates. Because turmeric does not produce seeds, it is propagated using rhizomes—underground stems that sprout new growth.

For home cultivation, turmeric can be grown in large containers or garden beds, planted from fresh rhizomes with visible buds. Once planted, it takes around eight to ten months to mature, with lush green leaves indicating active growth. When the foliage begins to yellow and die back—typically in late fall—the rhizomes are ready for harvest.

To harvest, the rhizomes are carefully dug from the soil, washed, and dried before use. Fresh turmeric can be stored in the refrigerator, while dried turmeric is typically ground into a fine powder for culinary and medicinal applications. Proper drying and storage ensure that its potent curcumin content remains intact, preserving its powerful anti-inflammatory and antioxidant benefits.

Fun Fact

In India, brides traditionally apply turmeric paste to their skin before weddings for its brightening and healing properties, symbolizing purity, health, and prosperity.

Golden Milk for Joint and Muscle Health

This warming, anti-inflammatory tonic has been used for centuries to ease joint stiffness, improve flexibility, and promote overall relaxation.

1 cup (240 ml) unsweetened coconut or almond milk (or milk of choice)

½ teaspoon (1.5 g) ground turmeric

¼ teaspoon (0.5 g) ground ginger

A pinch of black pepper (to enhance turmeric absorption)

A pinch of ground cinnamon (optional, for extra warmth and circulation support)

1 teaspoon (5 ml) raw honey or maple syrup (optional, for sweetness)

Preparation

In a small saucepan, combine the milk, turmeric, ginger, black pepper, and cinnamon. Heat over low to medium heat, stirring frequently to prevent scalding. Simmer gently for 5 to 7 minutes, ensuring all the ingredients are well incorporated. Remove from the heat and sweeten with honey or maple syrup if desired. Pour into a mug and enjoy warm as a calming, joint-nourishing beverage.

How to Use

Drink once daily to help manage inflammation, support joint mobility, and promote post-exercise muscle recovery. This tonic is ideal for sipping in the evening to wind down or as a nourishing boost in the morning.

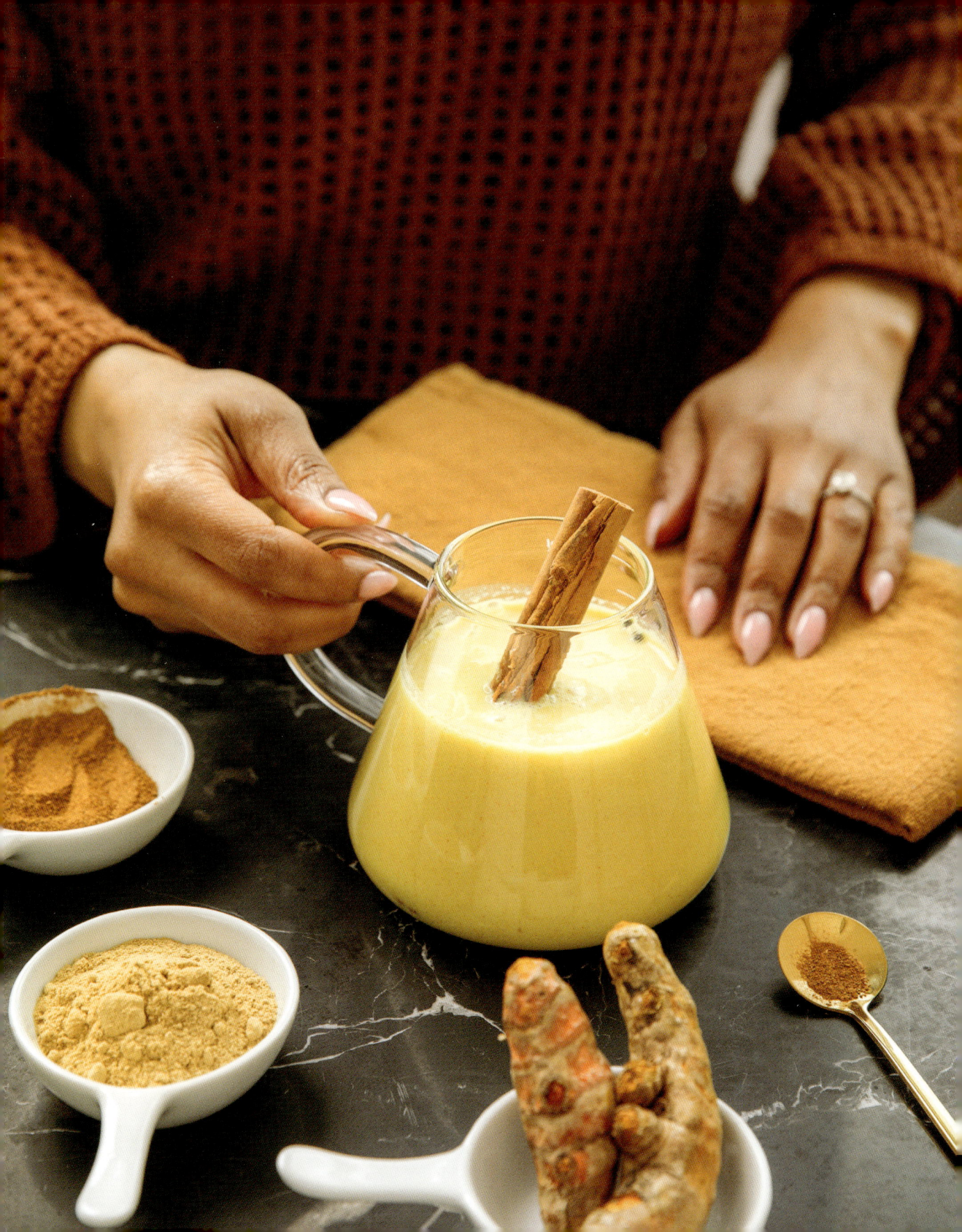

Nettle *(Urtica dioica)*
The Mineral-Rich Supporter

Nettle, valued for its rich mineral content and restorative properties, has been a cornerstone of traditional herbal medicine for centuries. In European folk medicine, it was often used as a spring tonic to replenish nutrients lost during the harsh winter months, supporting overall vitality and strengthening the body. Native American tribes also incorporated nettle into their healing traditions, using it to fortify the blood, support kidney function, and alleviate joint pain.

Herbalists throughout history have turned to nettle for its ability to enhance circulation, reduce inflammation, and support reproductive and adrenal health. Its reputation as a mineral powerhouse endures to this day, making it a staple for those seeking to nourish bones, muscles, and connective tissues.

What the Science Says

The medicinal strength of nettle *(Urtica dioica)* lies in its leaves, which contain an impressive profile of bioactive compounds essential for bone and muscle health. The leaves are rich in calcium, magnesium, and silica, all of which contribute to bone density and strength. These minerals play a key role in preventing conditions such as osteoporosis while supporting muscle contraction and relaxation.

One of nettle's standout compounds is silica, a trace mineral that enhances collagen production, strengthening bones, cartilage, and connective tissues. Silica works in synergy with calcium and magnesium to maintain skeletal integrity and prevent mineral depletion, making nettle an effective long-term tonic for bone health.

Nettle is also a natural anti-inflammatory, thanks to compounds such as **flavonoids** and **phenolic acids** that help modulate the body's inflammatory response. Modern studies support these claims. Research published in *Phytomedicine* (2007) found that nettle extract reduced markers of inflammation, showing promise for conditions such as arthritis and muscle stiffness, while another study published in *Heliyon* (2022) found that nettle extract effectively reduced joint pain and stiffness caused by inflammation in participants with osteoarthritis.

Nettle also contains iron and vitamin C, which work together to treat anemia or low energy levels. Iron supports red blood cell production, and vitamin C enhances iron absorption, ensuring optimal oxygen transport throughout the body. A study in *Biochemical and Cellular Archives* (2024) demonstrated nettle's role as a blood-building herb in participants who had mild anemia.

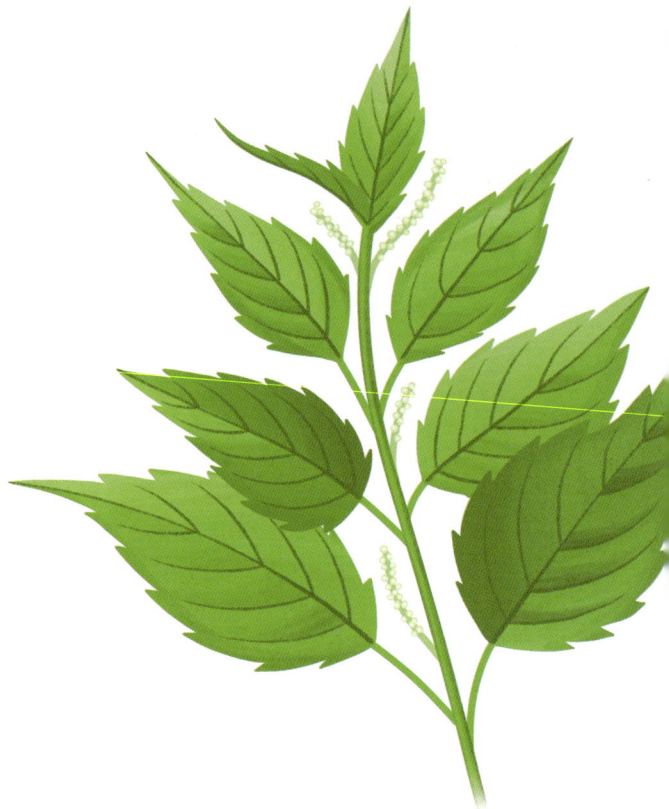

Beyond musculoskeletal support, nettle's mild diuretic properties encourage kidney function and toxin elimination, which can also help reduce inflammation in the body. Overall, nettle provides essential minerals, reduces inflammation, and supports circulation, making it a deeply nourishing herb for long-term skeletal and muscular health.

Uses and Indications

Use nettle for strengthening bones, reducing joint inflammation, and improving muscle function. It is an excellent choice if you're experiencing bone loss, joint pain, or muscle cramps because it helps replenish essential minerals and support overall tissue health.

Nettle is frequently found in herbal formulas for osteoporosis prevention and post-injury recovery. If you're an athlete, nettle can serve as a nourishing remedy to support endurance, muscle repair, and flexibility.

Nettle's ability to reduce inflammatory markers makes it particularly valuable if you suffer from arthritis or chronic joint discomfort. Regular use can help alleviate stiffness and promote greater mobility. Additionally, nettle's iron content makes it beneficial for individuals with fatigue or low energy, because it supports healthy red blood cell production.

Nettle Extract for Bone and Muscle Health

This mineral-rich extract provides deep nourishment for bones, muscles, and connective tissues, making it an excellent addition to your daily wellness routine.

Yield: About 2 cups (480 ml)

1 cup (89 g) dried nettle leaves

2 cups (480 ml) 80 to 100 proof vodka (for a tincture) OR a 50/50 blend of vegetable glycerin and distilled water (for a glycerite)

Preparation

In a quart-size (1 L) glass jar, add the dried nettle leaves. Pour in enough vodka or glycerite blend to fully cover the nettles, leaving about 1 inch (2.5 cm) of space at the top. Seal the jar tightly and shake well. Store in a cool, dark place for 4 to 6 weeks, shaking the jar daily to encourage extraction. Once the infusion is complete, strain the liquid through cheesecloth into a clean bottle, discarding the plant material. Label and store in a dark, cool place for up to 1 to 2 years.

How to Use

Take 15 to 30 drops (about ½ to 1 dropperful total) up to twice daily for bone and muscle support. This extract can be taken directly under the tongue or added to water, juice, or tea for easy consumption. Regular use over time can help nourish the body and maintain strong bones and flexible muscles.

Interactions and Safety

Nettle is generally well-tolerated and safe for long-term use. However, it is a mild diuretic, so if you have kidney disease or are taking diuretics, consult a healthcare provider before using it.

Nettle can also enhance iron absorption, so if you have an iron overload condition it's best to use caution. This herb may also interact with blood-thinning medications, so if you're on anticoagulants, seek medical advice before use. If you're pregnant, consult your healthcare provider before taking nettle, as its effects on uterine tone are not fully understood.

Growing and Harvesting

Nettle is a resilient, fast-growing perennial that thrives in temperate climates across Europe, North America, and Asia. It prefers nutrient-rich, moist soil and flourishes in partial to full sunlight. Often found along riverbanks, forest edges, and meadows, nettle has a reputation for spreading quickly, making it both a valuable herbal ally and an invasive species if left unchecked.

The best time to harvest nettle is from late spring to early summer when the young leaves are tender and rich in minerals. Wearing gloves to avoid the plant's stinging hairs, harvest the top 2 to 3 inches (5 to 7.5 cm) of the plant, leaving the lower sections intact to encourage regrowth. Multiple harvests can be taken throughout the growing season if cuttings are done carefully.

For medicinal use, nettle leaves are either used fresh or dried for long-term storage. Drying should be done in a shaded, well-ventilated area to retain its mineral content. Once dried, the leaves can be stored in airtight containers away from direct sunlight. The roots, which are sometimes used in tinctures, are best harvested in the fall when the plant's energy is concentrated belowground. Properly stored nettle retains its high nutritional value, making it a potent herb for mineral support, teas, and extracts year-round.

Boswellia *(Boswellia serrata)*
The Joint Soother

Boswellia, commonly known as "Indian frankincense," has been revered for centuries in Ayurvedic and traditional Middle Eastern medicine for its powerful anti-inflammatory and pain-relieving properties. Derived from the resin of the Boswellia tree, this healing botanical has been used to soothe aching joints, enhance mobility, and promote overall musculoskeletal health. Ancient practitioners from Ayurvedic, Egyptian, and Middle Eastern traditions recognized Boswellia as a potent remedy for arthritis, gout, and other inflammatory conditions. It was often combined with turmeric and ginger to amplify its effects and support overall joint health.

As knowledge of its healing potential spread, Boswellia became a popular remedy for those looking for a natural alternative to conventional pain relief. Boswellia offers a gentle yet effective approach to managing joint discomfort, unlike nonsteroidal anti-inflammatory drugs (NSAIDs), which may cause gastrointestinal irritation. With a growing body of scientific research supporting its benefits, Boswellia continues to be a trusted herbal remedy for individuals looking to maintain joint flexibility and overall well-being.

What the Science Says

The therapeutic power of Boswellia *(Boswellia serrata)* comes from its resin, which is rich in boswellic acids—plant compounds known for their strong anti-inflammatory effects. Unlike conventional NSAIDs like ibuprofen (Advil) or naproxen (Aleve), boswellic acids target a specific pathway in the body's inflammatory process, helping to reduce swelling without the gastrointestinal side effects often associated with synthetic drugs. Through this action, Boswellia helps protect cartilage, ease joint stiffness, and support more comfortable, fluid movement.

One of the standout features of Boswellia is its ability to protect joint tissues from damage caused by chronic inflammation. Studies show that boswellic acids block pro-inflammatory cytokines—chemical messengers released by immune cells that trigger inflammation and pain. By reducing these signals, Boswellia helps ease swelling and discomfort without the gastrointestinal side effects commonly associated with traditional anti-inflammatory medications.

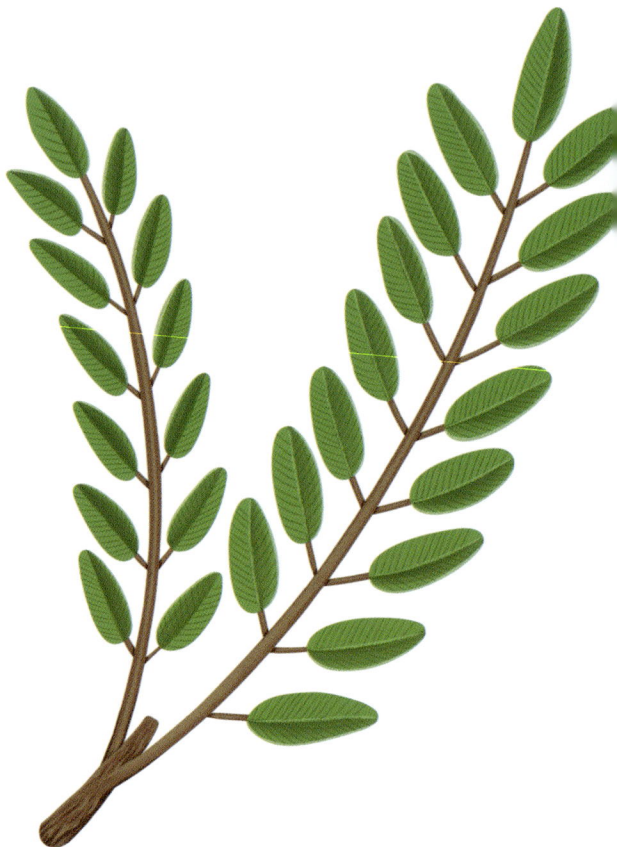

Scientific studies support Boswellia's effectiveness in managing joint pain and improving mobility. A clinical trial published in *Phytotherapy Research* (2019) found that patients with osteoarthritis who took Boswellia extract experienced significant improvements in pain relief and knee flexibility within just eight weeks. Another study in *Phytomedicine* (2003) demonstrated that Boswellia supplementation reduced joint stiffness and inflammation in individuals with rheumatoid arthritis, confirming its role as a natural alternative to conventional anti-inflammatories.

Beyond joint health, research suggests that Boswellia may have broader benefits, including support for gut health and cognitive function. These effects are largely attributed to its ability to reduce systemic inflammation—the kind of low-grade, chronic inflammation that can quietly disrupt multiple body systems over time. By inhibiting inflammatory enzymes and cytokines, Boswellia helps maintain the integrity of the gut lining and reduces neuroinflammation, which may enhance memory and focus. This makes Boswellia a valuable herb for conditions linked to chronic inflammation, including irritable bowel syndrome (IBS), ulcerative colitis, asthma, autoimmune disorders, and even age-related cognitive decline.

Uses and Indications

Boswellia is primarily used for joint and connective tissue health, making it an excellent choice for those with arthritis, sports injuries, or general joint stiffness. It helps reduce inflammation-related discomfort and supports long-term flexibility. Taken regularly, it may also help with tendonitis or other inflammatory musculoskeletal conditions.

In addition to joint support, you can take advantage of Boswellia's anti-inflammatory effects to improve digestive health and soothe inflammatory bowel conditions. Preliminary research suggests this herb may also offer potential neuroprotective effects to the brain by reducing inflammation-related cognitive decline.

Interactions and Safety

Boswellia is generally well-tolerated, but high doses may cause mild digestive discomfort. If you're taking blood thinners or anti-inflammatory medications, consult your healthcare provider before using Boswellia, because it may enhance the effects of these drugs. While it has traditionally been used in pregnancy for its warming properties, it's still best to consult a healthcare professional before using Boswellia if you're pregnant or breastfeeding.

Growing and Harvesting

Boswellia trees thrive in arid, rocky climates and are native to regions of India, North Africa, and the Middle East. The resin is harvested by making small incisions in the tree's bark, allowing the aromatic sap to ooze out and harden into tear-shaped resin drops. These hardened resins are then collected, cleaned, and processed into powders, extracts, and tinctures. Sustainable harvesting practices are crucial to protect Boswellia species, as overharvesting has led to concerns about declining tree populations in some regions.

Fun Fact

Ancient Egyptian priests valued Boswellia resin so highly that it was often burned in sacred temples as an offering to the gods. The resin's aromatic smoke was believed to purify the air, ward off disease, and elevate spiritual awareness.

Documenting Your Herbal Journey

Herbalism is a lifelong practice, and keeping track of your personal experiences with herbs in a journal can help deepen your understanding and intuition. Documenting how different herbs interact with the body can also reveal patterns, preferences, and what works best for you in different situations.

Your herbal journal can include notes on dosages, preparation methods, and personal observations. Tracking herbal use over time allows for adjustments and fine-tuning, ensuring the most effective support.

Journaling also fosters a deeper connection with plants. When you are able to reflect on how a certain herb feels in your body or how its effects change with the seasons, herbalism becomes more than just a remedy—it becomes a relationship.

Consider also including sketches of plants, recipes, and insights from research or traditional knowledge in your herbal journal. You'll find that over time, your herbal journal will become a valuable personal resource, as you chronicle your journey of herbal exploration and self-care.

Boswellia Joint-Soothing Cordial

This warming, anti-inflammatory cordial blends the resin's powerful joint-supporting properties with complementary herbs and spices to enhance its effectiveness and flavor. Note: *This syrup is not recommended for children under one year old, as infants should not consume honey.*

> *Yield: About 1 cup (240 ml)*

2 tablespoons (24 g) Boswellia resin (powdered or small pieces)

½ teaspoon (1.3 g) ground cinnamon (optional, for flavor and additional anti-inflammatory support)

½ teaspoon (1.5 g) dried orange peel (optional, for a citrus twist)

1 cup (240 ml) brandy or vodka (organic if possible)

¼ cup (60 ml) raw honey or Grade A maple syrup

Preparation

Place the Boswellia resin, cinnamon, if using, and orange peel, if using, in a clean glass jar. Pour the brandy or vodka over the ingredients, ensuring they are fully submerged. Seal the jar tightly and shake well. Store in a cool, dark place for 4 to 6 weeks, shaking the jar every few days to help extract the resin's active compounds. After the steeping period, strain through a fine-mesh sieve or cheesecloth to remove solids. Stir in the raw honey or maple syrup to sweeten the cordial. Transfer the finished cordial to a clean bottle for storage. Store in a cool, dark place for up to 6 months.

How to Use

Take 1 to 2 teaspoons (5 to 10 ml) daily, diluted in water or tea, to support joint health and reduce inflammation. Regular use provides the best results, especially during flare-ups or after intense physical activity.

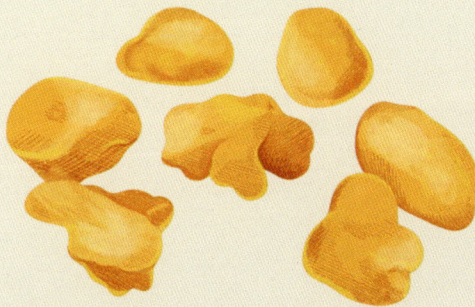

Chapter 8

Hormonal Harmony: Herbs for the Endocrine System

The endocrine system is like an internal orchestra, with each gland playing its part to regulate hormones that control energy, mood, metabolism, growth, and reproduction. This system operates with remarkable precision, using hormones as chemical messengers that travel through the bloodstream to influence cells, tissues, and organs. Key players like the pituitary, thyroid, and adrenal glands work in harmony, ensuring balance in processes like stress response and blood sugar regulation. However, modern stressors, poor diet, and aging can disrupt this balance, leading to mood swings, fatigue, and metabolic challenges.

Herbs provide gentle yet effective support for the endocrine system. Most of the herbs in this chapter are adaptogens—a unique class of herbs that help the body adapt to physical, emotional, and environmental stressors. Rather than pushing the body in one direction, they restore balance, supporting energy, focus, and endocrine harmony—without overstimulation or sedation.

Holy basil, revered as the "queen of herbs," lowers cortisol levels, helping the body manage stress. Shatavari, a staple in Ayurvedic medicine, balances female hormones and supports reproductive health, while Schisandra, an adaptogenic berry, fortifies adrenal function and helps the body adapt to stress. Though not a true adaptogen, fenugreek aids in stabilizing blood sugar by supporting insulin regulation and metabolic function.

This chapter includes recipes like a Holy Basil and Schisandra Berry Cordial for Adrenal Support to ease stress and a Fenugreek Seed Overnight Infusion for Blood Sugar Support. These herbal allies nurture the rhythms of the endocrine system, fostering resilience and harmony for both body and mind.

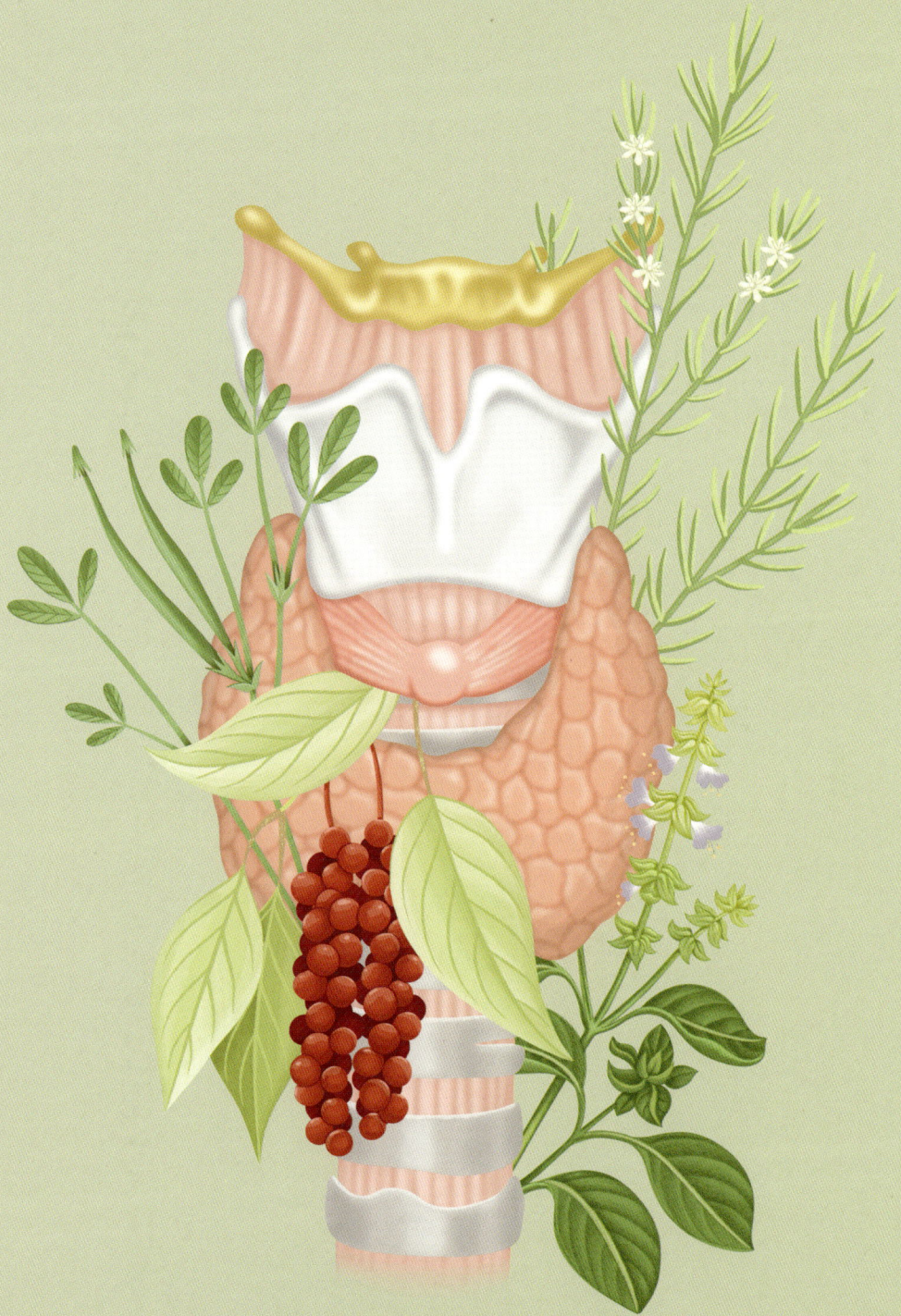

Fenugreek *(Trigonella foenum-graecum)*
The Blood Sugar Stabilizer

Fenugreek has been treasured for centuries in Indian, Middle Eastern, and Mediterranean medicine for its ability to support metabolic health and hormonal balance. It was used by the ancient Egyptians for medicinal purposes and mentioned in ancient Greek and Roman texts as a remedy for digestive issues and women's reproductive health. In Ayurveda and Unani medicine, fenugreek seeds were commonly prescribed to regulate blood sugar, enhance fertility, and support lactation. Beyond its medicinal uses, fenugreek has played an important role in culinary traditions, valued for its slightly bitter, nutty flavor in spice blends and tonics.

In more recent decades, fenugreek has gained attention in clinical research and integrative health circles for its potential to manage insulin resistance, ease polycystic ovary syndrome (PCOS) symptoms, and even support testosterone levels in men. Today it's commonly found in dietary supplements, protein powders, lactation teas, and metabolic health formulas, bridging traditional wisdom with modern functional wellness.

What the Science Says

Fenugreek seeds *(Trigonella foenum-graecum)* contain a wealth of bioactive compounds that contribute to their ability to regulate blood sugar, support metabolism, and enhance endocrine function. One of the most notable is 4-hydroxyisoleucine, a rare amino acid derivative found almost exclusively in fenugreek. It acts directly on the pancreas to stimulate insulin secretion in response to glucose, helping to stabilize blood sugar levels and enhance cellular glucose uptake.

Another key component, galactomannan, is a type of soluble fiber found in the inner part of the seed. It forms a gel-like substance in the digestive tract that slows down how quickly carbohydrates are digested and absorbed, helping to prevent post-meal blood sugar spikes and promote feelings of fullness. These compounds make fenugreek particularly beneficial for individuals managing insulin resistance, prediabetes, and type 2 diabetes.

Fenugreek's adaptogenic and endocrine-modulating properties also extend to reproductive health. By supporting balanced blood sugar levels, it indirectly promotes healthier hormone production, which is particularly beneficial for individuals with conditions such as PCOS, metabolic syndrome, and hormonal imbalances.

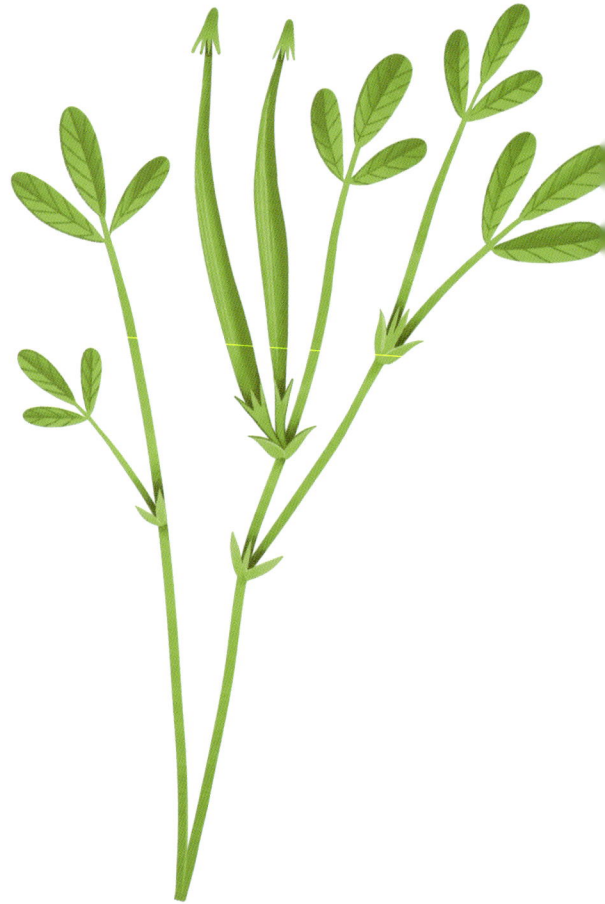

Fenugreek's benefits for blood sugar regulation and hormonal support have been well-documented in clinical research. A study in the *Journal of the Association of Physicians of India* (2001) found that fenugreek supplementation significantly improved fasting blood sugar levels and insulin sensitivity in individuals with prediabetes. Research in *Phytotherapy Research* (2017) showed that consuming fenugreek extract reduced post-meal glucose spikes in participants with type 2 diabetes. A review in *International Journal of All Research Education and Scientific Methods* (2024) highlighted fenugreek's role in hormonal balance, particularly for women with PCOS, as it was shown to improve menstrual regularity and reduce insulin resistance.

Fenugreek seeds also contain **saponins**, which support healthy lipid metabolism and contribute to the herb's cholesterol-lowering effects. Additionally, its high mineral content—including magnesium, zinc, and iron—aids in overall metabolic function and hormone balance. Altogether, fenugreek is multifunctional herb for metabolic, hormonal, and digestive support.

Uses and Indications

Use fenugreek to stabilize blood sugar, particularly if you have a metabolic disorder, insulin resistance, or PCOS. You can also use it to support digestion and appetite regulation, as its fiber content slows glucose absorption and promotes gut health. Finally, fenugreek may aid in cholesterol reduction, as studies suggest it can help lower LDL cholesterol while maintaining healthy triglyceride levels.

Interactions and Safety

When consumed in moderation, fenugreek is generally safe for most people. However, if you're taking diabetes medications, be advised that supplementing with fenugreek can cause hypoglycemia (low blood sugar). Use fenugreek cautiously if you're taking anticoagulants or blood-thinning medications, as it may have mild blood-thinning effects. Due to its potential uterine-stimulating properties, fenugreek is not recommended during pregnancy.

Growing and Harvesting

Fenugreek is an annual leguminous herb that thrives in warm, dry climates and well-drained soil. It grows best in regions with moderate temperatures, such as India, the Mediterranean, North Africa, and parts of the Middle East. This hardy plant is drought-resistant and can be cultivated in gardens, raised beds, or even containers.

Fenugreek seeds are directly sown into the soil in early spring once the risk of frost has passed. It requires full sun exposure and minimal watering, as overwatering can lead to root rot. The plant typically matures within 90 to 110 days, with small yellowish flowers developing before seedpods form.

Harvesting occurs when the seedpods turn golden brown and begin to dry out on the plant. Farmers and gardeners then handpick or thresh the pods to collect the seeds inside. Once harvested, the seeds are dried thoroughly to prevent spoilage and maintain their potency. Properly stored in an airtight container in a cool, dry place, fenugreek seeds remain viable for up to two years.

Although the seeds are the most commonly used part, fenugreek leaves are also edible and can be used fresh or dried in cooking. Known as methi leaves in Indian cuisine, they add a slightly bitter yet aromatic flavor to dishes, showcasing the versatility of this ancient medicinal plant.

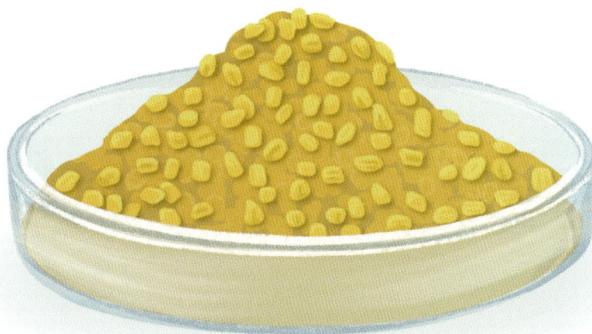

Fenugreek Seed Overnight Infusion for Blood Sugar Support

Yield: 1 cup (240 ml)

1 teaspoon (3.7 g) whole fenugreek seeds
1 cup (240 ml) warm filtered water

This gentle infusion provides a natural way to stabilize blood sugar levels and support insulin function because it enhances glucose uptake and digestion.

Preparation

Place the fenugreek seeds in a glass or cup and pour the warm water over them. Cover and let the seeds soak overnight (at least 8 hours) to allow full extraction of the active compounds. In the morning, strain the liquid and drink on an empty stomach for best results.

How to Use

Drink this infusion daily in the morning to support blood sugar balance and metabolic health. Regular use may improve insulin sensitivity, reduce sugar cravings, and promote digestive balance.

Fun Fact

Fenugreek seeds have a distinct maple-like aroma, and consuming it regularly can cause a person's sweat and urine to take on this scent, a harmless side effect that has been called "fenugreek syndrome."

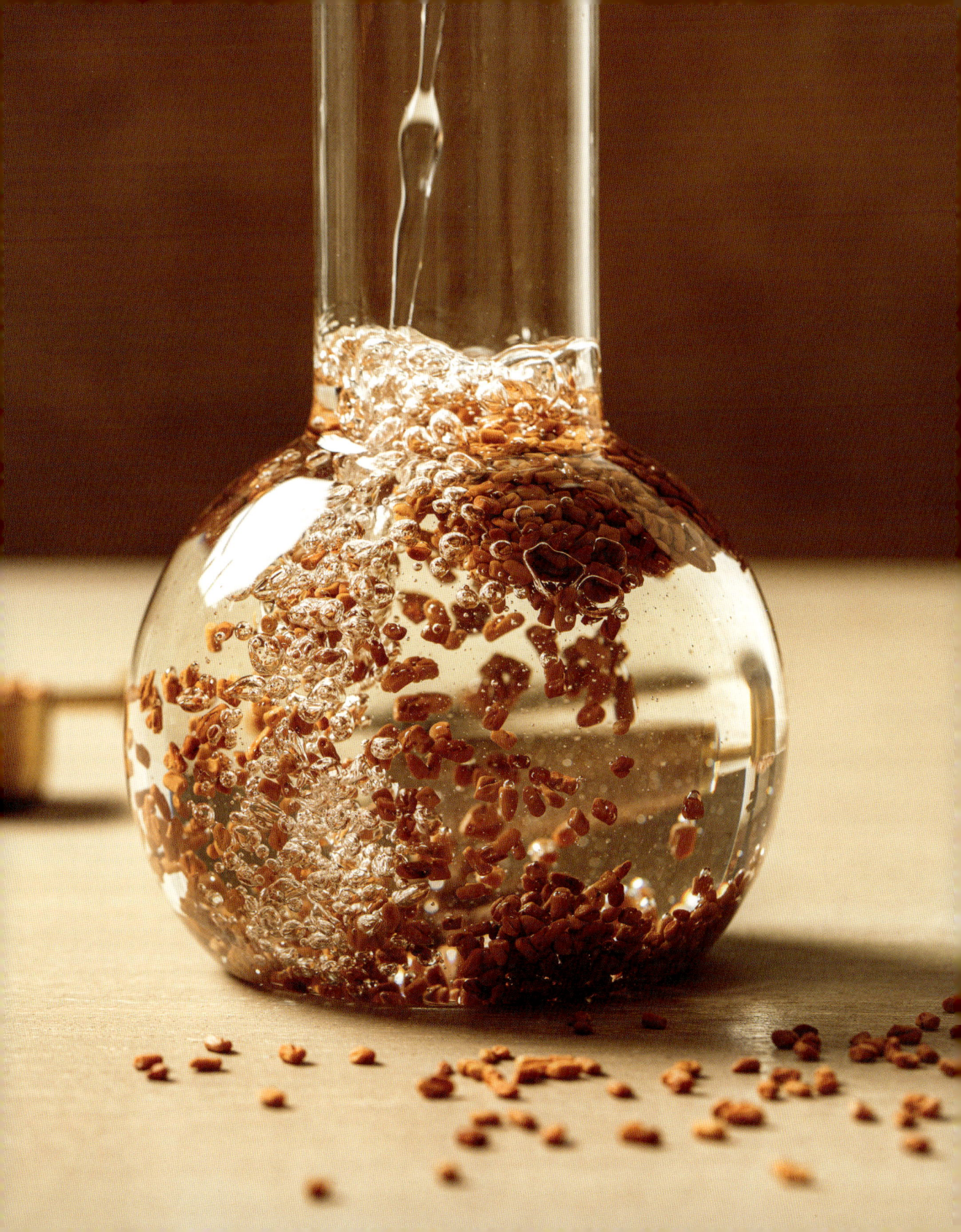

Holy Basil (*Ocimum sanctum*)
The Stress-Balancer

Holy basil, also known as tulsi, has been revered in Ayurvedic medicine for over three thousand years as a sacred and healing plant. Holy basil is classified as an adaptogen—a unique group of herbs that help the body respond to physical, emotional, and environmental stressors. In Ayurveda, tulsi is believed to promote *sattva*, a state of clarity and harmony, while strengthening the body's ability to adapt to change.

Traditionally, holy basil was used to support respiratory health, sharpen mental clarity, and protect the heart and mind during times of emotional upheaval. Its leaves were commonly brewed into teas and mixed into herbal preparations. Beyond India, holy basil has found its way into Southeast Asian healing systems and modern integrative medicine for its wide-ranging effects.

Today holy basil remains a trusted botanical for supporting adrenal balance, immune function, and mental calm, especially for those navigating chronic stress or burnout.

What the Science Says

The medicinal potency of holy basil (*Ocimum sanctum*) is concentrated in its leaves, which contain a rich array of bioactive compounds that support hormonal and adrenal function. Eugenol, one of its primary active compounds, acts as an anti-inflammatory agent while also helping to regulate blood sugar and cholesterol levels. Rosmarinic acid, a powerful antioxidant, protects the body from oxidative stress, which can otherwise disrupt hormonal signaling. Ursolic acid, another key compound, plays a role in reducing cortisol levels and supporting adrenal balance, making holy basil a key adaptogenic herb for endocrine health.

Holy basil works primarily by modulating the hypothalamic-pituitary-adrenal (HPA) axis, which governs the body's stress response. When stress levels rise and the body goes into fight-or-flight mode, the adrenal glands release cortisol to prepare the body for action. This is a good thing; it helps keep us alive in worst-case scenarios. Unfortunately, chronic stress can lead to chronically elevated cortisol levels, which can result in tiredness, fatigue, weight gain, and hormonal imbalances.

Not only does holy basil reduce excessive cortisol production, but it also improves the body's ability to respond to stress without overreacting—keeping stress hormones from spiking too high or staying elevated too long. This adaptogenic action helps the endocrine system work more efficiently, supporting steady energy, emotional stability, and protection against burnout or hormonal imbalances. In fact, a study published in the *Journal of Ayurveda and Integrative Medicine* (2017) found that holy basil supplementation significantly lowered cortisol levels associated with chronic stress, leading to improved mood and overall well-being.

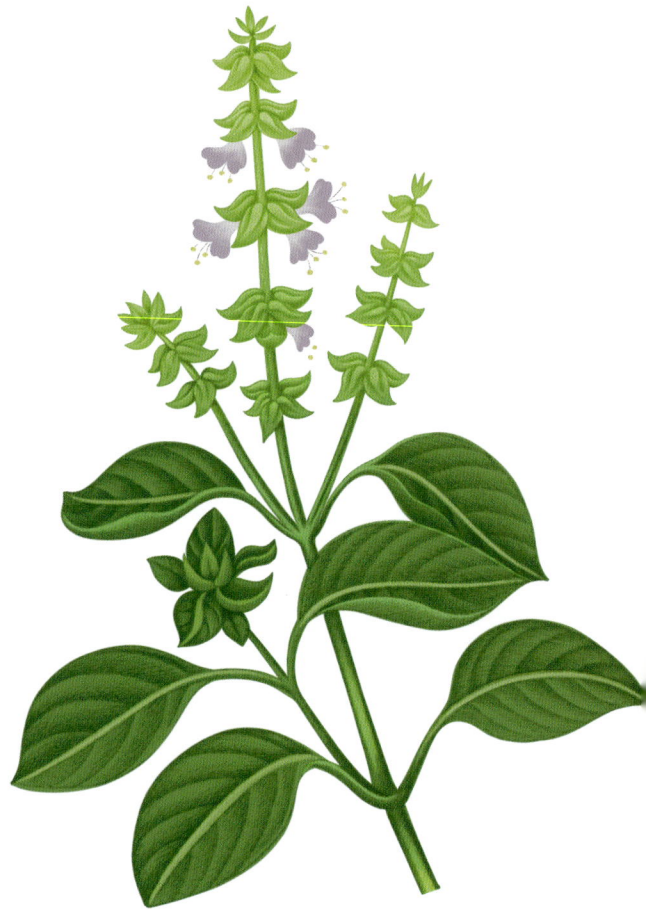

Beyond cortisol regulation, holy basil's bioactive compounds also influence neurotransmitter activity, helping to balance feel-good serotonin and dopamine hormone levels. This contributes to improved mood, reduced anxiety, and enhanced cognitive function. A study in *Frontiers in Nutrition* (2022) confirmed holy basil's effect on neurotransmitter activity and, in turn, its ability to ease anxiety and improve cognitive function.

Studies also show that holy basil may improve insulin sensitivity, which can help stabilize blood sugar fluctuations. A 2015 study in the *Indian Journal of Physiology and Pharmacology* highlighted its role in improving insulin sensitivity and reducing metabolic dysfunction, further validating its systemic benefits.

By acting as a regulator of stress hormones, neurotransmitters, and metabolic functions, holy basil serves as a powerful herbal ally for those seeking hormonal harmony and enhanced resilience in everyday life.

Holy Basil Tea for Stress Relief

This soothing tea is a simple and effective way to incorporate holy basil into your daily routine, promoting relaxation and hormonal balance.

Yield: 1 cup (240 ml)

1 teaspoon (0.7 g) dried holy basil leaves

1 cup (240 ml) boiling water

Raw honey or lemon (optional, for flavor and added relaxation benefits)

Preparation

Place the dried holy basil leaves into a tea infuser or directly into a mug. Pour the hot water over the leaves and let steep for 5 to 10 minutes. Strain, if necessary, and enjoy warm. Sweeten with honey or add a splash of lemon juice if desired.

How to Use

Drink 1 cup (240 ml) daily to help manage stress and promote hormonal balance. This tea is particularly beneficial when consumed in the morning to enhance resilience throughout the day or in the evening to encourage relaxation.

Uses and Indications

Holy basil is a popular herbal choice for managing stress, enhancing adrenal health, and supporting overall hormone balance. As an adaptogen, it is particularly beneficial if you experience chronic fatigue, mood fluctuations, or metabolic imbalances due to prolonged stress. It helps restore energy levels without overstimulation, making it ideal if you're feeling mentally or physically drained.

Holy basil helps regulate cortisol, which can be helpful for those who struggle with adrenal fatigue or have sleep disturbances. By balancing the body's response to stress, holy basil promotes a more restful and restorative sleep cycle. It may also help you deal with blood sugar fluctuations, metabolic disorders, or weight management concerns.

You can use holy basil in many ways, including as a tea, tincture, or extract. You can also combine it with other adaptogenic herbs such as ashwagandha or rhodiola for enhanced endocrine support.

Interactions and Safety

Holy basil is generally well-tolerated and safe in moderate amounts. However, if you're taking medications for diabetes or hypertension, consult a healthcare provider before using holy basil, which may influence blood sugar and blood pressure levels.

The same rule applies if you're taking blood thinners or are anticipating surgery, as holy basil has mild anticoagulant properties. Also, if you're pregnant or breastfeeding, consult a healthcare practitioner before using holy basil.

Growing and Harvesting

Holy basil thrives in warm, tropical climates but can also be grown in temperate regions as an annual. It prefers well-drained soil and full sunlight, making it an excellent addition to home herb gardens. The plant is highly aromatic and attracts pollinators, contributing to a vibrant and healthy garden ecosystem.

To grow holy basil, plant seeds or seedlings after the last frost in rich, well-aerated soil. It requires regular watering but should not be left in overly damp conditions. Pinching off flower buds encourages continued leaf production, ensuring a steady supply of medicinal foliage throughout the growing season.

Harvesting is best done in the morning when the essential oils are at their peak concentration. Leaves can be used fresh or dried for later use in teas, tinctures, or extracts. Dry leaves should be stored in an airtight container away from direct sunlight to preserve their potency. With proper care, holy basil provides an abundant and aromatic harvest that supports both body and mind.

Shatavari *(Asparagus racemosus)*
The Nourisher

Shatavari has been a cornerstone of Ayurvedic medicine for centuries. Ayurvedic practitioners consider it a *rasayana*, or rejuvenating herb, known to nourish the body, enhance longevity, and restore balance to the endocrine system.

The name *shatavari* translates to "she who possesses a hundred husbands," reflecting its traditional use in supporting female reproductive health and vitality. This revered adaptogen has long been valued for its ability to promote hormonal balance, increase fertility, and enhance overall well-being. Though often associated with women's health, shatavari is equally beneficial for men, aiding in stress resilience, reproductive function, and adrenal support.

Ancient texts describe shatavari as a cooling and hydrating tonic, making it especially useful in hot climates, where it helps the body retain internal moisture and combat inflammation. Traditionally, it was used in herbal formulations to support menstrual health, ease menopausal transitions, and promote post-partum recovery. Today shatavari continues to be widely used across the world in teas, tinctures, and powdered supplements for those seeking natural hormonal harmony.

What the Science Says
The root of shatavari contains a rich profile of bioactive compounds that contribute to its endocrine-supportive properties. Its most notable medicinal compounds are **steroidal saponins**, including shatavarins, which are thought to support hormone production and modulate estrogen levels. Unlike synthetic hormones that bind directly to hormone receptors and override the body's natural feedback loops, shatavari works more holistically by nourishing the endocrine system and supporting its ability to self-regulate. This gentle approach helps balance reproductive hormones over time without overriding the body's natural hormonal rhythms.

Shatavari has been shown to promote balanced estrogen levels, making it beneficial for managing irregular menstrual cycles, easing premenstrual syndrome (PMS) symptoms, and supporting menopausal transitions. It also supports lactation in postpartum women by enhancing prolactin, a hormone necessary for breast milk production. In men, shatavari has demonstrated the ability to support testosterone levels and improve sperm health, reinforcing its role as a reproductive tonic for both sexes.

Beyond reproductive health, shatavari supports adrenal function and helps the body adapt to stress. By modulating the body's response to cortisol, it promotes a more balanced stress reaction, reducing anxiety and fatigue often linked to hormonal imbalances. The herb's adaptogenic properties enhance energy levels, reduce mental burnout, and improve overall endurance, making it a valuable ally in managing modern-day stressors.

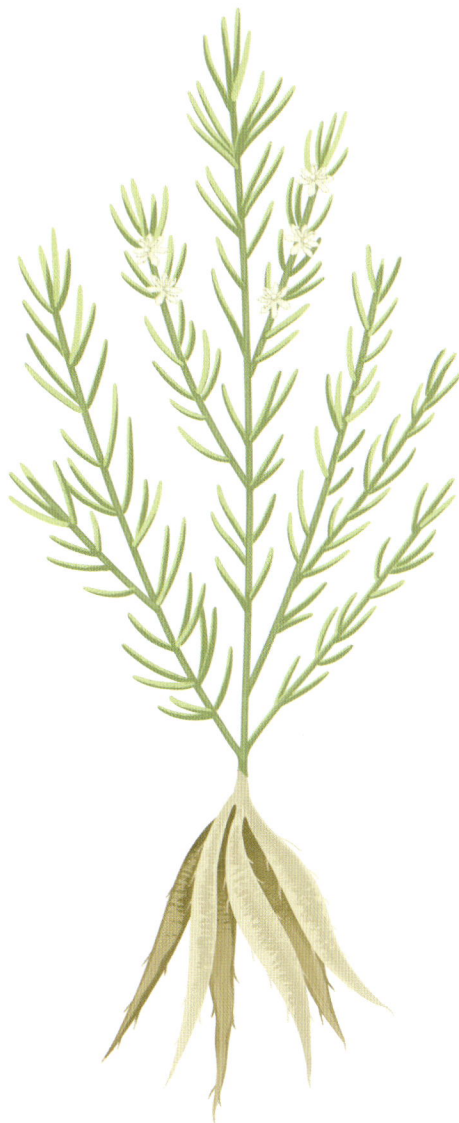

Studies suggest that shatavari exhibits antioxidant and anti-inflammatory properties, which help protect cells from oxidative stress, support immune function, and improve gut health. Research published in *Current Drug Metabolism* (2018) highlighted shatavari's anti-inflammatory and immune-modulating effects, while a clinical trial in *Antioxidants* (2025) demonstrated its potential to regulate estrogen and ease menopause-related symptoms.

By working on multiple pathways—hormonal, adrenal, immune, and digestive—shatavari offers a comprehensive approach to long-term endocrine and reproductive wellness.

Uses and Indications

Shatavari is widely used to promote hormonal balance, enhance fertility, and support overall reproductive health. Women can use shatavari to regulate menstrual cycles, reduce PMS discomfort, and ease the transition through menopause, while men can use it to enhance testosterone levels, improve sperm quality, and support sexual health.

Due to shatavari's ability to regulate cortisol levels, it can be a helpful herb if you're experiencing stress-related hormonal imbalances, adrenal fatigue, or low energy. Its cooling and hydrating properties also make it an excellent remedy for dry skin and even vaginal dryness. In addition, its role in immune support and gut health makes it a valuable herb for overall wellness.

Interactions and Safety

Shatavari is generally considered safe and well-tolerated. However, due to its estrogen-modulating effects, it should be used with caution if you have a hormone-sensitive condition such as estrogen-positive breast cancer. Consult with your healthcare provider before incorporating shatavari into a daily regimen if taking medications that affect hormone levels or blood sugar or if you're pregnant or breastfeeding. If you have diabetes or insulin sensitivity, you'll need to monitor your blood sugar levels while taking shatavari as it may lower them. If you have a known allergy to asparagus, it's best to avoid this herb, as it belongs to the same botanical family.

Growing and Harvesting

Shatavari is a climbing, perennial plant native to India, Sri Lanka, and parts of Southeast Asia, thriving in warm, humid climates with well-drained, sandy soil. It prefers partial to full sunlight and requires ample space to spread, often reaching heights of 6 to 7 feet (1.8 to 2.1 m) when mature. The plant produces small, white flowers and red, berry-like fruits, but its thick, tuberous roots hold the most medicinal value.

Cultivation requires patience, as shatavari takes eighteen to twenty-four months to fully mature before the roots are ready for harvest. Once harvested, the roots are washed, dried, and ground into a fine powder or used in tinctures and decoctions. Proper drying and storage in airtight containers help preserve its potency, ensuring its adaptogenic and reproductive-supporting properties remain intact.

As demand for shatavari grows globally, sustainable cultivation practices are essential to prevent overharvesting. Ethical sourcing from organic farms helps maintain the quality and long-term availability of this revered Ayurvedic herb.

Fun Fact

Shatavari is a type of wild asparagus! While it doesn't look like the kind you'd grill for dinner, it belongs to the same plant family and its root has been treasured in Ayurveda for over 3,000 years as the "queen of herbs."

Shatavari Powder Drink for Hormonal Support

This nourishing herbal drink provides gentle endocrine support, helping balance hormones while promoting relaxation and overall well-being.

Yield: 1 cup (240 ml)

1 teaspoon (2 g) shatavari powder

1 cup (240 ml) warm milk (dairy or plant-based, such as almond or oat milk)

¼ teaspoon (0.56 g) ground cinnamon (for warmth and flavor)

A pinch of nutmeg (for additional soothing properties)

1 teaspoon (5 ml) honey or maple syrup (optional, for natural sweetness)

Preparation

Add the shatavari powder to the warm milk, stirring until fully dissolved. Mix in the cinnamon and nutmeg, blending well to enhance flavor and therapeutic benefits. Sweeten with honey or maple syrup, if desired.

How to Use

Drink 1 cup (240 ml) per day as part of a hormonal support routine. It is best consumed before bed to promote relaxation and balance cortisol levels overnight. Regular use enhances long-term reproductive and adrenal health, making it a gentle yet powerful tonic for endocrine well-being.

Herbs for Different Life Stages

Your body's needs evolve throughout life, and herbalism provides a way to support well-being at every stage. Herbs are not one-size-fits-all; they can be tailored to suit the unique demands of childhood, adulthood, and elder years.

For children, gentle herbs help with digestion, sleep, and immunity. Chamomile and fennel soothe colic and aid digestion, while elderberry and echinacea provide immune protection. Oatstraw and lemon balm can help calm overstimulation, supporting restful sleep. These herbs are best given as teas, glycerites, or mild infusions that are safe for developing systems.

Adulthood brings a need for herbs that manage stress, enhance energy, and promote resilience. Adaptogens like ashwagandha, rhodiola, and holy basil help regulate cortisol levels, providing sustainable energy without overstimulation. For those managing reproductive health, herbs such as shatavari and vitex support hormone balance, while milk thistle and dandelion root aid in detoxification and liver function.

As the body ages, maintaining joint mobility, cardiovascular health, and cognitive function becomes a priority. Anti-inflammatory herbs like turmeric and Boswellia help ease arthritis and joint discomfort, while hawthorn and motherwort strengthen heart function. Gotu kola and ginkgo biloba support memory and circulation, helping to maintain mental clarity. Bone-strengthening herbs such as nettle and horsetail provide essential minerals for maintaining skeletal health.

By understanding how herbal support shifts with age, you can nourish the body through every phase of life, promoting long-term vitality and resilience.

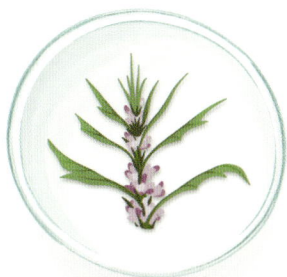

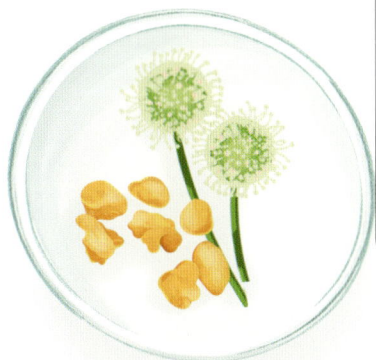

Schisandra *(Schisandra chinensis)*
The Adaptogenic Balancer

Schisandra is a highly regarded adaptogen that has been a staple in Traditional Chinese Medicine (TCM) for over two thousand years. It is often referred to as "five-flavor berry" due to its complex taste profile, which is said to include sweet, sour, salty, bitter, and pungent elements—each corresponding to different organ systems in TCM. Traditionally, Schisandra was used to boost longevity, improve mental clarity, and fortify the body's resilience against environmental stressors.

Beyond China, Schisandra has been used in Korean, Russian, and Japanese medicine to enhance physical stamina, support the liver, and improve overall well-being. It was even used by Soviet researchers in the twentieth century as part of their studies on natural performance enhancers for soldiers and athletes. Today Schisandra remains a powerful herbal ally for those looking to support adrenal health, improve mental focus, and build stress resilience.

What the Science Says

Schisandra (*Schisandra chinensis*) berries contain a wide range of bioactive compounds. These include schisandrins, a group of **lignans** unique to the plant that exhibit antioxidant, anti-inflammatory, and hepatoprotective effects, as well as other lignans, **flavonoids**, and essential oils. These compounds work together to protect the liver, regulate stress hormones, and improve endurance and cognitive function.

One of Schisandra's primary mechanisms is its ability to modulate the hypothalamic–pituitary–adrenal (HPA) axis, the body's central stress-response system. It does this by influencing key neuroendocrine signals that temper the release of cortisol from the adrenal glands. This balancing act helps prevent the overactivation of the stress response. Studies suggest that Schisandra can lower cortisol levels and help the body recover from prolonged stress while maintaining energy and mental clarity.

Schisandra also acts as a powerful liver protector. Its lignans stimulate liver detoxification enzymes, helping the body break down toxins more efficiently. A study published in the *Archives of Pharmacology and Therapeutics* (2024) confirmed that Schisandra extract significantly improves liver function and reduces inflammation in individuals with liver disorders.

Beyond stress and liver support, Schisandra is known for its cognitive-enhancing effects. A 2017 study in *Frontiers in Pharmacology* found that Schisandra extract improved memory, focus, and mental stamina, making it a valuable herb for those experiencing brain fog or cognitive fatigue. These nootropic effects are attributed in part to its lignans and flavonoids, which exhibit neuroprotective activity by reducing inflammation in the brain and enhancing neurotransmitter signaling.

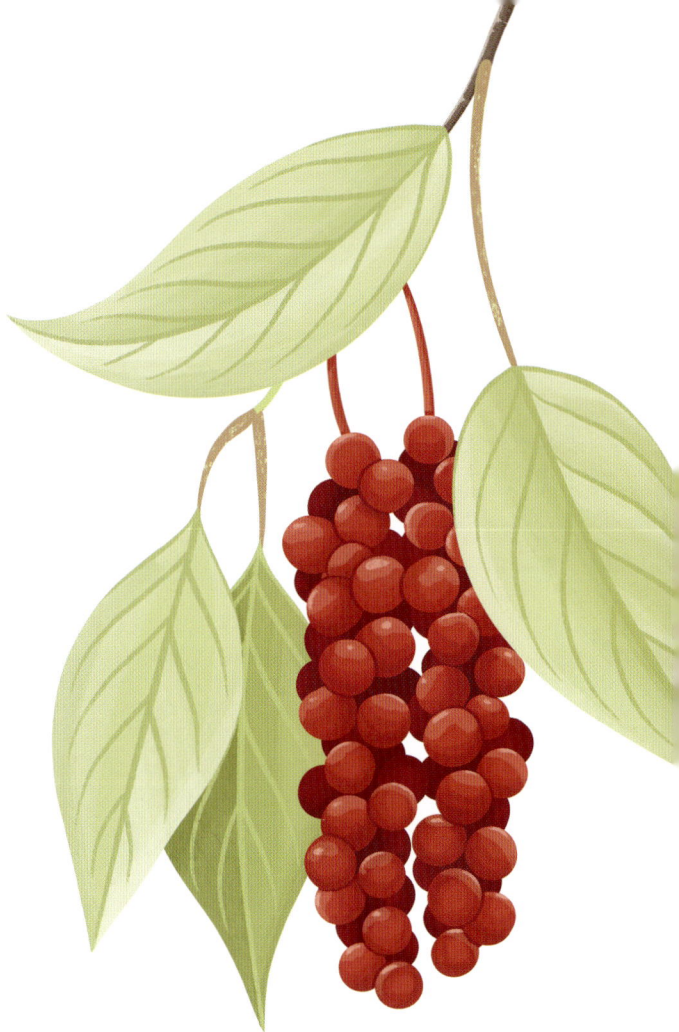

Schisandra's benefits extend to cardiovascular health as well. Research in *Fitoterapia* (2014) highlighted its role in supporting healthy circulation and reducing oxidative stress, which helps protect the heart from damage associated with chronic inflammation and elevated stress hormones. Flavonoids in Schisandra contribute to this antioxidant action by scavenging free radicals and supporting cellular function, while its essential oil compounds exhibit vasorelaxant, anti-inflammatory, and antimicrobial properties that complement the actions of its lignans.

With its multifaceted effects, Schisandra serves as a holistic adaptogen, helping the body recover from stress, enhance endurance, and maintain hormonal balance—all while supporting vital organ systems such as the liver, heart, and brain.

Uses and Indications

Schisandra is widely used to reduce stress, support adrenal function, and promote hormonal balance. As an adaptogen, it helps the body recover from chronic stress and fatigue, making it a valuable herb if you find yourself experiencing burnout or adrenal exhaustion. Its role in enhancing liver function makes it beneficial if you want to improve detoxification and metabolic health.

Schisandra is also known for its cognitive-enhancing effects, improving mental cvvlarity, focus, and memory, making it particularly useful if you're struggling with brain fog or cognitive fatigue. It also provides cardiovascular benefits. Many athletes and physically active individuals use Schisandra to increase endurance and stamina, while others rely on its immune-modulating properties to fortify overall well-being.

Interactions and Safety

Schisandra is generally well-tolerated and safe when used in moderate amounts. However, due to its ability to modulate liver enzymes, it may interact with medications that are metabolized by the liver, potentially altering their effects. If you have a pre-existing liver condition, consult a healthcare provider before using Schisandra regularly. If you're taking sedatives or blood pressure medications, exercise caution as Schisandra may enhance or alter their effects.

While traditionally used in pregnancy-supporting formulas in Chinese medicine, the effects of Schisandra during pregnancy and breastfeeding have not been extensively studied in modern clinical trials, so it is best to seek guidance from a qualified practitioner before using it. Though rare, some individuals may experience mild digestive discomfort or allergic reactions, particularly if taken in high doses. As with all adaptogens, consistency in use is key, and it is best to start with a lower dose and adjust as needed based on how you feel.

Growing and Harvesting

Schisandra is a deciduous woody vine that thrives in cool, temperate climates in China, Korea, Russia, and parts of North America. It requires moist, well-drained soil and partial to full sun exposure to flourish. The plant produces clusters of bright red berries that ripen in late summer to early fall, typically August to October.

Harvesting Schisandra berries involves handpicking them at peak ripeness, when they are deep red and slightly soft to the touch. After harvesting, the berries are traditionally sun-dried or low-heat dehydrated to preserve their medicinal compounds. Once dried, they can be used in teas, tinctures, cordials, and powdered extracts.

Schisandra vines are fast-growing and resilient, making them an excellent addition to home gardens in regions with cooler climates. With proper care, they can produce berries for years, offering a sustainable source of this valuable adaptogenic herb.

Holy Basil and Schisandra Berry Cordial for Adrenal Support

This restorative cordial blends the adaptogenic power of holy basil and Schisandra berries, creating a warming and revitalizing elixir to support the adrenal glands, ease stress, and enhance resilience. Note: *This syrup is not recommended for children under one year old, as infants should not consume honey.*

> *Yield: About 2 cups (480 ml)*

¼ cup (8 g) dried holy basil leaves

¼ cup (100 g) dried Schisandra berries

1 tablespoon (1.5 g) dried rose petals (optional, for a subtle floral note)

1-inch (2.5 cm) piece fresh ginger, sliced (for warmth and digestion support)

2 cups (480 ml) brandy or vodka (organic if possible)

¼ cup (60 ml) raw honey or Grade A maple syrup (to sweeten, adjust to taste)

Preparation

Place the dried holy basil leaves, Schisandra berries, rose petals, and ginger in a clean glass jar. Pour the brandy or vodka over the ingredients, ensuring they are fully submerged. Seal the jar tightly and shake well. Store in a cool, dark place for 4 to 6 weeks, shaking the jar every few days to enhance the infusion.

After the steeping period, strain the cordial through a cheesecloth or fine-mesh strainer into a clean bottle, discarding the solids. Stir in the raw honey or maple syrup to add natural sweetness and balance the flavors. Store the cordial in a cool, dark place.

How to Use

Take 1 to 2 teaspoons (5 to 10 ml) daily, either straight or diluted in a small amount of water, to support adrenal function, enhance stress resilience, and promote overall vitality. This cordial is best enjoyed in the morning or early afternoon, as Schisandra may be stimulating for some individuals.

Fun Fact

For an extra cooling and restorative effect, mix the cordial with sparkling water and ice for a refreshing adaptogenic tonic.

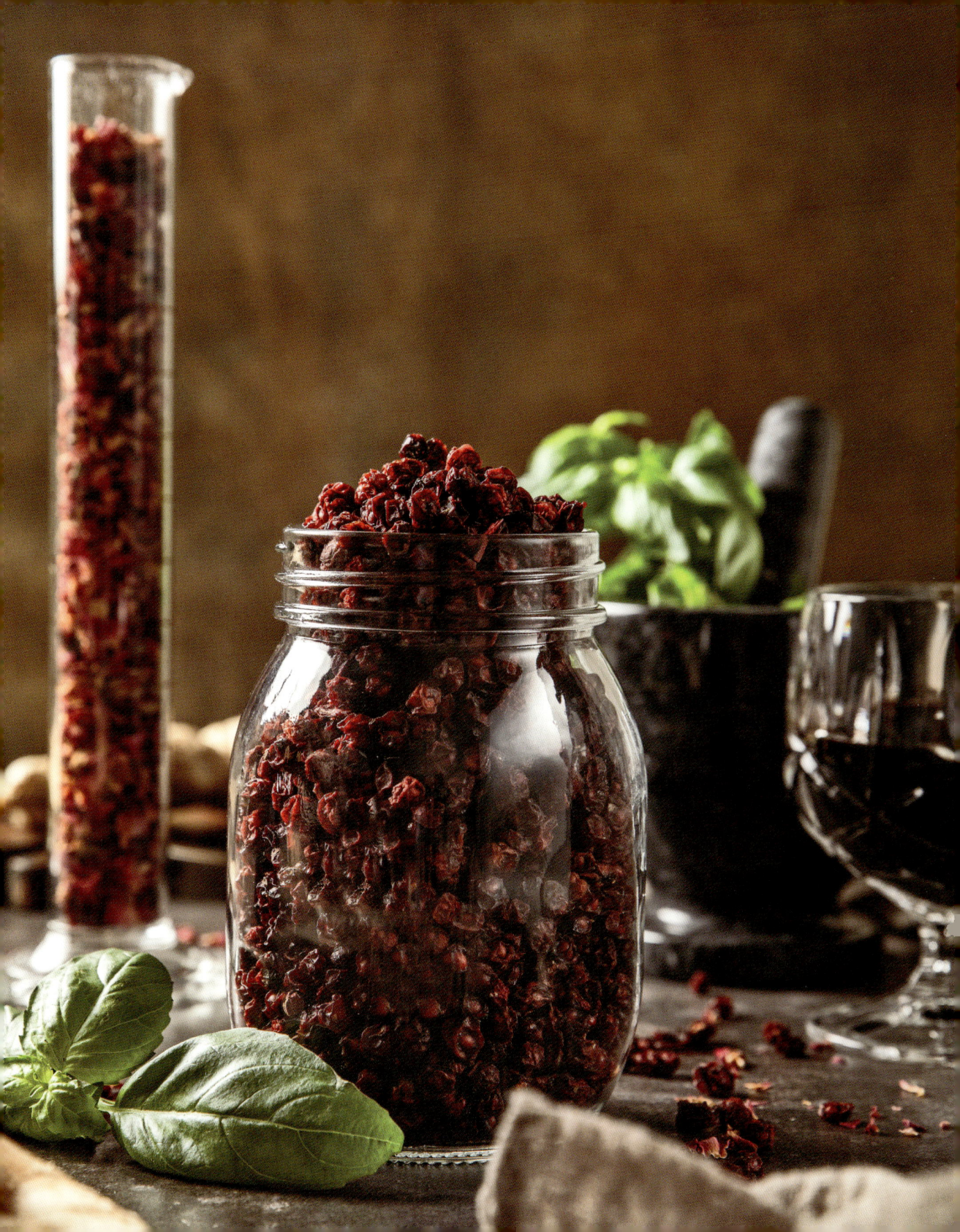

Chapter 9

Nature's Detox: Herbs for Liver Health and Detoxification

The liver is the body's central hub for detoxification, metabolism, and energy storage, performing an astonishing array of vital tasks daily. This largest internal organ has a number of jobs: filtering blood, processing nutrients, neutralizing toxins, and helping to regulate hormones. Think of the liver as a bustling factory: it receives raw materials like nutrients and compounds from food and breaks them down or transforms them into forms the body can use or safely eliminate.

Liver cells, or hepatocytes, are the biochemical powerhouses driving these processes. They convert excess glucose into glycogen for storage, metabolize fats, produce clotting proteins, and generate bile—a fluid crucial for digesting fats and carrying away waste. The liver also houses Kupffer cells, immune sentries that act as scavengers, removing pathogens, worn-out blood cells, and debris from the bloodstream.

Modern life places heavy demands on the liver. Pollutants, alcohol, processed foods, medications, and high-fat or high-sugar diets burden this essential organ, leading to fatty liver deposits, oxidative stress, and inflammation. Over time, this can disrupt metabolism, hormonal balance, and overall health. Supporting the liver's resilience is key to sustaining energy, clarity, and vitality.

Herbs offer gentle yet powerful support for liver health. Milk thistle, rich in silymarin, protects liver cells from damage and encourages regeneration. Dandelion root stimulates bile production, aiding toxin removal and fat metabolism. Burdock root acts as a natural blood purifier, while yellow dock enhances bile flow for efficient waste elimination.

This chapter features recipes like a Milk Thistle and Dandelion Detox Decoction and "Three Roots" Herbal Detox Tonic to nourish and support the liver's essential functions. These herbs don't just "detox"—they also harmonize with the body's rhythms, fostering balance, resilience, and renewal. Let's explore how to give this vital organ the care it deserves.

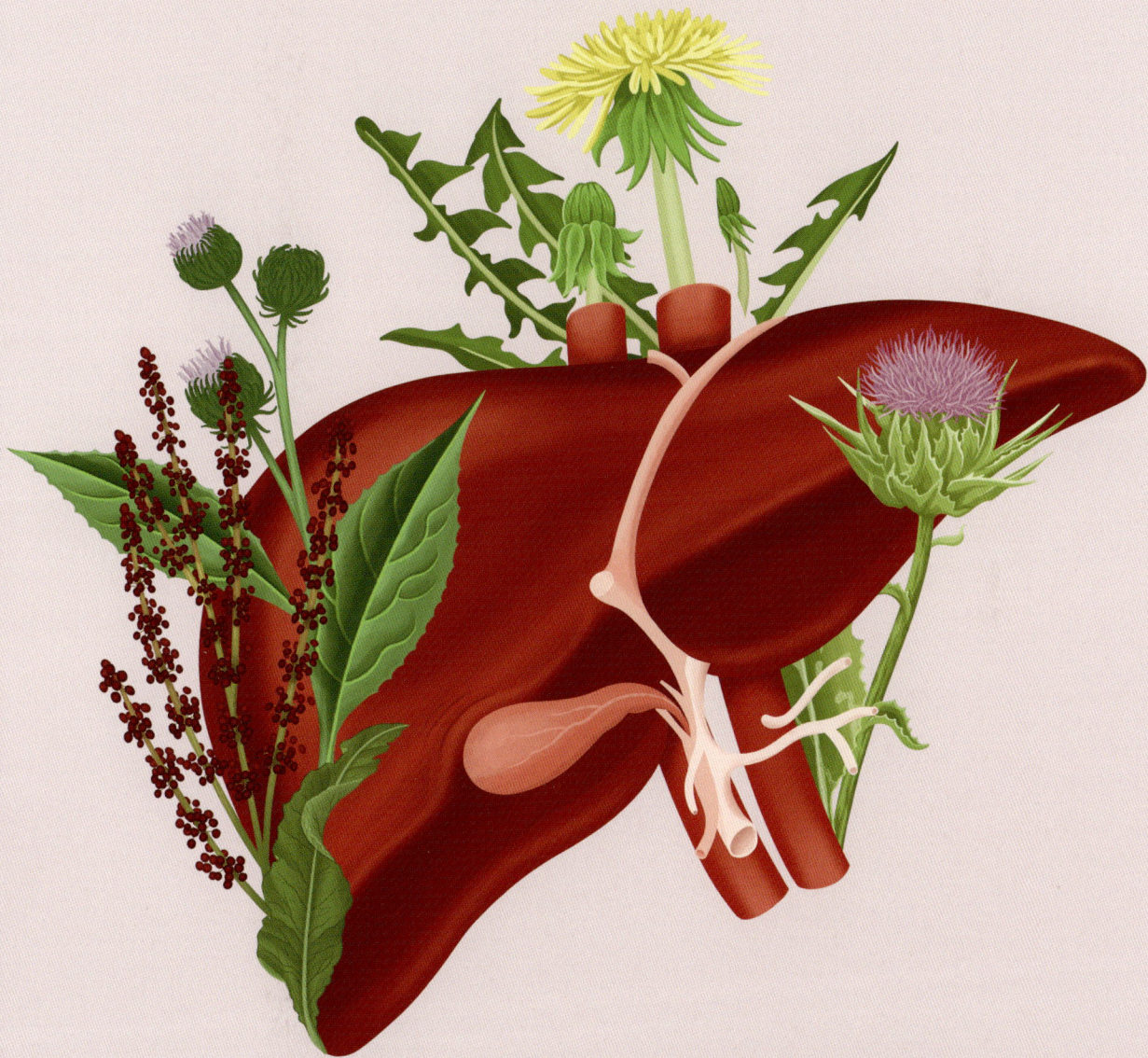

Burdock Root *(Arctium lappa)*
The Blood Cleanser

Burdock root has been used as a blood purifier and detoxifying herb in traditional medicine systems for centuries. In Traditional Chinese Medicine (TCM), burdock is known as *niu bang zi* and is used to remove toxins from the body, clear heat, and promote skin health. European herbalists valued burdock for its ability to support liver function, aid digestion, and improve skin clarity. Native American healers used burdock root in tonics to cleanse the bloodstream and support overall vitality.

By the nineteenth century, burdock became a key ingredient in Western "blood-purifying" formulas, when it was often combined with herbs like yellow dock and dandelion. These traditional remedies were used to address chronic skin conditions, digestive sluggishness, and systemic inflammation.

Today burdock is known as a powerful aid for detoxification, celebrated for its ability to cleanse the liver, support lymphatic function, and promote overall health and wellness.

What the Science Says

Burdock root (*Arctium lappa*) is rich in bioactive compounds that have detoxifying, anti-inflammatory, and antimicrobial properties.

One key compound is inulin, a prebiotic fiber that helps regulate blood sugar levels by slowing digestion and reduces systemic inflammation by promoting a healthy balance of gut bacteria. A study published in *Phytotherapy Research* (2010) found that burdock root extract significantly reduced inflammation and oxidative stress, suggesting its potential for supporting liver health and reducing chronic inflammatory conditions. Another study in *Cosmetics* (2023) showed that burdock root improved skin hydration and elasticity in individuals with dry or irritated skin, likely due to its high antioxidant and anti-inflammatory content.

In addition to inulin, burdock contains unique compounds called **polyacetylenes**, which exhibit strong antibacterial and antifungal properties, making the herb useful for fighting skin infections and supporting immune function. Research in *Frontiers in Pharmacology* (2018) showed that burdock root was able to inhibit the growth of *Staphylococcus aureus* and *Cutibacterium acnes*, two bacteria commonly associated with skin infections and acne, respectively.

Burdock root also supports liver detoxification by stimulating bile production and promoting the elimination of toxins through the kidneys and digestive system. By enhancing liver and lymphatic function—the lymphatic system is essentially a drainage network for the body—burdock helps clear metabolic waste, leading to improved digestion, clearer skin, and increased energy levels.

By supporting detoxification, balancing blood sugar levels, reducing inflammation, and fighting bacteria, burdock root provides a holistic approach to overall wellness.

Uses and Indications

Use burdock root to support liver health, reduce inflammation, and promote skin wellness, particularly if you have dry or irritated skin. It may also be helpful for acne and minor skin infections, as it targets bacteria associated with those conditions.

You can also use burdock root to support a healthy gut microbiome through its prebiotic fiber, inulin. This in turn helps modulate inflammation and improve overall immune function. As a detoxifier, burdock may enhance the body's ability to process and eliminate waste through both the digestive and immune systems. This herb is especially helpful if you're looking to support overall detoxification, improve the gut-skin connection, or maintain immune resilience through gentle, plant-based interventions.

Interactions and Safety

Burdock root is generally well-tolerated, but if you have an allergy to plants in the Asteraceae family (such as daisies, ragweed, or marigolds), use with caution. Due to burdock root's mild diuretic properties, it may interact with diuretics and blood pressure medications that alter kidney function or fluid balance. If you're taking diabetes medication, be sure to monitor blood sugar levels because burdock root may lower glucose levels. If you're pregnant or breastfeeding, consult your healthcare provider before using this herb as its effects on pregnancy and lactation are not well studied. People undergoing treatment for kidney or liver disease should also speak to their doctor before using burdock root.

Growing and Harvesting

Burdock is a biennial plant that thrives in well-drained, loamy soil and full to partial sun. In its first year, burdock develops a deep taproot, which is the most medicinally valuable part of the plant. By the second year, the plant produces tall flowering stalks and eventually goes to seed.

For medicinal use, the roots should be harvested in the fall of the first year or early spring of the second year before the plant flowers. To harvest, dig deep into the soil to extract the long taproot, taking care not to break it. Once harvested, the root should be washed, sliced, and dried for later use in teas, tinctures, or decoctions. Properly dried burdock root can be stored in an airtight container for up to a year.

Recipe

"Three Roots"
Herbal Detox Tonic

This nourishing tonic combines burdock root with yellow dock (page 154) and dandelion root (page 148) to support liver health, lymphatic function, and overall vitality.

Yield: 2 cups (480 ml)

2 cups (480 ml) filtered water

1 tablespoon (7 g) dried burdock root

1 tablespoon (7 g) dried dandelion root

1 teaspoon (0.75 g) dried yellow dock root (optional, for enhanced detoxification)

½ teaspoon (2.5 ml) fresh lemon juice (optional, to support digestion)

Raw honey or maple syrup (optional)

Preparation

In a small saucepan, bring the water to a gentle boil. Add the burdock root, dandelion root, and yellow dock root (if using), then reduce the heat to low. Simmer for 15 to 20 minutes to allow the herbs to release their beneficial compounds. Remove the tonic from the heat and allow it to cool slightly. Strain the liquid through a fine-mesh strainer or cheesecloth. Add lemon juice and sweetener if desired.

How to Use

Drink 1 cup (240 ml) daily in the morning or between meals to support liver detoxification and overall vitality. This tonic is particularly beneficial after periods of dietary excess, medication use, or environmental toxin exposure.

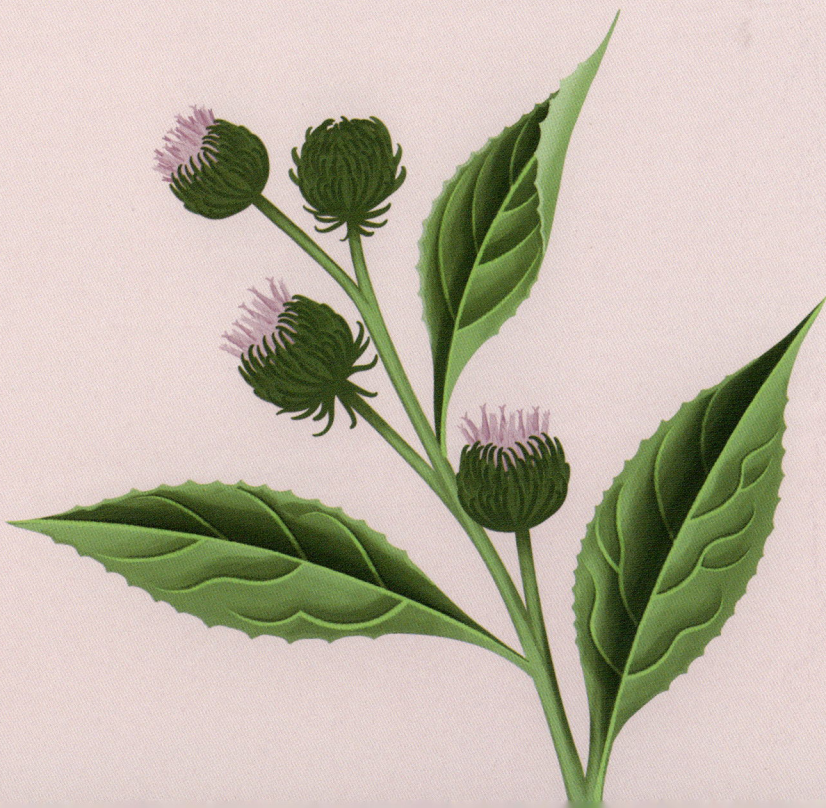

Dandelion Root (*Taraxacum officinale*)
The Gentle Detoxifier

Dandelion root has been valued for centuries in both Western herbalism and Traditional Chinese Medicine (TCM) as a natural blood purifier and detoxification herb. Historically, it was used by ancient Greek, Roman, and Middle Eastern practitioners to support bile production, liver and digestive health, and overall vitality. Native American tribes used it as a tonic to promote kidney and liver function. In traditional European medicine, dandelion root was a staple in spring tonics, consumed to cleanse the body after winter's heavier diet.

Today dandelion root remains one of the most respected herbs for liver health thanks to its ability to gently stimulate detoxification and support overall health and wellness. It's commonly found in detox teas, tinctures, and capsule blends aimed at digestive support and skin clarity. Unlike harsh detoxifiers, dandelion root encourages the body's natural elimination processes without overstimulating or depleting vital nutrients, making it a well-tolerated choice for long-term use. Its versatility and safety profile have helped it remain a cornerstone in both clinical and at-home herbal practice to this day.

What the Science Says

Dandelion root (*Taraxacum officinale*) is packed with bioactive compounds that support liver detoxification, digestion, and overall metabolic health. It contains **sesquiterpene lactones**, bitter compounds that stimulate bile flow, aiding digestion and helping the liver process and eliminate toxins more efficiently. A study in the *Journal of Molecular Sciences* (2025) confirmed dandelion root's role in promoting bile production and enhancing fat metabolism. These properties make it a valuable ally for individuals dealing with sluggish digestion or fatty liver concerns.

Dandelion root's antioxidant properties are largely attributed to its high content of **polyphenols**, **flavonoids** (such as luteolin and apigenin), and **phenolic acids** (including chlorogenic and caffeic acids). These compounds work together to neutralize free radicals and protect liver cells from oxidative stress. Research published in *Evidence-Based Complementary and Alternative Medicine* (2011) found that dandelion root extract supports liver function by increasing antioxidant activity and reducing inflammation within liver cells. A study in the *Journal of Chemical and Pharmaceutical Research* (2016) further confirmed dandelion root's liver-protective effects, showing that its antioxidant-rich profile helps reduce oxidative stress—a major contributor to liver damage.

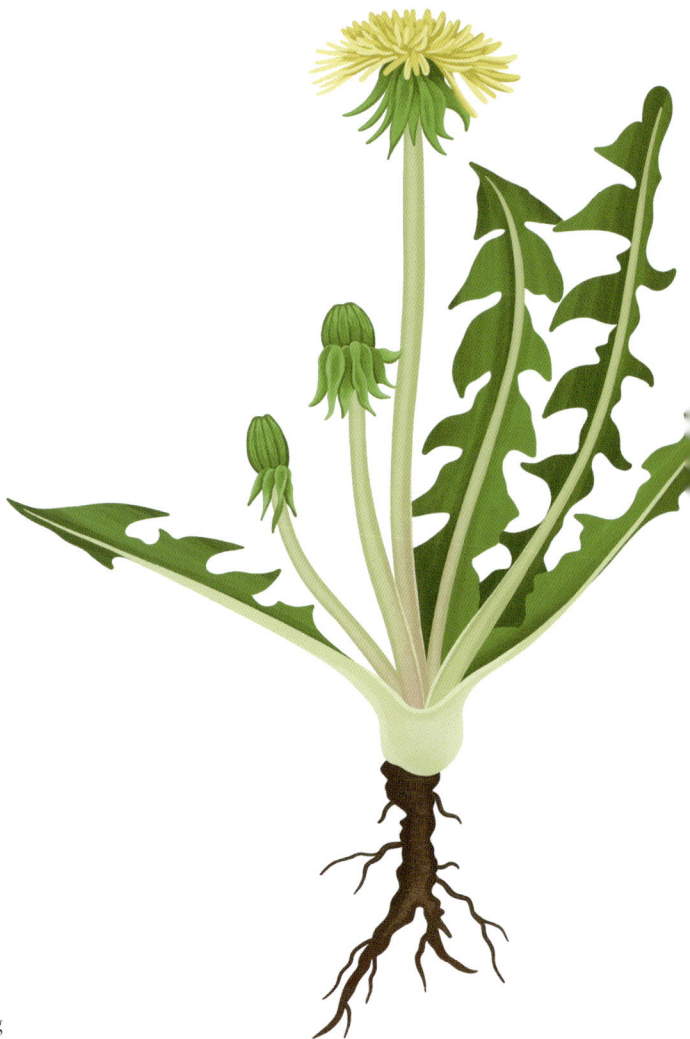

Dandelion root is rich in inulin, a prebiotic fiber that nourishes beneficial gut bacteria, promoting a balanced microbiome. It also offers mild diuretic effects, which support kidney function by helping the body flush excess fluids and metabolic waste.

A versatile herb that increases bile flow, reduces inflammation, and protects liver cells from oxidative damage, dandelion root is a valuable remedy for gentle detoxification and liver and digestive health.

Uses and Indications

Use dandelion root to promote liver detoxification, support digestion, and enhance bile production. It's particularly beneficial if you're experiencing sluggish digestion, bloating, or mild liver congestion. Its ability to stimulate bile flow makes it helpful if you have gallbladder or fat metabolism issues. In addition, dandelion root's prebiotic content aids gut health, making it useful for individuals looking to balance their microbiome.

Interactions and Safety

Dandelion root is generally well-tolerated and safe. However, if you have a bile duct obstruction or gallstones, consult a healthcare provider before using dandelion root, as its bile-stimulating effects could cause discomfort. Due to its mild diuretic properties, it may also increase the excretion of certain medications, including diuretics and lithium, which can limit the effectiveness of the drugs. If you have ragweed allergies, use caution as dandelion belongs to the same plant family. If you're pregnant or breastfeeding, consult your healthcare provider before use.

Growing and Harvesting

Dandelion is a hardy, resilient plant that grows abundantly in meadows, gardens, and even cracks in sidewalks. It thrives in a variety of soils, particularly well-drained, nutrient-rich environments with full sun exposure. The roots are best harvested in the fall when they are at peak potency, containing the highest concentration of inulin and other beneficial compounds.

To harvest dandelion root, dig deep into the soil to extract the long taproot intact. Wash the roots thoroughly, then slice and dry them for later use in teas, tinctures, or decoctions. Properly dried dandelion roots can be stored in an airtight container for up to a year, maintaining their medicinal properties.

See page 152 for a recipe for Milk Thistle and Dandelion Detox Decoction, an excellent daily tonic for liver health and detoxification.

Fun Fact

Dandelion root was once roasted and brewed as a caffeine-free coffee substitute during wartime shortages in Europe and North America. Its naturally bitter compounds give it a rich, earthy flavor that mimics the roastiness of coffee without the jitters—plus, it supports liver function and digestion, making it a win-win for herbal coffee lovers.

Milk Thistle *(Silybum marianum)*
The Liver Protector

Milk thistle has been celebrated as a liver-supporting herb for centuries, with historical roots tracing back to ancient Greek and Roman medicine. The Greek physician Dioscorides first documented its use for liver ailments in the first century AD, highlighting its role in protecting against toxins. In Traditional Chinese Medicine, milk thistle was used to clear "liver heat" to detoxify the body and reduce inflammation.

Throughout medieval Europe, milk thistle was relied upon as a tried-and-true remedy for jaundice and liver inflammation. Herbalists regularly prescribed it to support digestion and bile production. Today it remains one of the most extensively studied herbs for liver health, recognized for its ability to safeguard liver cells, stimulate regeneration, and improve detoxification pathways.

What the Science Says

Milk thistle *(Silybum marianum)* gets its healing reputation from its seeds, which are packed with silymarin—a powerful antioxidant compound. Silymarin isn't just one thing; it's a group of plant-based chemicals called flavonolignans (a fusion of **flavonoids** and **lignans**—both known for their antioxidant and anti-inflammatory effects). The main players in this group are silybin, silydianin, and silychristin, with silybin doing most of the heavy lifting when it comes to liver protection.

These compounds act like a cellular shield: they neutralize free radicals, which are unstable molecules that can damage liver cells over time. But silymarin doesn't stop there. It also strengthens the outer layer (membrane) of liver cells—called hepatocytes—making it harder for toxins, alcohol, and drugs to get inside and cause harm.

At the same time, silymarin stimulates protein production within liver cells, encouraging them to repair themselves and even grow new healthy tissue. This means that milk thistle not only protects your liver but also supports its natural ability to regenerate after damage.

One of milk thistle's primary benefits is its protective effect on the liver. Research in *Biomedicine & Pharmacotherapy* (2022) confirmed that silymarin reduced liver enzyme levels in participants who had liver disease, indicating decreased liver inflammation and improved function. Another study published in *Metabolism Open* (2022) demonstrated that silymarin supplementation reduced fat accumulation and oxidative stress, two markers of liver health in participants who had non-alcoholic fatty liver disease (NAFLD).

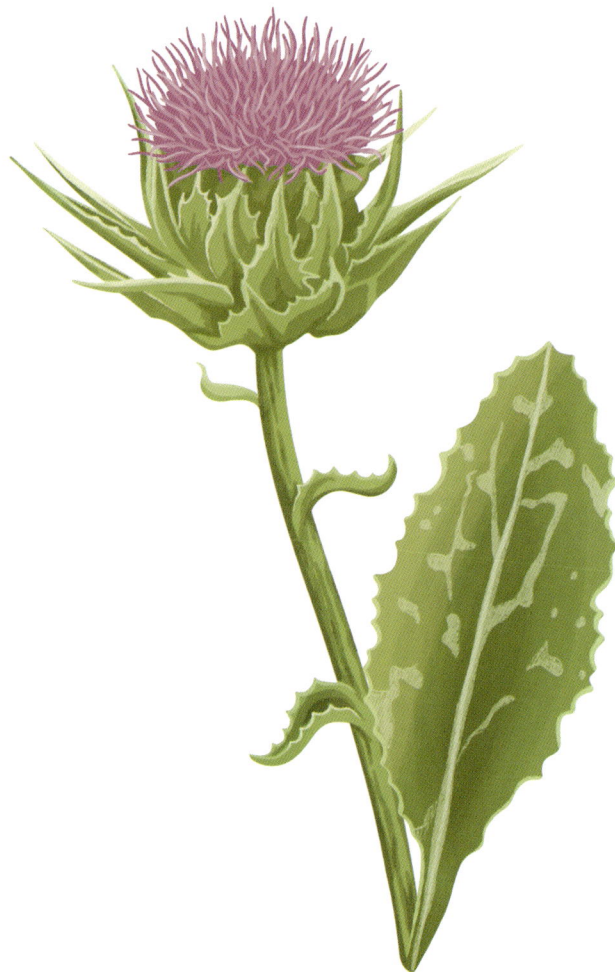

Beyond its role in liver detoxification, milk thistle also supports bile production, which aids digestion and promotes efficient fat metabolism. Bile helps break down fats into smaller droplets, making them easier to digest and absorb, while also carrying waste products and toxins out of the liver for elimination.

In addition, silymarin helps regulate immune function, reducing liver inflammation triggered by viral infections or autoimmune conditions. In fact, research published in *Molecules* (2022) suggested that silymarin exhibits antiviral activity against hepatitis C, helping slow disease progression and reduce viral load.

By enhancing detoxification, protecting against liver damage, and stimulating regeneration, milk thistle provides comprehensive support for liver health, making it a key herb for anyone looking to maintain optimal liver function.

Uses and Indications

Use milk thistle to support liver detoxification and protect against liver damage caused by toxins, alcohol, medications, and environmental pollutants. It's a helpful herbal remedy if you have a liver condition such as non-alcoholic fatty liver disease (NAFLD), cirrhosis, or hepatitis; are recovering from liver stress due to excessive alcohol consumption; or are taking medicines like ibufprofen that tax the liver. The herb also improves digestion by promoting bile flow, if you have sluggish digestion or gallbladder issues. Some research suggests that milk thistle may support skin health by reducing inflammation and oxidative stress, particularly in conditions linked to liver function, such as acne and eczema.

Interactions and Safety

Milk thistle is generally considered safe when taken in moderate amounts. However, because it affects liver enzyme activity, it may alter the metabolism of certain medications, including blood thinners, statins, and antidepressants. Since milk thistle has mild estrogenic effects, consult a healthcare provider before using it if you have a hormone-sensitive condition such as endometriosis, fibroids, or breast, ovarian, or uterine cancer. If you're pregnant or breastfeeding, seek medical advice before using this herb.

Some may experience mild digestive discomfort, such as bloating or diarrhea, when first using milk thistle. To minimize discomfort, start with a low dose and gradually increase. Taking it with food or diluting it in teas and tinctures can also help. Monitor your body's response, and consult a healthcare provider if symptoms persist.

Growing and Harvesting

Milk thistle is a hardy, drought-resistant plant that thrives in well-drained soil with full sun exposure. It is native to the Mediterranean region but has since naturalized across North America and parts of Asia. The plant produces striking purple flowers with spiky green leaves that have characteristic white veins, believed to resemble "milk," giving the herb its name.

Milk thistle is best grown from seeds sown in early spring. Once mature, the flower heads produce small, black seeds containing the highest concentration of silymarin. These seeds are harvested in late summer or early fall when the flower heads dry and turn brown. To collect the seeds, the flower heads are cut, dried, and threshed to separate the seeds from the chaff. Proper drying and storage in airtight containers help preserve the potency of the medicinal compounds.

Fun Fact

Milk thistle has been studied for its ability to counteract mushroom poisoning from the deadly death cap mushroom. Silymarin is believed to block the toxin's uptake by liver cells, reducing damage and potentially preventing fatal liver failure.

Milk Thistle and Dandelion Detox Decoction

Yield: 2 cups (480 ml)

This herbal decoction combines the liver-protective properties of milk thistle with the bile-stimulating effects of dandelion root, making it an excellent daily tonic for liver health and detoxification.

2 cups (480 ml) filtered water

1 tablespoon (14.3 g) milk thistle seeds, crushed

1 tablespoon (7 g) dried dandelion root

½ teaspoon (2.5 ml) fresh lemon juice (optional, for added detox support)

Raw honey or maple syrup (optional)

Preparation

In a small saucepan, bring the water to a gentle boil. Add the crushed milk thistle seeds and dandelion root, then reduce the heat to low. Simmer for 15 to 20 minutes, allowing the herbs to infuse fully. Remove from the heat and let the decoction cool slightly. Strain the liquid through a fine-mesh strainer or cheesecloth into a mug. Add fresh lemon juice and sweetener if desired.

How to Use

Drink 1 cup (240 ml) daily in the morning or between meals to support liver detoxification and overall digestive health. This decoction is especially beneficial after periods of dietary excess, medication use, or alcohol consumption.

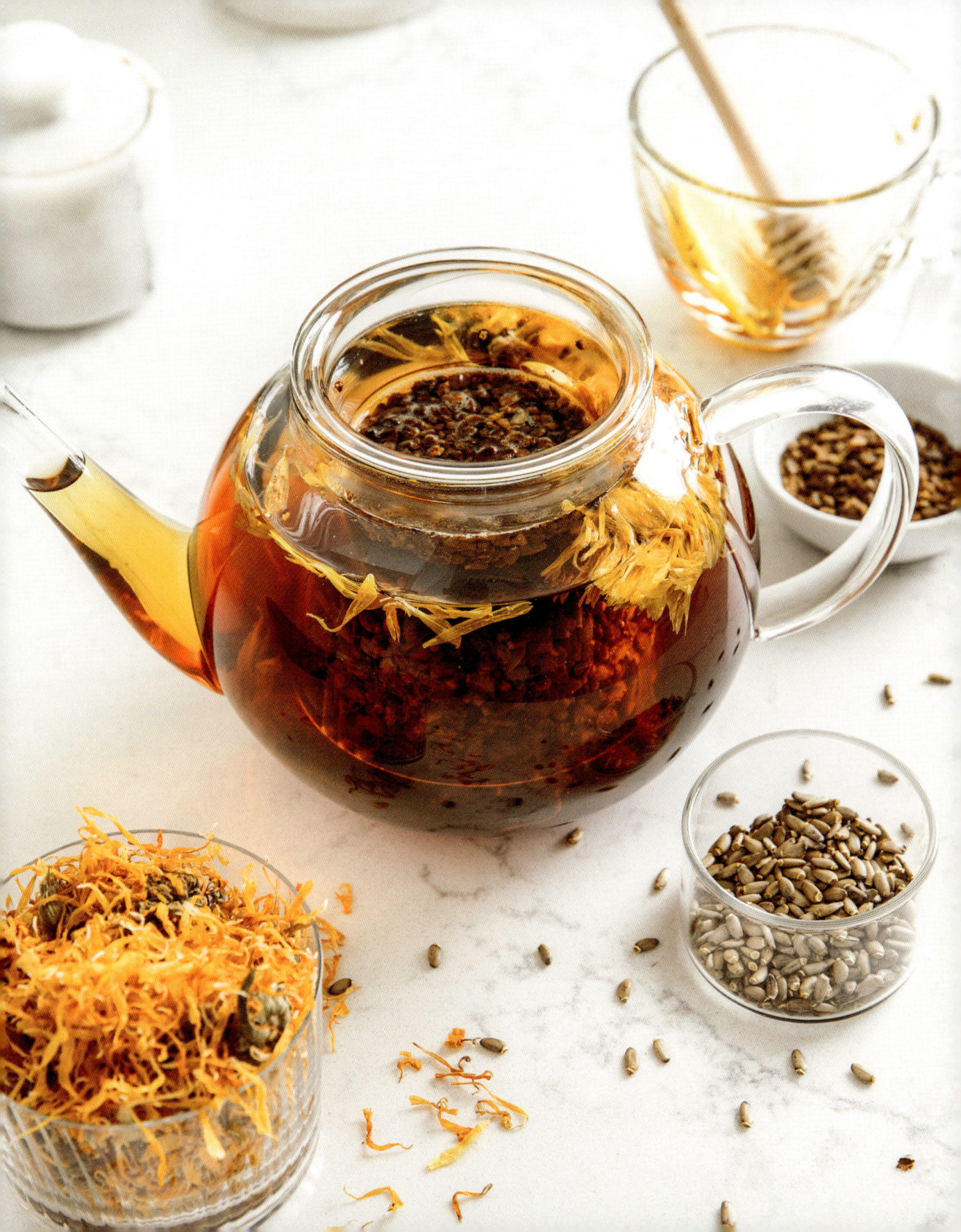

Yellow Dock (*Rumex crispus*)
The Bile Stimulator

Yellow dock has a well-deserved reputation as a potent detoxifying herb, valued for centuries in both Western herbalism and Traditional Chinese Medicine (TCM). Indigenous North American tribes used yellow dock as a blood purifier and digestive aid, while European herbalists incorporated it into formulas to support liver function and bile production. It was often used to alleviate skin conditions, which were thought to be caused by sluggish digestion and toxins in the body.

By the nineteenth century, yellow dock became a key ingredient in "alternative" herbal remedies—formulas designed to gradually restore proper function to the body by supporting elimination, cleansing the blood, and promoting overall metabolic balance. Herbalists of the Eclectic tradition frequently prescribed it as a gentle laxative and liver stimulant. Today yellow dock continues to be used for its ability to promote bile flow, enhance digestion, and support detoxification pathways.

What the Science Says

The medicinal benefits of yellow dock (*Rumex crispus*) are thanks to its rich composition of bioactive compounds that aid digestion, enhance bile production, and support liver detoxification. The root contains **anthraquinones**—plant-derived compounds known for their laxative properties—including emodin and chrysophanol, which stimulate peristalsis and encourage bowel regularity. These compounds also help improve the elimination of metabolic waste, preventing toxin buildup that can contribute to skin and digestive issues.

Yellow dock is also rich in **tannins**, which help tighten and strengthen the mucous membranes in the intestines, reduce inflammation, and promote gut health. A study published in the Korean *Journal of Pharmacognosy* (2007) confirmed that yellow dock reduced liver cell inflammation and improved liver enzyme activity. In addition, yellow dock's **flavonoids** and **phenolic acids** exhibit antioxidant properties that protect liver cells from oxidative stress and support overall metabolic function.

One of yellow dock's most important properties is its ability to stimulate bile production in the liver. By increasing bile flow, yellow dock supports the body's natural detoxification processes, ensuring that harmful substances are processed and excreted easily and efficiently.

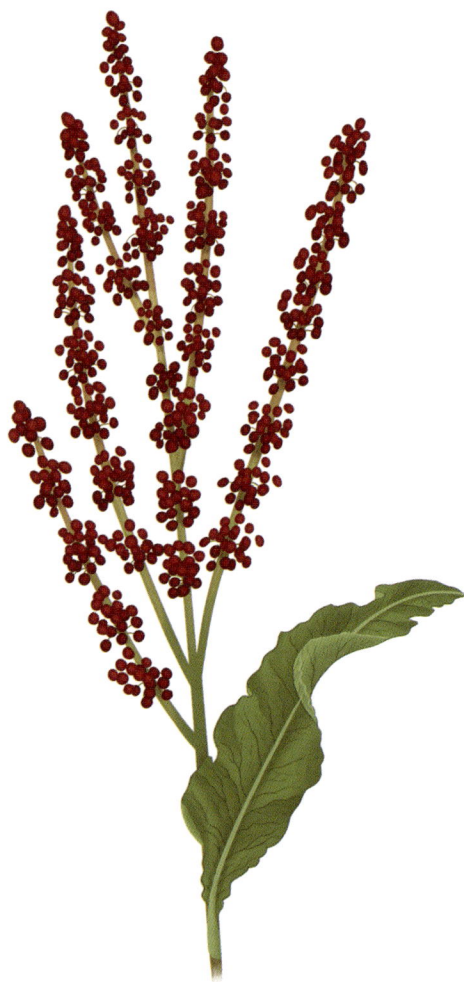

In addition to its liver-supportive properties, yellow dock is a natural source of iron, making it beneficial for individuals with anemia or low iron levels. The presence of bioavailable iron, combined with its ability to promote mineral absorption, has made it a valuable herb for improving energy levels and addressing nutritional deficiencies. Yellow dock has traditionally been used to support iron levels, especially when paired with herbs rich in vitamin C to enhance absorption. While this practice is common in herbalism, current scientific studies confirming its ability to increase iron bioavailability are limited, and more research is needed to validate its effectiveness in addressing anemia.

By promoting bile flow, improving digestion, and supporting detoxification, yellow dock serves as a powerful herb for maintaining metabolic balance and overall vitality.

Uses and Indications

Yellow dock is commonly used to support liver and gallbladder function, which can be especially beneficial if you're experiencing sluggish digestion, bloating, or difficulty breaking down fats. By stimulating bile secretion, it enhances nutrient absorption and supports the body's natural elimination processes. This improved waste clearance may also indirectly benefit skin health, particularly when imbalances in digestion or detoxification are contributing to issues like breakouts or irritation.

Due to its mild laxative properties, yellow dock is frequently included in herbal detox formulas designed to promote regularity and improve gut health. In addition, yellow dock's natural iron content makes it useful for those with anemia or low energy levels because it helps improve iron absorption and overall blood health.

Beyond digestion, yellow dock can help cool inflammatory skin conditions. Herbalists often recommend it for people who are struggling with chronic acne, hives, or other skin flare-ups that may be linked to sluggish liver function. Its combination of blood-cleansing, bile-stimulating, and mild laxative properties make it a well-rounded herb for metabolic and skin health.

Interactions and Safety

Yellow dock is generally considered safe for short-term use. However, its anthraquinone content means it should not be used long term as a laxative on a daily basis. This can lead to dependency and electrolyte imbalances. If you have a history of kidney stones, use caution because yellow dock contains oxalates, which may contribute to stone formation.

Due to its mild iron-binding properties, yellow dock may interact with iron supplements, so it's best to take them at different times of day to avoid interference with absorption. If you're on diuretics or medications that affect electrolyte balance, consult a healthcare provider before using yellow dock because its mild laxative effects can contribute to potassium depletion. If you're pregnant or breastfeeding, seek medical advice before using yellow dock because its stimulant effects on digestion can impact uterine health.

Growing and Harvesting

Yellow dock is a hardy, perennial herb that thrives in disturbed soils, roadsides, and meadows across North America and Europe. It prefers well-drained, slightly acidic to neutral soil and full to partial sun exposure. The plant produces long, lance-shaped leaves and a tall flowering stalk that turns reddish-brown as it matures.

The medicinal part of the plant—its root—is best harvested in the fall of its first year or early spring of its second year before it flowers. Harvesting the root requires deep digging, as yellow dock develops a long taproot that extends deep into the soil. Once harvested, the root should be cleaned, chopped, and dried for later use in teas, tinctures, or decoctions. Properly dried yellow dock root can be stored in an airtight container in a cool, dark, and dry place for up to a year. To preserve its potency, avoid exposure to moisture, heat, and direct sunlight. When stored correctly, the root retains its bitterness and therapeutic properties, making it ideal for use in herbal preparations such as teas, tinctures, syrups, or decoctions whenever needed.

See page 147 for "Three Roots" Herbal Detox Tonic, which combines yellow dock with other liver-friendly herbs to support healthy detoxification.

Chapter 10

Clean and Clear: Herbs for the Urinary System and Kidney Health

The urinary system and kidneys are the body's essential filtration units, tirelessly purifying blood, balancing electrolytes, and maintaining fluid harmony. These unsung heroes of detoxification flush out metabolic waste, regulate blood pressure, and ensure cells receive the right balance of nutrients. The kidneys, with their intricate nephrons, work as precision instruments, filtering blood, removing toxins, and reabsorbing vital water and nutrients. This delicate balance keeps the body hydrated, free of harmful buildup, and ready for daily life.

Modern lifestyles, however, can strain this critical system. High-sodium diets, caffeine, and environmental toxins, combined with inadequate hydration, challenge the kidneys and urinary tract. Over time, these factors can lead to imbalances, dehydration, or kidney strain. Supporting this system with water and herbs can enhance its resilience and efficiency, ensuring long-term health.

Herbal allies provide natural and effective support. Parsley, a nutrient-packed herb, helps the kidneys flush out toxins while promoting gentle fluid elimination. Corn silk soothes the urinary tract lining, reducing inflammation and promoting comfort. Cranberry prevents bacteria from adhering to the bladder wall, making it indispensable for urinary health. Marshmallow root, rich in mucilage, acts as a protective balm for the urinary tract, shielding and soothing vital tissues.

This chapter explores recipes like a Parsley Kidney-Cleansing Cordial and a gentle Corn Silk and Herbal Infusion, offering daily support for urinary wellness. These herbs act as gifts to your body's filtration system, promoting clarity, balance, and resilience. Let's give our kidneys and urinary system the care they deserve.

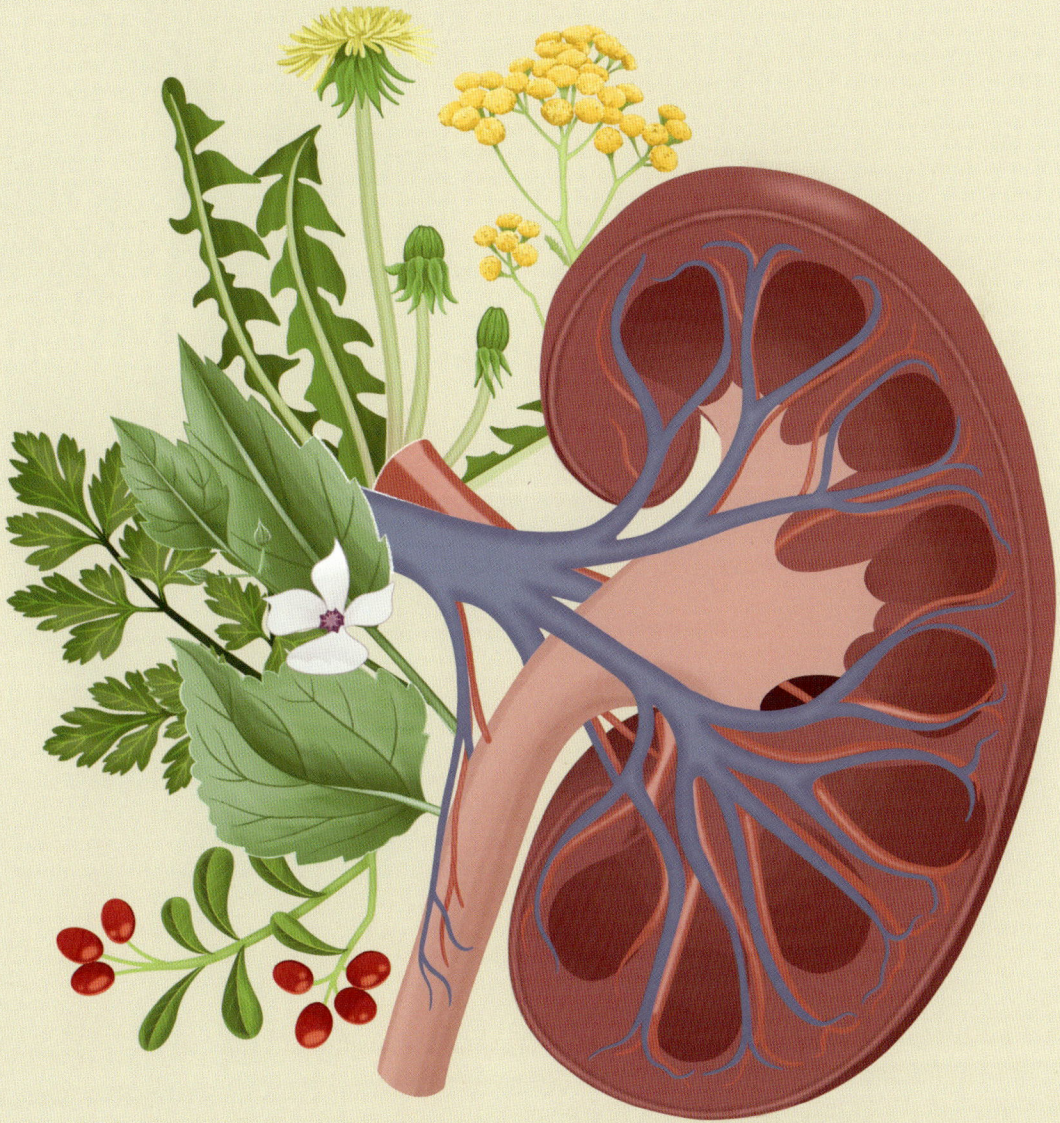

Parsley *(Petroselinum crispum)*
The Kidney Cleanser

Parsley has long been valued in herbal medicine for its ability to promote kidney health and support natural detoxification. Traditionally used in ancient Greece, Rome, and throughout Europe, parsley was often incorporated into cleansing remedies to "flush" the kidneys and urinary tract. In medieval herbal traditions, it was considered a key herb for balancing fluids in the body, reducing water retention, and preventing kidney-related ailments. In addition to its medicinal uses, parsley was widely cultivated as a culinary staple, prized for its fresh, invigorating flavor and nutrient-dense profile.

Parsley's reputation as a natural diuretic has made it a go-to remedy for promoting kidney function, particularly in cases of mild urinary discomfort or fluid retention. Today herbalists continue to recommend parsley for its gentle, effective ability to support kidney health, making it a simple but powerful herb for everyday wellness.

What the Science Says

The medicinal benefits of parsley *(Petroselinum crispum)* are thanks to its rich composition of bioactive compounds that enhance kidney function and promote urinary health. The leaves and stems are chock-full of helpful **flavonoids** such as apigenin and luteolin, which exhibit potent antioxidant and anti-inflammatory properties, helping to protect kidney cells. A study in *Frontiers in Medicine* (2024) showed parsley's protective effects against kidney damage, demonstrating its ability to reduce oxidative stress and inflammation in renal tissue. Parsley is also a source of chlorophyll, which aids in detoxification by binding to toxins and facilitating their elimination through the urinary system.

One of parsley's most well-known effects is its natural diuretic action, attributed to its **volatile oils**—aromatic compounds that easily evaporate and are responsible for the herb's distinct fragrance and many of its therapeutic effects—particularly apiol and myristicin. These compounds increase urine production, helping to flush out excess fluids and metabolic waste while maintaining electrolyte balance. Unlike synthetic diuretics, which can deplete the body of essential minerals, parsley is naturally rich in potassium, which helps prevent electrolyte imbalances and supports overall kidney function. Research published in *Phytomedicine* (2013) confirmed parsley's diuretic effects, showing that it significantly increased urinary output while preserving essential minerals such as potassium and sodium, making it a safe and effective choice for supporting kidney function.

Beyond its role in kidney health, parsley has been studied for its potential antimicrobial properties. Its flavonoids and volatile oils have been shown to inhibit the growth of harmful bacteria in the urinary tract, further supporting its traditional use for urinary health. Research in *Journal of Traditional Chinese Medicine* (2013) found that parsley extracts exhibited antibacterial activity against common urinary pathogens, suggesting its role in promoting a healthy urinary system.

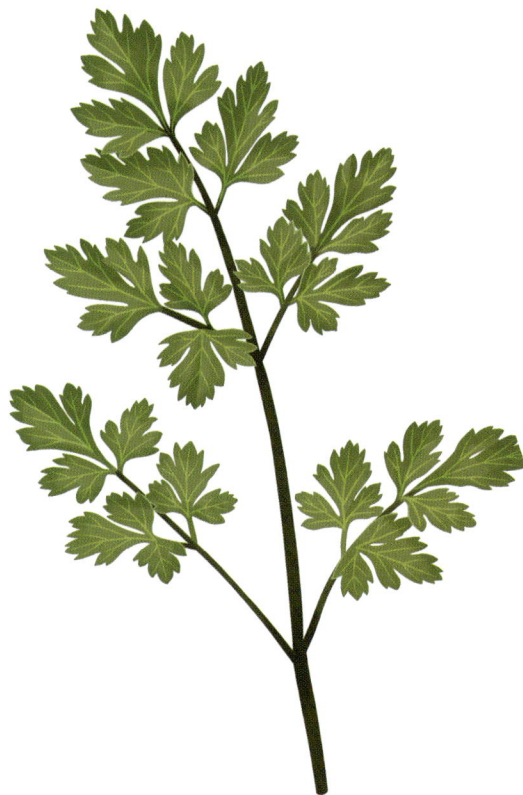

Parsley is also a highly nutritious food, offering a concentrated source of vitamins A, C, and K, as well as essential minerals like iron, calcium, and magnesium. Incorporating fresh parsley into the diet not only provides kidney-supportive compounds but also contributes to overall wellness through its dense nutrient profile.

By enhancing urine flow, reducing inflammation, and supporting the body's natural detoxification pathways, parsley serves as a gentle yet effective kidney cleanser, making it a valuable herb for long-term renal support.

Uses and Indications

You'll find parsley in many formulas designed to bolster urinary tract health. You can use the herb to naturally support kidney function, encourage fluid balance, and assist the body in eliminating waste products. Its mild diuretic properties make it a useful herb if you're experiencing occasional bloating or water retention.

In addition, parsley helps rid the body of toxins that can contribute to sluggish digestion or skin imbalances. It can be particularly beneficial if you're looking for a way to detoxify

Parsley Kidney-Cleansing Cordial

This herbal cordial combines parsley's kidney-cleansing properties with the warming and detoxifying benefits of ginger and lemon zest, creating a delicious and effective tonic for urinary health.
Note: *This syrup is not recommended for children under one year old, as infants should not consume honey.*

> *Yield: 1 cup (240 ml)*

¼ cup (15 g) fresh parsley leaves (washed and chopped)

½ teaspoon (1 g) fresh lemon zest

¼ teaspoon (0.68 g) grated ginger root

1 cup (240 ml) vodka or brandy

¼ cup (60 ml) raw honey or Grade A maple syrup

Preparation

Place the chopped parsley, lemon zest, and ginger in a clean glass jar. Pour the vodka or brandy over the ingredients, ensuring they are fully submerged. Seal the jar tightly and shake well. Store in a cool, dark place for 2 to 4 weeks, shaking the jar every few days to enhance the infusion. After the steeping period, strain through a fine-mesh strainer or cheesecloth to remove solids. Stir in the raw honey or maple syrup to sweeten the cordial. Transfer the finished cordial to a clean bottle for storage.

How to Use

Take 1 teaspoon (5 ml) diluted in water or tea, up to twice daily, as part of a kidney-supportive regimen. This cordial is best used in moderation to support kidney function and gentle detoxification.

---

without the harsh effects of stronger diuretics. Some herbalists also recommend parsley for mild cases of urinary discomfort, as its diuretic and antimicrobial properties may help promote a balanced urinary environment.

Interactions and Safety

Parsley is generally safe and well-tolerated when consumed in moderate amounts, whether as an herbal remedy or in food. However, if you have kidney disease or are taking diuretics, consult a healthcare provider before using parsley medicinally, as its diuretic effects may interact with medications or conditions that affect fluid balance.

Due to its volatile oil content, large amounts of parsley should be avoided during pregnancy, because it has potential uterine-stimulating effects. If you're on anticoagulants, use caution, as parsley is rich in vitamin K, which plays a role in blood clotting and may interact with blood-thinning medications.

Growing and Harvesting

Parsley is a hardy, biennial herb that thrives in a variety of climates, making it an easy addition to home gardens and kitchen windowsills. It prefers well-drained, nutrient-rich soil and full to partial sun exposure. While parsley is often grown as an annual, it will produce seeds in its second year if left to mature.

The leaves can be harvested throughout the growing season, with fresh leaves offering the highest potency for both culinary and medicinal use. For a more concentrated medicinal effect, parsley can be dried and stored in an airtight container, preserving its essential oils and bioactive compounds. The best time to harvest is in the morning when the plant's volatile oils are at their peak.

Parsley can also be grown indoors in pots, providing a year-round source of fresh greens. Regular harvesting encourages continued growth, ensuring a steady supply of this powerful kidney-supportive herb.

Marshmallow Root *(Althaea officinalis)*
The Soothing Diuretic

Marshmallow root has been prized for its soothing and protective properties for centuries, with historical use dating back to ancient Egypt, Greece, and Rome. The Greek physician Hippocrates recommended marshmallow root for wound healing and respiratory ailments, while Dioscorides, a Roman herbalist, noted its use for soothing mucous membranes and urinary discomfort.

In medieval European medicine, marshmallow root became a staple remedy for bladder irritation, kidney support, and digestive complaints. Traditional healers across cultures valued its ability to calm inflamed tissues, particularly in the urinary and digestive systems. Marshmallow root was often used as a tea or poultice to relieve irritation and promote healing.

Today marshmallow root remains a go-to herb for soothing inflammation, particularly in the urinary tract. It's a natural effective remedy for easing discomfort caused by irritation, infections, or excessive acidity in the urine.

What the Science Says

The medicinal power of marshmallow root *(Althaea officinalis)* lies in its mucilage-rich composition. Mucilage is a gel-like **polysaccharide** that forms a protective barrier over inflamed mucous membranes, reducing irritation, preventing further damage, and promoting healing. This demulcent (soothing) effect makes marshmallow root particularly beneficial for urinary tract infections (UTIs), bladder inflammation, and kidney irritation. Research published in the *American Journal of Nephrology* (2014) found that marshmallow root extract reduced inflammation and protected tissues from oxidative damage, reinforcing its traditional use to soothe irritation in the bladder and kidneys.

Beyond its mucilage content, marshmallow root also contains **flavonoids** and polysaccharides, which contribute to its immune-supportive and diuretic effects. A study in the *Indian Journal of Research in Pharmacy and Biotechnology* (2013) showed that marshmallow root promoted gentle diuresis, which means it encouraged fluid elimination without excessive dehydration or mineral loss. By increasing urine flow, marshmallow root helps flush out irritants, bacteria, and toxins from the urinary tract, which promotes overall kidney and bladder health.

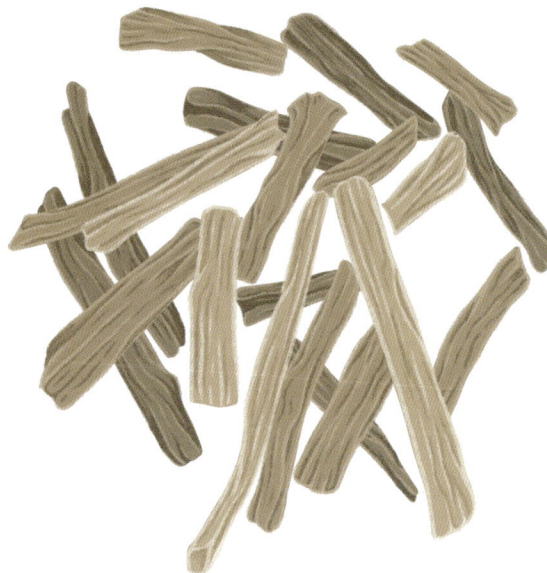

In addition, marshmallow root's antioxidant compounds help combat oxidative stress, which is linked to chronic inflammation and tissue damage. These protective effects make marshmallow root a valuable herb for those experiencing recurrent UTIs or kidney irritation.

Uses and Indications

Marshmallow root is a reliable natural remedy that relieves inflammation and irritation in the urinary tract. It is particularly beneficial if you're experiencing discomfort from UTIs, bladder irritation, or kidney stress. Due to its mild diuretic properties, marshmallow root can also help reduce water retention and support kidney function. You will often find it in formulas combined with other urinary-supportive herbs like corn silk and dandelion root to enhance its effects.

Beyond urinary health, marshmallow root can support the digestive system by coating the stomach lining, easing acid reflux, and reducing irritation from gastritis.

Interactions and Safety

Marshmallow root is generally considered safe with no known toxic effects when consumed in moderation. However, due to its mucilage content, it may interfere with the absorption of medications by coating the digestive tract. To prevent interactions, it is best to take marshmallow root separately from medications by at least one to two hours.

If you're pregnant or breastfeeding, consult a healthcare provider before using marshmallow root as research on its effects during pregnancy is limited. If you have diabetes, it's important to monitor your blood sugar levels while taking marshmallow root, as it may have a mild blood sugar–lowering effect.

Growing and Harvesting

Marshmallow (*Althaea officinalis*) is a hardy perennial herb that thrives in damp, marshy environments, as its name suggests. Native to Europe, Western Asia, and North Africa, it prefers rich, moist soil and full to partial sunlight. The plant grows tall, with soft, velvety leaves and pale pink flowers that bloom in midsummer.

The medicinal root is best harvested in the fall after the plant has completed its growing cycle, as this is when its mucilage content is at its peak. Once harvested, the roots are cleaned, sliced, and dried for use in teas, infusions, and tinctures. Proper drying ensures the preservation of its soothing properties, allowing for long-term storage and use.

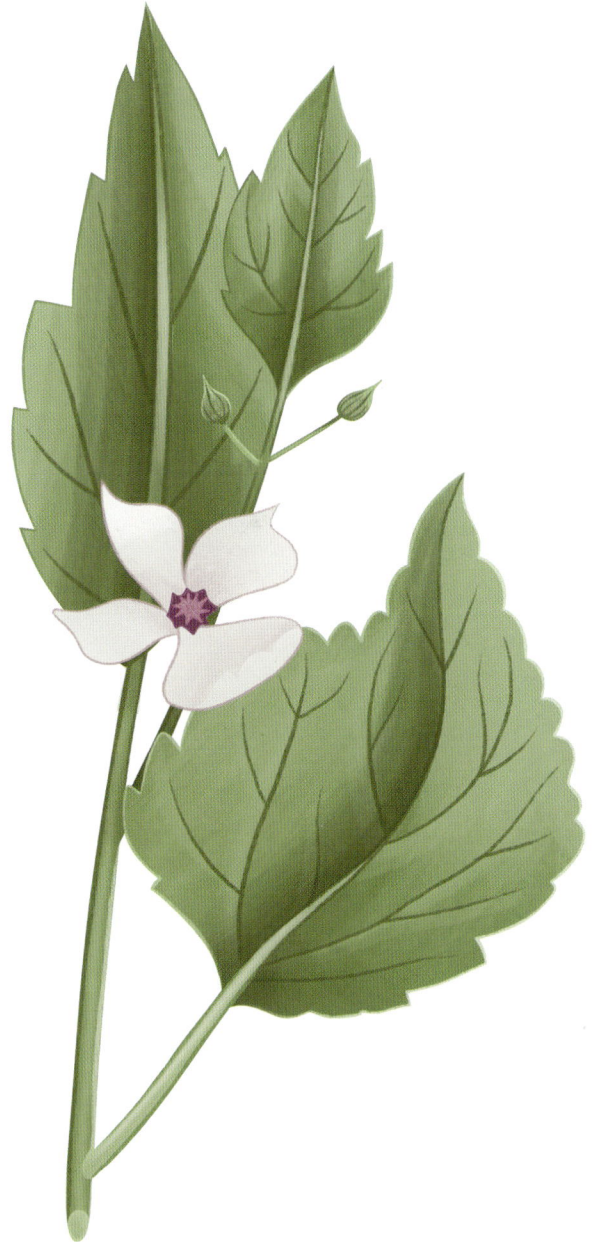

Marshmallow Root Cold Infusion

Yield: 1 quart (1 L)

This gentle cold infusion is the best way to extract marshmallow root's mucilaginous compounds, creating a smooth, soothing drink that helps coat and protect the urinary tract.

1 to 2 tablespoons (3 to 6 g) dried marshmallow root

1 quart (1 L) cold, filtered water

Preparation

In a clean quart-size glass (1 L) jar, add the dried marshmallow root. Fill the jar with the cold water, ensuring the herb is fully submerged. Seal the jar with a lid and let it sit at room temperature for 4 to 8 hours or overnight to create a thick, mucilaginous infusion. Once infused, strain the mixture through a fine-mesh strainer or cheesecloth into a clean jar or pitcher, discarding the marshmallow root.

How to Use

Drink 1 to 2 cups (240 to 480 ml) daily to support urinary tract health and hydration. The resulting infusion has a smooth, slightly thick texture and can be enjoyed plain or with a touch of honey for sweetness. Store any remaining infusion in the refrigerator for up to 2 days.

Fun Fact

Marshmallow root was the original ingredient in the marshmallow confection we know today. In ancient Egypt, the root was mixed with honey and used as a medicinal treat for sore throats and digestive issues. Over time, the medicinal use faded, and modern marshmallows are now made with gelatin instead of plant-based mucilage.

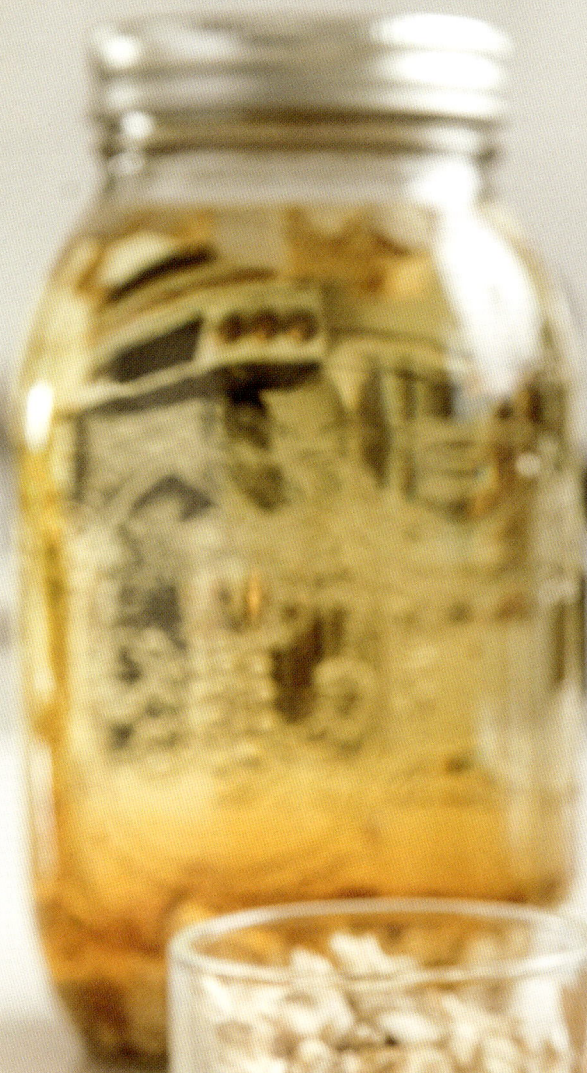

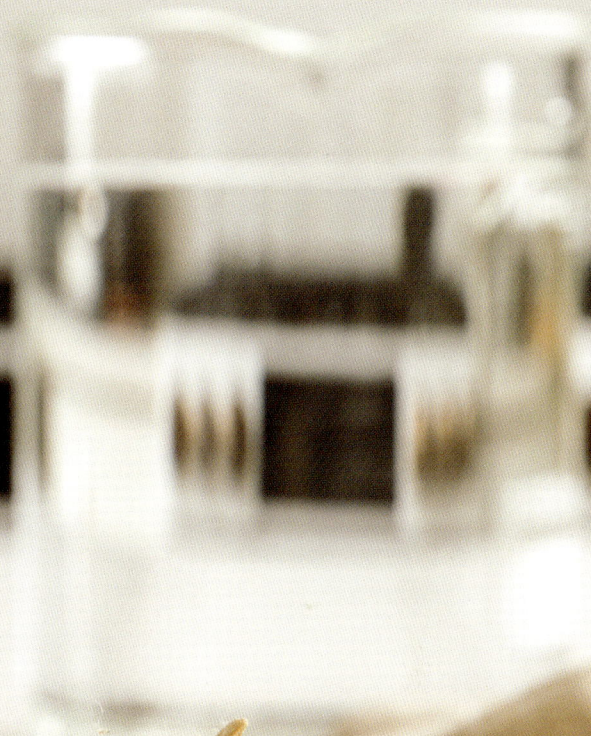

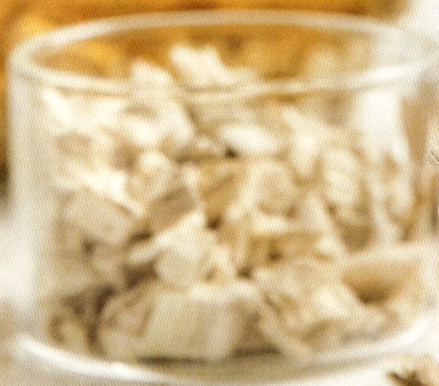

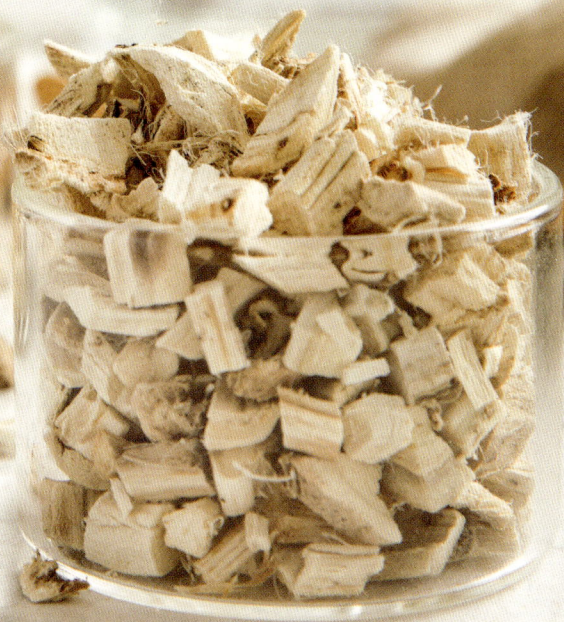

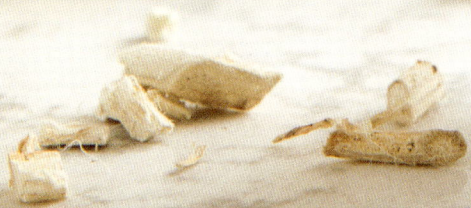

Corn Silk (*Zea mays*)
The Urinary Tract Soother

Corn silk, the delicate golden threads found beneath the husks of corn, has long been prized in traditional medicine for its ability to support urinary health. Native American tribes used corn silk as a remedy for urinary tract discomfort, bladder irritation, and kidney-related issues, often preparing it as a tea to promote a gentle diuretic effect and soothe inflammation. Traditional Chinese Medicine (TCM) also recognized corn silk's benefits, using it to clear damp heat from the bladder, support kidney function, and encourage detoxification.

By the early twentieth century, corn silk appeared in several American and European herbal pharmacopeias and Eclectic medical texts as a natural treatment for cystitis, nephritis, and bedwetting. In more recent decades, corn silk has remained a mainstay in Western herbalism and naturopathic protocols for managing mild urinary tract infections, fluid retention, and bladder irritation. It's commonly included in herbal tea blends and tinctures focused on urinary health, and it's even found in some over-the-counter herbal formulas in Europe and North America. Today it continues to be embraced for its soothing effects on the urinary tract, making it an essential remedy for those seeking gentle, natural support for bladder and kidney wellness.

What the Science Says

The medicinal properties of corn silk (*Zea mays*) stem from its rich composition of bioactive compounds that provide soothing, anti-inflammatory, and diuretic effects. It contains mucilage, a gel-like, plant-based fiber that forms a protective coating over irritated tissues, helping to reduce inflammation in the urinary tract. This soothing, slippery quality is what makes corn silk an effective demulcent—a type of herb that calms and protects mucous membranes, offering relief for individuals experiencing mild urinary discomfort.

Corn silk also contains **tannins**, which help tighten and tone the bladder lining, reducing excessive irritation and supporting bladder strength. **Saponins** present in the silk contribute to its mild diuretic action, helping to increase urine output while maintaining electrolyte balance. Additionally, its **flavonoids** and **volatile oils** offer gentle antimicrobial properties, which may help protect against bacterial overgrowth in the urinary tract.

A study published in the *Journal of Food Chemistry and Nanotechnology* (2023) highlighted corn silk's diuretic and anti-inflammatory effects, showing its ability to promote fluid balance while reducing inflammation in the bladder and kidneys. Another study in *International Journal of Science and Research Archive* (2024) found that corn silk extract helped decrease symptoms of bladder irritation, supporting its historical use as a urinary tract soother.

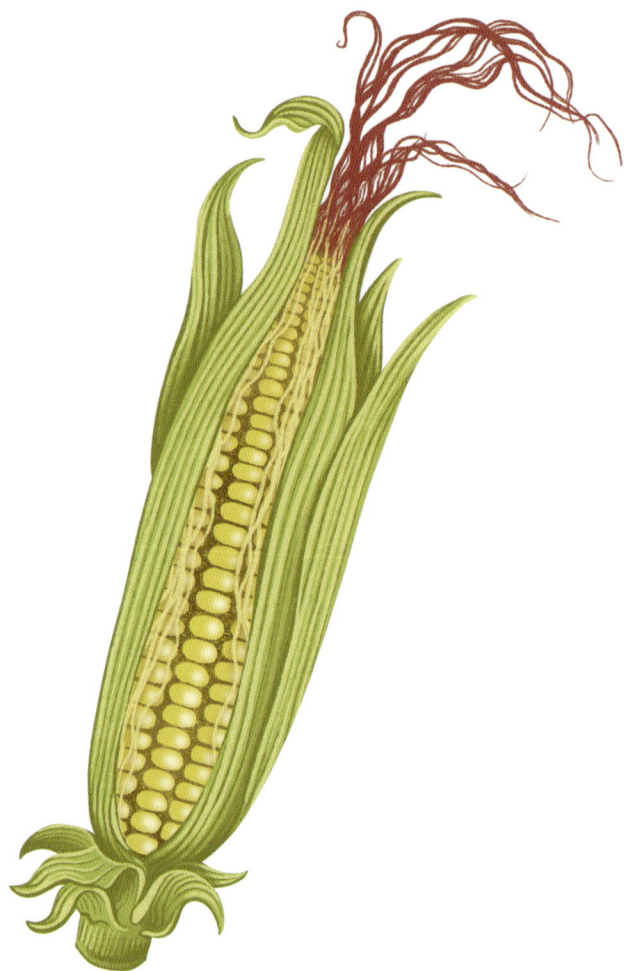

By combining its anti-inflammatory, mucilaginous, and mild diuretic properties, corn silk offers comprehensive support for urinary tract health. Its gentle yet effective nature makes it a preferred herbal remedy for those experiencing urinary discomfort, fluid retention, or mild bladder irritation.

Uses and Indications

Use corn silk to soothe irritation in the urinary tract and promote bladder health. It is particularly useful for easing mild discomfort in the bladder caused by inflammation or irritation. Corn silk's soothing effects on mucous membranes may be beneficial if you experience occasional urinary urgency or sensitivity. As a mild diuretic, it may also help with mild water retention or bloating.

Herbalists also recommend corn silk for those recovering from urinary tract infections (UTIs) or bladder irritation, as its

Corn Silk and Herbal Infusion

This gentle urinary-supportive infusion combines corn silk with dandelion leaf for added diuretic benefits and peppermint for a refreshing flavor.

Yield: 4 cups (1 L)

2 tablespoons (24 g) dried corn silk

1 tablespoon (2 g) dried dandelion leaf (for additional urinary support)

1 teaspoon (0.5 g) dried peppermint (for a refreshing taste and digestive benefits)

4 cups (1 L) boiling water

Preparation

In a clean quart-size glass (1 L) jar, add the corn silk, dandelion leaf, and peppermint. Pour the boiling water over the herbs, ensuring they are fully submerged. Seal the jar and let the infusion steep for 4 to 6 hours, or overnight for a stronger extraction. Once ready, strain the liquid into a pitcher, discarding the herbs.

How to Use

Drink 1 to 2 cups (240 to 480 ml) daily, either warm or cold, to support urinary tract health and fluid balance. Store any leftover infusion in the refrigerator for up to 2 days. This mild, earthy infusion provides gentle hydration while soothing and nourishing the urinary system.

soothing and hydrating properties help restore comfort and function to the urinary system. It pairs well with other urinary-supportive herbs such as dandelion leaf and marshmallow root for a synergistic effect.

Interactions and Safety

Corn silk is generally well-tolerated and safe when used in moderate amounts. However, if you have a known allergy to corn it's best to avoid it, because it may trigger an allergic reaction. If you're pregnant or breastfeeding, consult a healthcare provider before using corn silk medicinally.

Since corn silk has mild diuretic properties, use caution if you're taking prescription diuretics or blood pressure medications because it may enhance the effects of these drugs. If you are managing kidney-related conditions, seek medical advice before incorporating corn silk into your routine.

Growing and Harvesting

Corn silk is readily available as a by-product of fresh corn harvests, making it one of the easiest herbal remedies to collect. It thrives in warm, temperate climates and is grown worldwide as part of standard corn cultivation.

To harvest corn silk, simply gather the long, silky threads from freshly husked corn ears. The silk should be light golden to pale green in color, indicating freshness. Avoid using silk that appears dry, brown, or wilted.

Once collected, the silk can be used fresh or dried for later use. To dry, spread the silk in a single layer on a clean surface in a warm, well-ventilated area, avoiding direct sunlight. Once fully dried, store it in an airtight container away from heat and moisture. Properly dried corn silk retains its potency for up to a year, making it a convenient and accessible remedy for urinary health.

Cranberry *(Vaccinium macrocarpon)*
The UTI Defender

Cranberries have long been celebrated for their ability to support urinary tract health, particularly in Indigenous American herbal traditions. Native American tribes, including the Wampanoag and Algonquin, used cranberries as both food and medicine, recognizing their effectiveness in preventing infections and promoting overall well-being. They often prepared cranberries as poultices for wounds, used them as a natural dye, and consumed them as a tart, nutrient-rich fruit to maintain health during harsh winters.

With European colonization, cranberries gained further recognition as a valuable remedy for urinary and digestive health. By the nineteenth century, physicians began recommending cranberry juice for urinary tract infections (UTIs), a practice that continues today. Overall, cranberry has become a staple in both folk remedies and seasonal preparations, bridging cultural traditions and continuing to play an important role in herbal wellness today.

What the Science Says
The medicinal benefits of cranberries stem from their unique composition of bioactive compounds, particularly **proanthocyanidins** (PACs)—a class of **polyphenols** known for their antioxidant and anti-adhesion properties—along with **flavonoids** and **organic acids**. These compounds work together to support urinary tract health by preventing harmful bacteria, such as *Escherichia coli* (*E. coli*), from attaching to the bladder walls. This anti-adhesion effect makes it difficult for bacteria to colonize the tissue and cause infection. In other words, unlike antibiotics that kill bacteria directly, cranberries reduce the likelihood of infections before they begin.

Cranberry's anti-adhesion mechanism has been extensively studied, with research published in *Research Review* (2024) confirming that regular cranberry consumption significantly lowers the risk of recurrent UTIs, particularly in women with a history of infections.

Cranberries also contain quinic acid, which helps acidify urine, creating an environment less hospitable to bacterial overgrowth. Additionally, their high antioxidant content provides protection against oxidative stress and inflammation, further supporting bladder and kidney function.

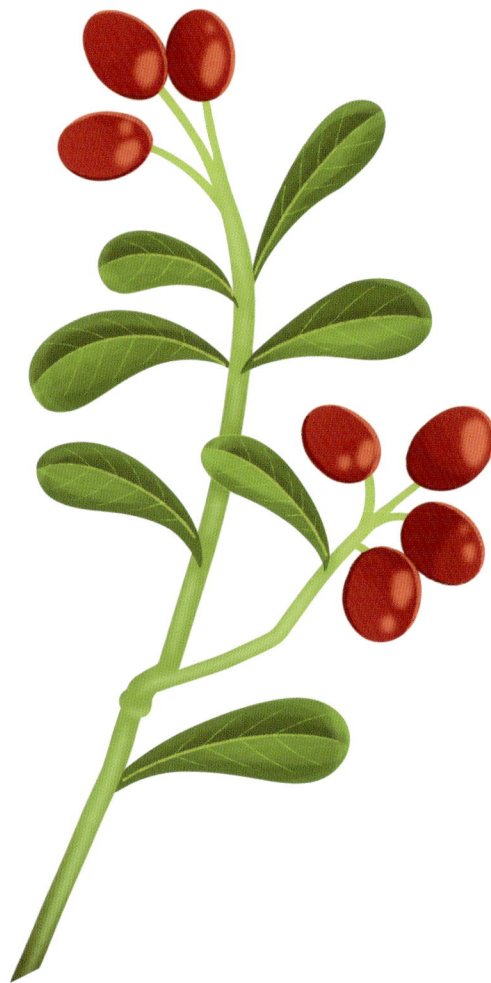

By reducing bacterial adhesion, lowering inflammation, and supporting microbial balance, cranberries provide a safe and effective means of preventing UTIs and maintaining long-term urinary health.

Uses and Indications
Use cranberries as a go-to remedy if you're prone to recurrent UTIs. Their ability to prevent bacterial attachment to the bladder lining helps reduce the frequency of infections without contributing to antibiotic resistance.

Beyond UTI prevention, you can use cranberries to support overall bladder and kidney health by reducing inflammation and oxidative stress. Their mild diuretic properties encourage hydration and natural detoxification, helping to flush out irritants and maintain urinary comfort. Cranberries also provide cardiovascular benefits, as their high antioxidant content supports healthy blood vessels and circulation.

Cranberry can be consumed as an extract or supplement, or you can simply drink fresh cranberry juice. You can also pair cranberries with other urinary-supportive herbs such as corn silk and dandelion for a comprehensive approach to bladder health.

Interactions and Safety

Cranberries are generally safe when consumed in moderate amounts, whether as juice, whole fruit, or extract. However, due to their natural acidity, excessive consumption may cause mild stomach upset or acid reflux in sensitive individuals.

If you're taking blood-thinning medications, such as warfarin, consult a healthcare provider before consuming large amounts of cranberry products as this may enhance the effects. If you're prone to kidney stones, exercise caution because cranberries contain oxalates, which may contribute to stone formation in susceptible individuals.

When choosing cranberry juice, it's important to opt for pure, unsweetened varieties, as many commercial cranberry drinks contain added sugars that diminish their health benefits.

Growing and Harvesting

Cranberries thrive in cool, acidic wetlands and are primarily cultivated in North America, particularly in regions like Wisconsin, Massachusetts, and Canada. The plants grow low to the ground, forming dense vines that spread across sandy or peat-rich soils.

Harvesting typically takes place in the fall when the berries turn a deep red color, indicating peak ripeness. Two primary harvesting methods are used: dry harvesting, where berries are collected directly from vines, and wet harvesting, which involves flooding cranberry bogs and using specialized machinery to gather floating berries.

Once harvested, cranberries can be stored fresh, dried, or processed into juice and extracts. Proper storage in a cool, dry place helps preserve their potency and nutritional benefits for long-term use.

Fun Fact

Cranberries can bounce when they're fresh—and that's not just fun trivia, it was once a quality control test. Early cranberry farmers used wooden "bounce boards" to sort ripe berries from spoiled ones. Because of their internal air pockets and firm structure, the best berries literally bounced, while bruised or overripe ones stayed put. That natural buoyancy also explains why cranberries float during harvest, making water harvesting possible. Nature's little red balloons, engineered for flotation and fermentation.

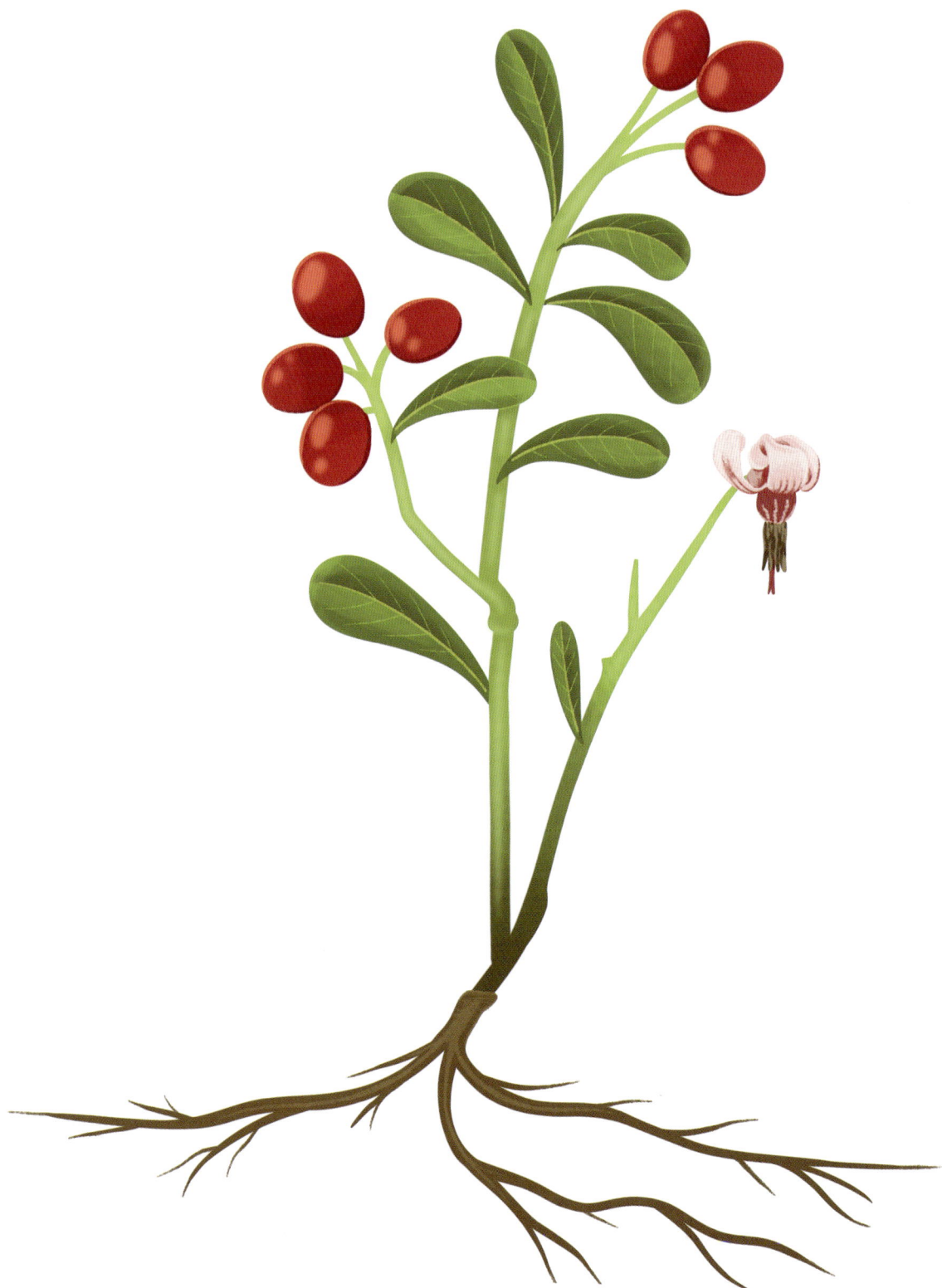

Fresh Cranberry Juice for Urinary Health

This tart and refreshing juice provides natural support for urinary tract health by preventing bacterial adhesion and promoting hydration.

Yield: 2 cups (480 ml)

1 cup (150 g) fresh cranberries

2 cups (480 ml) water

Juice of half a lemon
(for added cleansing support)

1 to 2 teaspoons (5 to 10 ml)
honey or maple syrup (optional,
for natural sweetness)

Preparation

Add the cranberries, water, and lemon juice to a blender. Blend on high speed until the cranberries are fully broken down and the mixture is smooth. If desired, add honey or maple syrup and blend again to incorporate. Strain the juice through a fine-mesh strainer or cheesecloth into a pitcher, pressing the pulp to extract as much liquid as possible.

How to Use

Drink ½ to 1 cup (120 to 240 ml) daily as part of a urinary health routine. Serve immediately over ice or store in the refrigerator for up to 3 days. For best results, use fresh or unsweetened cranberry juice to maximize its UTI-preventive properties.

Fun Fact

Cranberries are one of the few commercially grown fruits native to North America. Early European settlers referred to them as "craneberries" due to the flower's resemblance to the head and beak of a sandhill crane.

Chapter 11

Gut Check:
Herbs for the Digestive System

Welcome to the core of your vitality: the digestive and metabolic systems! Think of your digestive system as a dynamic food-processing plant, breaking down every bite into the nutrients that fuel and rebuild your body, while your metabolic system transforms those nutrients into energy. Together, they drive your body's wellness, influencing immunity, mood, energy, and clarity.

The digestive system is more than a conveyor belt—it's a "second brain," filled with enzymes, beneficial microbes, and immune cells working in harmony to break down food, produce vitamins, and protect against threats. When digestion falters due to stress or poor diet, the result can be discomfort, nutrient deficiencies, and a weakened immune response.

Your metabolic system operates like a well-tuned engine. Cellular workers transform carbohydrates, fats, and proteins into adenosine triphosphate (ATP), the energy currency that powers every thought and movement. Hormones like insulin and molecules such as AMPK (adenosine monophosphate–activated protein kinase), a key energy-sensing enzyme, help regulate this process by balancing energy production and usage throughout the body. However, stress, oxidative damage, and sedentary habits can disrupt this delicate balance, leaving you fatigued and out of sync.

Herbs offer valuable support to these vital systems. Ginger and fennel ease digestion and reduce discomfort, while gymnema helps regulate blood sugar and curb sugar cravings, supporting metabolic balance. *Coleus forskohlii*, a traditional Ayurvedic herb, stimulates cellular energy production and supports thyroid function, making it a useful ally for enhancing metabolism and vitality.

This chapter includes energizing, metabolism-supportive recipes like Fermented Ginger Honey for Nausea and Digestion, Fennel Digestive Oxymel, and Gymnema-Infused Elixir for Sugar Cravings—each crafted to gently awaken your body's natural energy rhythms. Let's dive in and nurture the systems that ensure robust immunity, a positive mood, sustained energy, optimal brain function, and overall health and well-being.

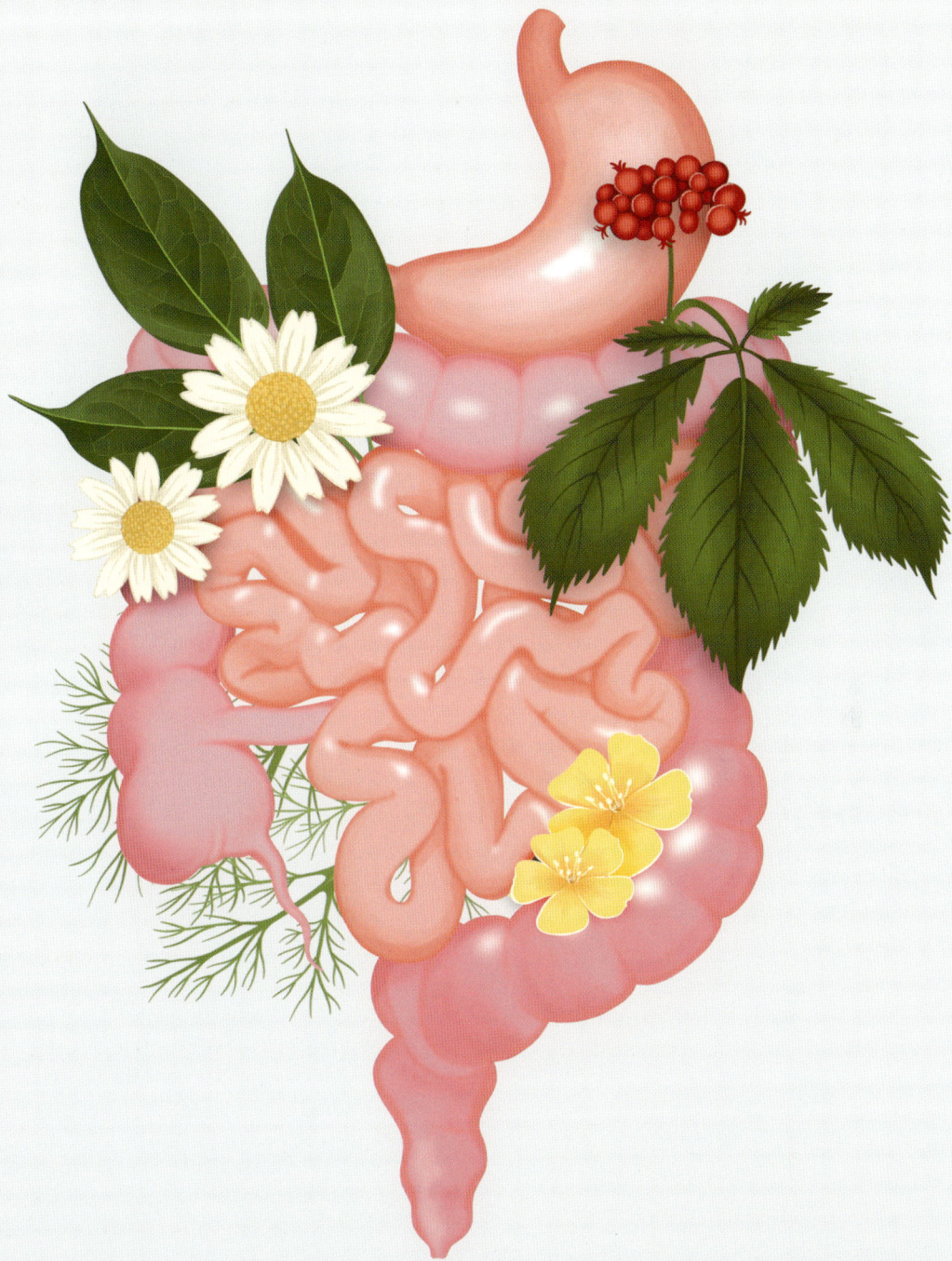

Coleus (*Coleus forskohlii*)
The Metabolic Booster

Coleus, a vibrant member of the mint family, has been used for centuries in Ayurvedic medicine, to promote digestive health, cardiovascular and respiratory function, metabolic balance, and overall vitality. In Sanskrit, it was referred to as *Makandi* or *Pashanabhedi*, meaning "stone breaker," suggesting its use in supporting kidney health and breaking down urinary stones. Beyond Ayurveda, traditional healers in Southeast Asia and Africa also used the plant for skin conditions, inflammation, and digestive disorders.

Even though coleus had been a staple in traditional medicine for centuries, it wasn't until the twentieth century that researchers began to uncover its unique metabolic properties, leading to increased interest in coleus as a natural metabolic booster and fat-burning aid. Today it is widely studied for its potential to support weight management, cardiovascular health, and athletic performance, making it a popular supplement in modern herbal and sports nutrition.

What the Science Says
The root of coleus (*Coleus forskohlii*) contains a rich medicinal compound known as forskolin, a powerful **diterpene**—a type of plant-based compound made of two terpene units, often involved in hormone signaling and metabolic processes. Unlike stimulants that artificially accelerate metabolism, forskolin works by increasing the production of cyclic adenosine monophosphate (cAMP), a messenger molecule that plays a critical role in fat breakdown, energy regulation, and cellular communication.

Here's how it works: Forskolin activates cAMP, which promotes the release of stored fat from fat cells, making it easier for the body to burn fat for energy. A study published in *Obesity Research* (2005) found that forskolin supplementation helped reduce body fat percentage and increase lean muscle mass in overweight men without altering total body weight. This suggests that coleus may help improve body composition—meaning it supports a healthier ratio of muscle to fat—rather than acting simply as a weight-loss agent.

Beyond fat metabolism, forskolin has shown promise in cardiovascular health by promoting vasodilation (widening of blood vessels), which can help regulate blood pressure and improve circulation. A study in the *Journal of the International Society of Sports Nutrition* (2005) demonstrated that forskolin enhances heart function and oxygen delivery while reducing arterial resistance. These findings show this herb's potential role in supporting cardiovascular resilience and maintaining optimal heart function.

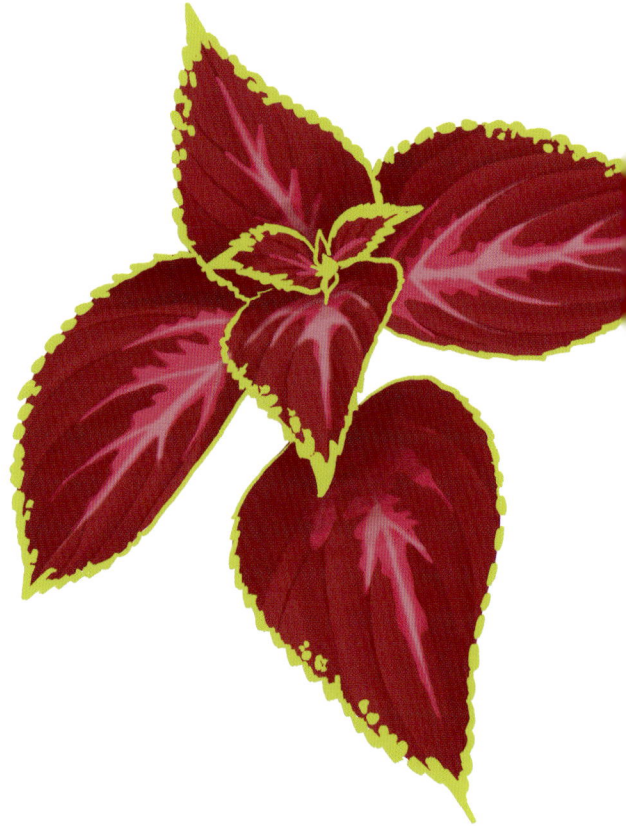

Researchers have also explored coleus's role in thyroid function. A study in *Die Pharmazie–An International Journal of Pharmaceutical Sciences* (2012) suggested that forskolin may help regulate thyroid hormones, potentially benefiting individuals with sluggish metabolism due to hypothyroidism.

Coleus is a multifunctional herb that enhances fat metabolism, cardiovascular function, and energy production, supporting overall metabolic health and vitality.

Coleus Metabolic Extract

This stimulating extract supports metabolic health by encouraging fat breakdown and promoting cellular energy. Traditionally used in Ayurvedic medicine, coleus offers gentle support without overstimulating the nervous system.

> *Yield: 1 cup (240 ml)*

¼ cup (11 g) dried *Coleus forskohlii* root (chopped or powdered)

½ cup (120 ml) vodka (at least 40% alcohol, organic if possible)

½ cup (120 ml) distilled water

Preparation

In a clean glass jar, combine the dried coleus root, vodka, and distilled water. Seal the jar tightly and shake well to mix the ingredients. Store the jar in a cool, dark place for 4 to 6 weeks, shaking it gently every few days to enhance the extraction process. After the infusion period, strain the liquid through a fine-mesh strainer or cheesecloth into a clean dropper bottle, discarding the root material. Label and store in a dark place for up to a year.

How to Use

Take 15 to 30 drops (about ½ to 1 dropperful total) once or twice daily in a small amount of water or herbal tea to support metabolism and energy levels. For best results, use consistently as part of a balanced lifestyle that includes proper nutrition and physical activity.

Uses and Indications

Use coleus to enhance metabolic function, support fat breakdown, and promote cardiovascular health. It may be particularly beneficial if you want to improve body composition, boost energy levels, and optimize cellular function. Its ability to stimulate cAMP production also makes it a valuable herb for supporting thyroid function, athletic endurance, and overall vitality.

Interactions and Safety

Coleus is generally well-tolerated, but if you're taking blood pressure medication or an anticoagulant, use caution because this herb can enhance blood vessel dilation and circulation. If you have low blood pressure or a heart condition, consult a healthcare provider before use. Some people may experience mild digestive discomfort or increased stomach acidity when taking coleus in high doses.

Growing and Harvesting

Coleus forskohlii is a tropical perennial that thrives in warm, humid climates with well-drained soil and ample sunlight. It is primarily cultivated in India, Thailand, and Sri Lanka, where it grows in rocky hillsides and subtropical forests. The plant produces thick, fleshy roots, which are the most medicinally valuable part.

The roots are typically harvested in late summer or early fall after the plant reaches full maturity. Once harvested, they are washed, sliced, and dried for use in herbal extracts, powders, and tinctures. Proper drying is essential to preserve the potency of forskolin and ensure maximum bioavailability.

Ginger (*Zingiber officinale*)
Nature's Digestive Aid

Ginger has long been a cornerstone of traditional medicine thanks to its natural ability to support digestion and ease nausea. Its documented use dates back over five thousand years to ancient China and India, where it was prescribed for digestive ailments, respiratory conditions, and overall vitality. In Ayurveda, ginger was revered as a "universal medicine," often used to kindle digestive fire, or *agni*, improving food assimilation and metabolism.

The spice made its way to the Mediterranean through trade routes, becoming a prized remedy in ancient Greek and Roman medicine. Dioscorides, a renowned Greek physician, recorded its use for stomach discomfort and motion sickness. Later, medieval European healers would use ginger in tonics for similar maladies.

Today ginger remains one of the most widely used natural digestive aids worldwide. It is commonly taken as a tea, tincture, or supplement to relieve nausea, bloating, and indigestion. Whether used fresh, dried, or fermented, ginger's warming and carminative properties continue to make it a staple in herbal medicine.

What the Science Says

The medicinal power of ginger (*Zingiber officinale*) lies in its rhizome—the thick, underground stem of the plant that stores nutrients and produces new shoots. This part of the plant contains potent bioactive compounds that support digestive function. The most notable of these are gingerols and shogaols—compounds responsible for ginger's distinctive pungency and its ability to stimulate digestion, reduce nausea, and combat inflammation. Research published in *Phytotherapy Research* (2018) found that gingerols enhance gastric motility by stimulating peristalsis, the wave-like contractions that move food through the digestive tract. This action helps prevent bloating, indigestion, and sluggish digestion.

Ginger is also a natural remedy for nausea. A clinical study in the *American Journal of Obstetrics and Gynecology* (2020) confirmed that ginger effectively reduces nausea and vomiting in pregnancy, making it a safe and effective remedy for morning sickness. An earlier study in *Critical Reviews in Food Science and Nutrition* (2013) demonstrated ginger's ability to prevent motion sickness by inhibiting the neurotransmitter signals that trigger nausea.

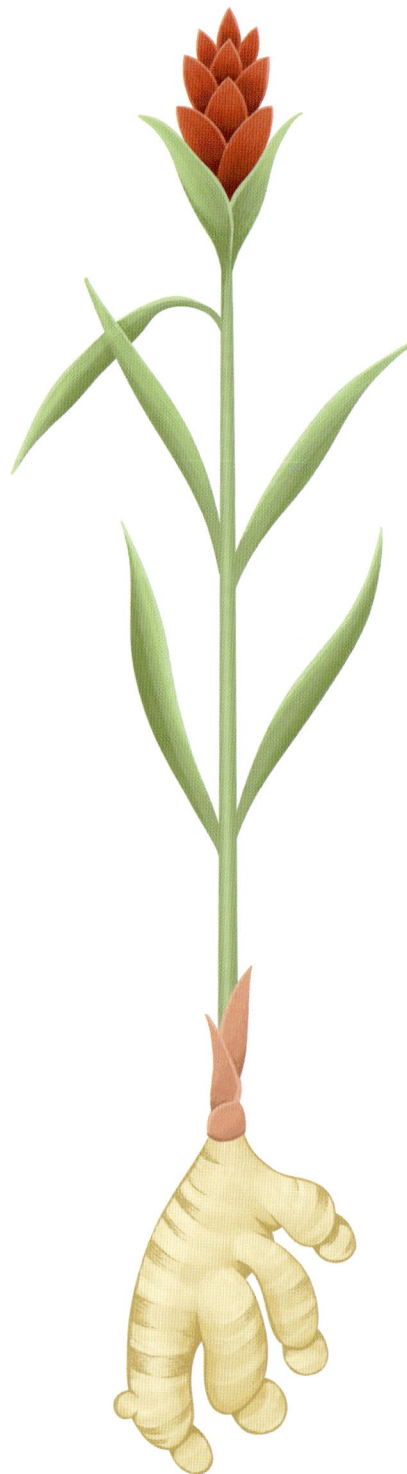

Additionally, ginger exhibits anti-inflammatory properties that protect the stomach lining and reduce irritation caused by acid reflux or gastritis. Its ability to regulate inflammatory pathways has made it a valuable remedy for conditions like irritable bowel syndrome (IBS) and functional dyspepsia.

Ginger has also been studied for its role in supporting immune function and reducing oxidative stress. The presence of antioxidants helps neutralize free radicals, preventing cellular damage and promoting overall well-being. With its wide-ranging benefits, ginger remains a cornerstone herb for digestive health, immune support, and everyday resilience.

Uses and Indications

Ginger is best known for its ability to ease nausea, whether caused by motion sickness, pregnancy, chemotherapy, or digestive upset. You can also use it to improve appetite, stimulate digestive enzymes, and rev up sluggish digestion after a heavy meal. In addition, ginger is a carminative herb, which means that it helps expel gas from the digestive tract, making it useful if you struggle with bloating or discomfort.

If you're prone to acid reflux or mild gastritis, ginger's anti-inflammatory compounds help calm irritation while promoting proper digestion. Regular consumption may also support gut health by enhancing microbial balance in the digestive tract.

Interactions and Safety

Ginger is generally safe when consumed in moderate amounts. However, if you're taking blood-thinning medications, use caution as ginger may enhance anticoagulant effects. If you have gallbladder issues or a history of ulcers, consult with a health-care provider before using ginger in large amounts because its stimulating effects can increase bile production.

If you have a sensitive stomach, you may experience mild heartburn or stomach upset from high doses of ginger. If this occurs, smaller amounts or pairing ginger with food can help mitigate any discomfort. If you're pregnant, limit ginger intake to no more than 1 gram per day to ensure safety while still benefiting from its anti-nausea effects.

Growing and Harvesting

Ginger (*Zingiber officinale*) thrives in warm, tropical climates with well-drained, loamy soil. It is a perennial plant that grows from rhizomes rather than seeds, making propagation simple. This is because cultivated ginger rarely produces viable seeds—so the plant naturally relies on its rhizomes (underground stems) to spread and regenerate. Each segment of rhizome contains growing points, or "eyes," that develop into new shoots.

In home gardens, ginger is best planted in early spring, allowing it to establish before the growing season. The rhizomes take about eight to ten months to mature and can be harvested once the leaves begin to yellow and die back—signaling that the plant has stored enough energy belowground for future growth.

To harvest, gently dig up the rhizomes, wash them thoroughly, and allow them to dry before storage. Fresh ginger can be stored in the refrigerator or dried for long-term use in teas, powders, and herbal preparations.

For optimal potency, ginger should be harvested before the rhizomes become too fibrous. Young ginger has a milder, more delicate flavor, making it ideal for culinary and medicinal use.

Fermented Ginger Honey for Nausea and Digestion

> *Yield: About 1 cup (240 ml)*

½ cup (50 g) thinly sliced fresh ginger root

1 lemon, thinly sliced

1 cup (240 ml) raw local honey

This delicious honey infusion combines the soothing properties of ginger with the probiotic benefits of fermentation, which encourages a healthy gut microbiome, making this a potent remedy for digestive health and nausea relief. Note: *This syrup is not recommended for children under one year old, as infants should not consume honey.*

Preparation

In a clean glass jar, layer the sliced ginger and lemon. Pour the raw honey over the ingredients, ensuring they are fully submerged. Seal the jar loosely with a lid to allow fermentation gases to escape. Let the mixture sit at room temperature for 3 days, opening the jar daily to release any built-up gas and gently stirring to mix the ingredients.

After 3 days, store in the refrigerator to slow the fermentation process. The honey will take on a rich, syrupy consistency infused with the warming, digestive-supportive properties of ginger.

How to Use

Take 1 teaspoon (5 ml) as needed for nausea relief, digestive support, or sore throats.

Stir into warm chamomile, peppermint, or lemon balm tea for added soothing effects, drizzle over fruit, or mix with warm water for a soothing elixir.

Fun Fact

Ginger was so highly valued in the Middle Ages that a single pound (455 g) of ginger could cost as much as an entire sheep!

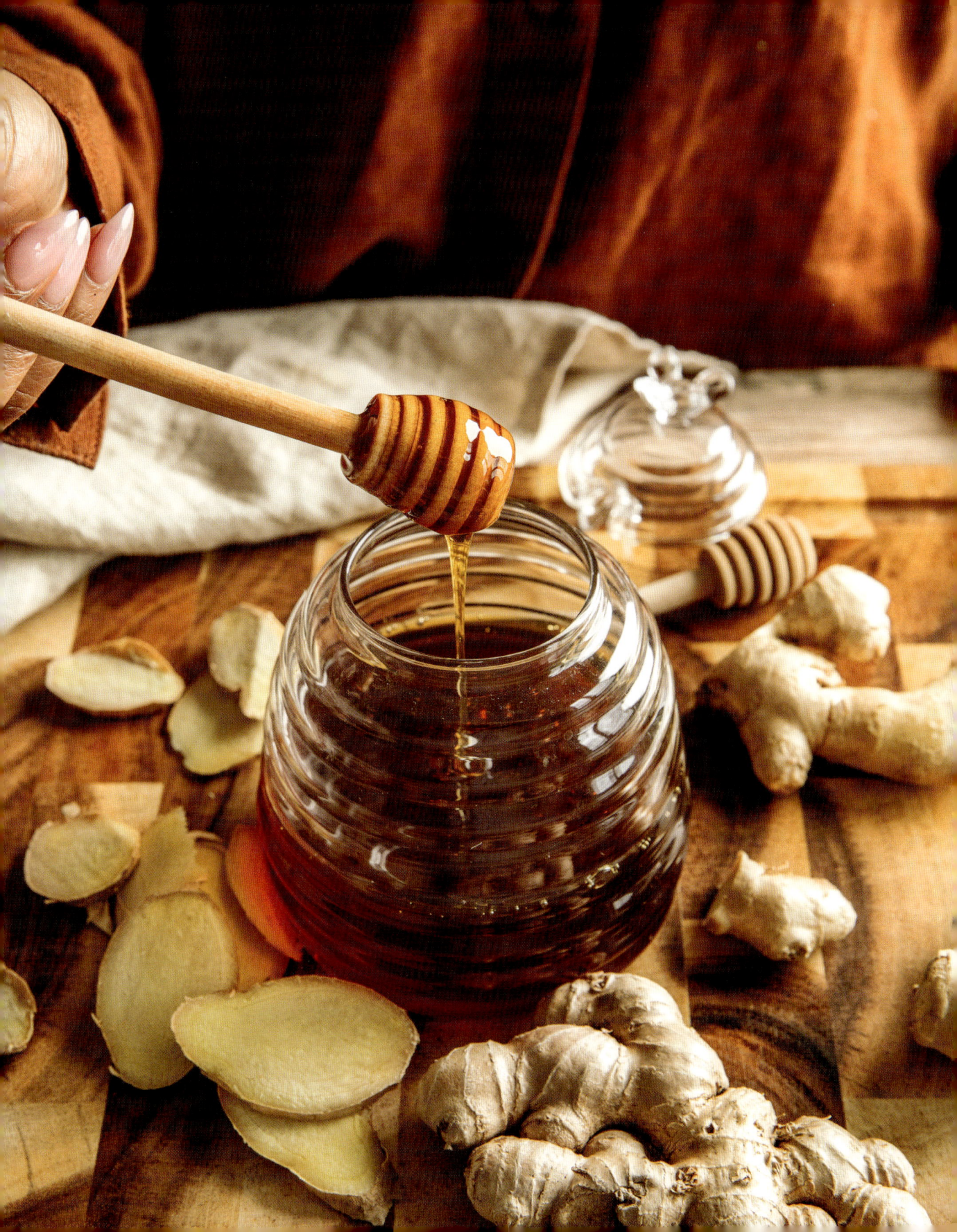

Fennel (*Foeniculum vulgare*)
The Gut Soother

Fennel has been revered for centuries as both a culinary spice and a medicinal herb, valued for its ability to promote digestion and ease gastrointestinal discomfort. Originating in the Mediterranean, fennel was widely used by ancient Egyptians, Greeks, and Romans for its carminative properties—meaning its ability to reduce bloating and gas. Roman soldiers chewed fennel seeds to aid digestion and maintain strength, while Ayurvedic and Traditional Chinese Medicine (TCM) practitioners incorporated fennel into formulas for soothing digestive distress.

During the Middle Ages, fennel was a staple in European households, often placed on dining tables for guests to chew after meals to prevent indigestion. In Indian culture, it remains a common practice to chew fennel seeds after meals for fresh breath and digestive ease. Today fennel continues to be a trusted remedy for bloating, cramping, and sluggish digestion, enjoyed in teas, tinctures, and more.

What the Science Says
The medicinal power of fennel (*Foeniculum vulgare*) lies in its seeds, which are rich in bioactive compounds that support digestive function. The most notable of these is anethole, an aromatic compound that relaxes the smooth muscles of the gastrointestinal tract, helping to ease bloating, cramping, and gas. Anethole also has mild antispasmodic properties, making fennel useful for relieving intestinal discomfort associated with irritable bowel syndrome (IBS) and colic.

A study published in the *Jundishapur Journal of Natural Pharmaceutical Products* (2024) found that fennel extract significantly reduced bloating and cramping in individuals with functional dyspepsia, a condition marked by persistent indigestion. A later study in *Phytotherapy Research* (2024) demonstrated fennel's ability to alleviate colic in infants, showing a reduction in crying episodes compared to a placebo.

Fennel also contains **phytoestrogens**, plant-based compounds that mimic estrogen's effects in the body. These compounds help balance hormonal fluctuations that can contribute to digestive discomfort, especially in individuals with menstrual-related bloating. Research in the *Journal of Complementary and Integrative Medicine* (2021) found that fennel's phytoestrogenic properties contributed to reduced bloating and improved digestion in individuals experiencing hormonal digestive disruptions.

Additionally, fennel supports overall gut health by stimulating the production of digestive enzymes, which enhance the breakdown of food and improve nutrient absorption. This helps prevent sluggish digestion and promotes a more comfortable post-meal experience. With its long-standing reputation as a gentle yet effective digestive aid, fennel remains a go-to herb for easing discomfort and supporting everyday gut balance.

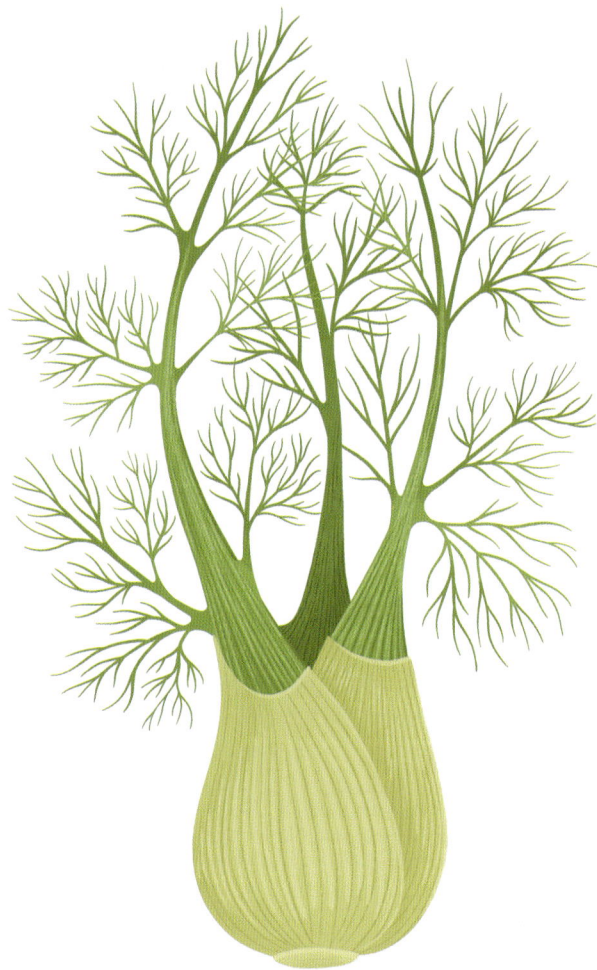

Uses and Indications
You can use fennel (*Foeniculum vulgare*) to alleviate bloating, indigestion, or gas. It works by relaxing the digestive tract muscles and encouraging the smooth passage of food, making it useful if you experience discomfort after meals.

Beyond digestion, fennel can also support hormonal balance thanks to its phytoestrogens. Many people find it helpful for easing menstrual-related bloating and digestive discomfort. It is also commonly used in herbal preparations for soothing colic in infants and relieving mild stomach discomfort in children.

Gymnema-Infused Elixir for Sugar Cravings

This infused elixir combines the sugar-craving-blocking power of gymnema with cinnamon, fenugreek, and ginger—herbs known for their ability to support blood sugar balance and digestion.

> *Yield: About 1 quart (1 L)*

2 tablespoons (4 g) dried gymnema leaves

1 tablespoon (15 g) dried cinnamon chips

½ tablespoon (5.6 g) dried fenugreek seeds

1 teaspoon (3 g) dried orange peel

1-inch (2.5 cm) piece fresh ginger, sliced

2 cups (480 ml) water, at room temperature

2 cups (480 ml) raw apple cider vinegar

Raw honey or maple syrup to sweeten (optional)

Preparation

In a clean, quart-size (1 L) glass jar, combine the dried gymnema leaves, cinnamon chips, fenugreek seeds, orange peel, and ginger. Pour the water and apple cider vinegar over the herbs, ensuring they are fully submerged. Seal the jar tightly and shake well. Let the mixture infuse at room temperature for 1 to 2 weeks, shaking the jar every day to distribute the herbal properties evenly. After the infusion period, strain the liquid through cheesecloth or a fine-mesh strainer into a clean bottle, discarding the herbs. If desired, sweeten with a small amount of raw honey or maple syrup to balance the tartness of the vinegar. Store the elixir in the refrigerator in a sealed glass bottle. When properly stored, it will keep for up to 3 months. Shake well before each use.

How to Use

Take 1 to 2 tablespoons (15 to 30 ml) of elixir before meals to help reduce sugar cravings and support balanced blood sugar levels. It can be consumed as is or diluted in a small amount of water or herbal tea.

For best results, incorporate this elixir into a consistent routine, particularly if managing sugar cravings or blood sugar fluctuations. When used alongside a balanced diet and lifestyle, gymnema can help naturally curb your desire for sweets while supporting overall metabolic health.

Peppermint (*Mentha × piperita*)
The Cooling Comforter

Peppermint has been revered for centuries as a medicinal and culinary herb, with its cooling, soothing properties making it a staple in both traditional and modern healing practices. Thought to be a natural hybrid between watermint (*Mentha aquatica*) and spearmint (*Mentha spicata*), peppermint has a long and rich history spanning multiple cultures.

Ancient Egyptian texts dating back to 1000 BCE reference peppermint as a digestive aid, while Greeks and Romans used it to relieve headaches, respiratory ailments, and bad breath. In Traditional Chinese Medicine (TCM), peppermint was used to release heat from the body, soothe sore throats, and aid digestion. In Ayurveda, it was known for its cooling energy, often combined with warming herbs such as ginger to balance digestive fire and promote gut health.

By the Middle Ages, European monks cultivated peppermint in monastery gardens, using it to treat nausea, colds, and headaches. It was a common remedy in English folk medicine, often brewed as tea or distilled into peppermint oil for stomach ailments and muscle pain.

By the nineteenth century, peppermint was commonly used by physicians to ease colic, indigestion, and bloating. Today peppermint remains one of the most widely used herbal remedies, incorporated into teas, essential oils, and digestive aids worldwide.

What the Science Says

The medicinal properties of peppermint (*Mentha × piperita*) are largely concentrated in its leaves, which are rich in menthol, rosmarinic acid, and **flavonoids**. Menthol is responsible for peppermint's signature cooling sensation and plays a crucial role in its anti-inflammatory and antispasmodic effects. Research has shown that menthol helps relax the smooth muscles of the digestive tract, reducing spasms that contribute to bloating, cramping, and discomfort. This makes peppermint an effective natural remedy for irritable bowel syndrome (IBS) and other digestive disorders. In addition, peppermint stimulates bile flow, enhancing the breakdown of fats and improving overall digestion.

Peppermint has antimicrobial, expectorant, and anti-inflammatory properties. The first two stem from its essential oil constituents—particularly menthol, menthone, and 1,8-cineole—which help inhibit the growth of bacteria and thin mucus to ease respiratory congestion and soothe irritated airways. Its antioxidant properties are primarily due to rosmarinic acid, flavonoids like eriocitrin and luteolin, and other **phenolic compounds**, which help neutralize free radicals and reduce inflammation in the gastrointestinal tract, further promoting gut health. Studies in *Complementary Therapies in Medicine* (2021) highlight peppermint's ability to reduce nausea, particularly in postoperative patients and those undergoing chemotherapy.

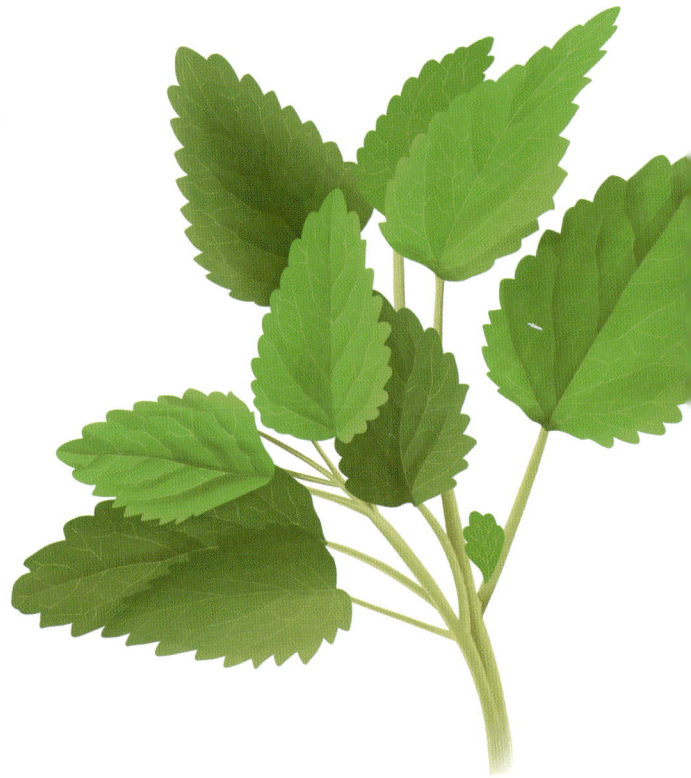

Beyond its role in digestive health, peppermint has been studied for its ability to relieve headaches. A study published in *Evidence-Based Practice* (2023) found that topical application of peppermint oil helped reduce tension headaches by improving blood circulation and relaxing muscles. With its multifaceted benefits, peppermint continues to be a cornerstone of herbal medicine for digestive wellness.

Uses and Indications

Peppermint is a versatile herb widely used to relieve digestive discomfort, including bloating, cramping, and nausea. It's especially effective if you have IBS or sluggish digestion because it helps relax gastrointestinal muscles and promote smoother digestion. Peppermint is also valued for its headache-relieving properties. The menthol it contains provides a cooling effect that helps alleviate tension headaches and migraines. Peppermint's decongestant and expectorant actions also support respiratory health, making it a go-to remedy for colds and sinus congestion.

Fermented Peppermint Honey for Digestive Comfort

> *Yield: About 1 cup (240 ml)*

This simple fermented honey infusion captures peppermint's soothing digestive properties while enhancing its benefits with natural probiotics from raw honey. Note: *This syrup is not recommended for children under one year old, as infants should not consume honey.*

1 cup (25.6 g) fresh peppermint leaves, lightly bruised

1 cup (240 ml) raw honey (preferably local and unpasteurized)

Preparation

Place the fresh peppermint leaves into a clean glass jar. Pour the raw honey over the leaves, ensuring they are fully submerged. Stir gently to release air bubbles and coat the leaves evenly. Cover the jar loosely with a lid to allow gases to escape, and let it ferment at room temperature for 3 to 5 days. Open the jar daily to release any gas buildup, stirring gently to mix. After fermentation is complete, store the peppermint honey in the refrigerator with a tightly sealed lid for up to 3 months, though flavor and potency are best within the first 4 to 6 weeks.

How to Use

Take 1 teaspoon (5 ml) directly as a digestive aid or mix it into warm water or tea. This fermented peppermint honey can also be drizzled over fresh fruit, added to smoothies, or used as a natural sweetener in herbal remedies. Always use a clean, dry spoon to avoid introducing moisture.

Interactions and Safety

Peppermint is generally safe when used in moderate amounts. However, if you have severe acid reflux or gastroesophageal reflux disease (GERD), avoid peppermint because it may relax the lower esophageal sphincter and make symptoms worse. If you have gallbladder disease or bile duct obstruction, consult a healthcare provider before using peppermint due to its bile-stimulating effects. While peppermint is safe for children in small amounts, concentrated peppermint oil should not be used on infants or young children due to potential respiratory risks.

Growing and Harvesting

Peppermint is an easy-to-grow perennial herb that thrives in moist, well-drained soil and partial to full sunlight. It spreads rapidly, so planting it in containers can prevent it from overtaking the garden.

Peppermint leaves are most potent just before flowering, usually in late spring to early summer. Harvest leaves in the morning when their essential oil content is highest. You can use fresh peppermint immediately, or store dried leaves in an airtight container away from direct sunlight to maintain their potency.

> ### *Fun Fact*
>
> In ancient Rome, peppermint was so highly regarded for its refreshing and invigorating properties that scholars and philosophers wore peppermint wreaths on their heads to enhance concentration and mental clarity.

Ginseng *(Panax* spp.)
The Vitality Booster

Ginseng has been revered for thousands of years as one of the most powerful adaptogenic herbs, prized for its ability to enhance energy, stamina, and overall vitality. Indigenous to East Asia and North America, ginseng has been a cornerstone of Traditional Chinese Medicine (TCM), Korean herbalism, and Indigenous American healing traditions. The name *panax*, derived from the Greek word for "all-healing," reflects its broad therapeutic applications.

In TCM, ginseng was classified as a supreme tonic, believed to restore *qi* (vital energy) and strengthen the body's resilience against stress, fatigue, and disease. It was also used to enhance cognitive function, support longevity, and improve sexual vitality.

North American ginseng (*Panax quinquefolius*) was used by Indigenous tribes such as the Iroquois and Cherokee for its medicinal properties, particularly in treating fatigue, respiratory conditions, and digestive issues. When European settlers discovered its value, American ginseng became a major export to China during the eighteenth and nineteenth centuries, creating a thriving trade that persists today.

Modern herbal medicine recognizes several varieties of ginseng, including Asian ginseng (*Panax ginseng*), American ginseng (*Panax quinquefolius*), and Siberian ginseng (*Eleutherococcus senticosus*), which, though not a true ginseng, is often grouped with these varieties due to its similar adaptogenic benefits. Ginseng remains one of the most studied and widely used herbs in the world, valued for its ability to enhance physical and mental endurance, support immune function, and promote overall well-being.

What the Science Says

The root of ginseng (*Panax* spp.) is rich in bioactive compounds called ginsenosides, which contribute to its adaptogenic, anti-fatigue, and cognitive-enhancing effects. These compounds influence multiple physiological pathways, making ginseng a well-rounded herbal ally for energy, stress management, and immune support.

Scientific research supports ginseng's role in improving energy levels and reducing fatigue. A 2013 study published in the *Journal of Clinical Oncology* found that cancer patients experiencing fatigue showed significant improvements in energy levels after supplementing with American ginseng for eight weeks. Another study in *Foods* (2021) demonstrated that Asian ginseng (*Panax ginseng*) supplementation enhanced endurance and reduced exercise-induced fatigue in athletes, likely due to its effects on mitochondrial energy production.

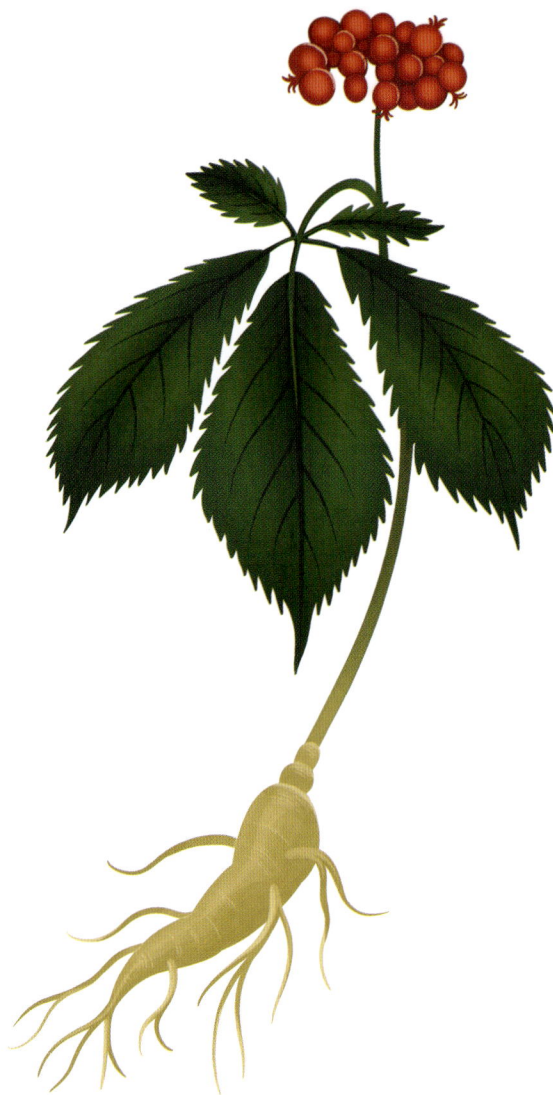

Research shows that ginseng also offers cognitive benefits. Scientists have found that ginsenosides help modulate neurotransmitter activity, increasing dopamine and serotonin levels, which can enhance focus and reduce mental fatigue. A 2005 study published in *Psychopharmacology* found that Panax ginseng improved mental performance, reaction time, and working memory in healthy adults.

Ginseng's adaptogenic properties make it a valuable herb when it comes to dealing with stress. A study in *PLOS One* in 2013 found that Panax ginseng helps regulate the hypothalamic-pituitary-adrenal (HPA) axis, reducing cortisol levels and mitigating the effects of chronic stress on adrenal function and overall hormonal balance. Additionally, ginseng's immune-boosting effects have been highlighted in research showing increased resistance to infections, including respiratory illnesses.

By supporting energy metabolism, cognitive function, and stress adaptation, ginseng remains one of the most comprehensive herbs for vitality and endurance.

Uses and Indications

Ginseng is widely used to promote energy, stamina, and resilience to stress. You can use it to reduce fatigue, increase endurance, and improve cognitive function, including memory, focus, and mental clarity. It also supports immune function and reduces susceptibility to infections.

Many turn to ginseng for its ability to enhance vitality and libido, especially as one ages. Whether used as a daily tonic or an occasional energy booster, ginseng is a trusted herb for maintaining strength and endurance.

Interactions and Safety

Ginseng is generally safe for most individuals, but some precautions should be noted. If you have high blood pressure or a heart condition, it's important to consult a healthcare provider before using ginseng because it may stimulate cardiovascular activity. Ginseng may interact with blood-thinning medications, such as warfarin, and should be used with caution if you're taking anticoagulants. If you have insomnia or are sensitive to stimulants, you may experience restlessness when taking high doses of ginseng, particularly in the evening. If you're pregnant or breastfeeding, consult a healthcare provider before using ginseng as its safety in these populations is not well-established.

Growing and Harvesting

Ginseng is a slow-growing perennial that thrives in shaded, forested environments with rich, well-draining soil. It requires several years to mature before the roots develop their full medicinal potency, typically taking five to seven years for cultivated ginseng and up to twenty years for wild varieties.

The best time to harvest ginseng roots is in the fall, after the plant has gone dormant. Harvesting is done carefully to preserve the integrity of the root, as mature roots fetch higher value in herbal medicine. After harvesting, the roots are washed, dried, and sometimes steamed to enhance their medicinal properties before being used in teas, extracts, and supplements.

Due to overharvesting, wild ginseng populations have declined significantly, leading to regulations in many regions to protect this valuable plant. Sustainable cultivation practices ensure the continued availability of ginseng for future generations.

Potent Ginseng Elixir for Energy

This energizing ginseng elixir combines the adaptogenic power of ginseng with warming spices and immune-supporting honey to create a revitalizing tonic.

Yield: About 1 cup (240 ml)

1 cup (240 ml) filtered water

1 tablespoon (11 g) dried ginseng root (sliced or powdered)

1 teaspoon (5 g) cinnamon chips (for warmth and blood circulation)

½ teaspoon (1 g) dried ginger root (for digestive support and added energy)

1 teaspoon (5 ml) raw honey or maple syrup (optional, for sweetness)

Preparation

In a small saucepan, bring the water to a boil. Add the dried ginseng, cinnamon chips, and ginger. Reduce the heat and let simmer for 20 to 30 minutes to extract the beneficial compounds. Strain the mixture into a cup and stir in the honey or maple syrup if desired.

How to Use

Drink 1 cup (240 ml) in the morning or early afternoon to enhance energy and focus. Consume before physical activity or demanding mental work for increased endurance. Use as part of a daily routine for sustained vitality and immune support. This warming elixir provides a natural, sustained energy boost without the jitteriness associated with caffeine.

Fun Fact

The world's most expensive ginseng roots can sell for thousands of dollars per pound.

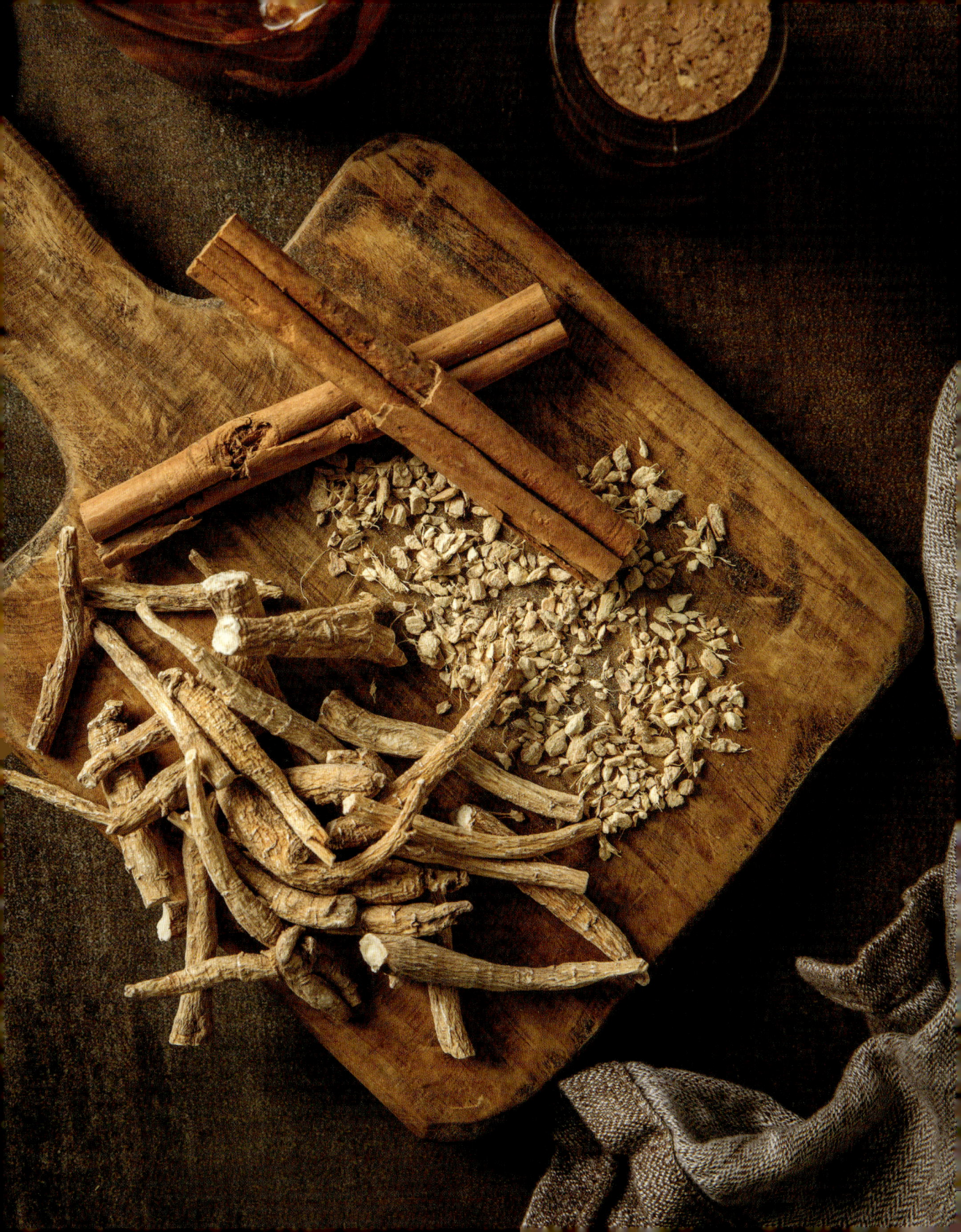

Glossary

Alkaloids: Nitrogen-rich compounds that can affect mood, pain perception, or blood pressure. Found in plants like motherwort, alkaloids often interact with the nervous or cardiovascular systems.

Alkamides: Natural compounds that help support the immune system and reduce inflammation. They work by interacting with parts of the body that regulate immunity.

Anthocyanins: Pigments that give dark fruits their deep color. They are rich in antioxidants and help protect cells from damage.

Anthraquinones: Laxative compounds found in herbs like senna and cascara. They work by stimulating the muscles of the colon and increasing fluid secretion to support elimination.

Caffeic Acid Derivatives: Natural compounds that support immune function and help reduce inflammation.

Carotenoids: Nutrients that give plants their bright colors and support overall health, including the immune system.

Coumarins: Aromatic plant chemicals that may thin blood, calm inflammation, or increase sensitivity to sunlight. Chasteberry contains small amounts that contribute to its hormonal effect.

Diterpene: A type of plant compound that supports immune health, eases inflammation, and protects brain function. Their effects vary widely depending on structure. Holy basil contains certain diterpenes believed to modulate stress responses.

Diterpene Lactones: The main active compounds in certain plants that contribute to their bitter taste and powerful immune-boosting effects.

Ferulic Acid: A strong antioxidant that protects cells from aging and environmental damage. Often found in plant cell walls, where it supports tissue strength and resilience.

Flavonoids: Natural antioxidants found in many plants that help reduce inflammation and support immune health.

Ganoderic Acids: Unique compounds from reishi mushrooms that support liver health, modulate the immune system, and help the body adapt to stress.

Hydrogen Sulfide (H_2S): A gas that helps relax blood vessels and improve circulation, which supports heart health.

Iridoid Glycosides: Bitter-tasting compounds that reduce inflammation and support stress recovery. They're part of what gives certain herbs their adaptogenic and calming effects.

Lignans: Plant compounds that help with hormone balance and have antioxidant properties.

Monoterpene: Tiny aromatic molecules that give herbs their scent and flavor. Many have antimicrobial, mood-lifting, or digestive benefits.

Organic Acids: Naturally acidic compounds that support digestion, help balance pH, and may aid in gentle detoxification. They can also improve mineral absorption.

Phenolic Acids: Compounds that help fight infections and reduce inflammation.

Phenolic Compound: Plant-based molecules known for their antioxidant activity. They help protect cells from damage and calm chronic inflammation.

Phytocompounds: A broad term for the active chemicals found in plants. This includes everything from calming terpenes to hormone-balancing saponins.

Phytoestrogens: Plant-based compounds that weakly mimic estrogen in the body. They can support hormonal balance without replacing natural hormones.

Polyacetylenes: Compounds with antimicrobial and anti-inflammatory properties. More active in fresh plants than dried, they help defend against infections.

The Practical Science of Herbs

Polyphenolic Compound: Another name for polyphenols—plant-based defenders that support graceful aging and protect the skin, brain, and heart.

Polyphenols: A group of antioxidants that help fight free radicals, protect the heart, and reduce inflammation. Known for their deep pigments and healing power.

Polysaccharides: Natural sugars found in plants that help boost the immune system.

Polysulfides: Sulfur-rich compounds that support detoxification and heart health. They also help fight microbes and regulate inflammation.

Saponins: Natural compounds that help the body absorb nutrients, support the immune system, and sometimes act as natural cleansers.

Sesquiterpene Lactones: Bitter compounds that can calm the immune system and reduce inflammation. Especially helpful for skin issues and allergy-prone systems.

Sesquiterpenes: Naturally occurring molecules with anti-inflammatory, antimicrobial, and calming properties. Often found in essential oils and plant resins.

Steroidal Lactones: Compounds that look and act like natural hormones in the body. They help regulate stress, energy, and reproductive function.

Steroidal Saponins: Foaming plant compounds that support hormone production and cholesterol balance. They also improve absorption of other nutrients.

Sulfur Compounds: Powerful compounds that help fight infections, support heart health, and reduce inflammation.

Tannins: Astringent compounds in plants that help tighten tissues and have antimicrobial properties.

Terpenes: Aromatic oils that give herbs their signature scent. Many support immune health, calm the nerves, or improve mood.

Terpenoids: Terpenes with slight modifications that make them more bioactive. Found in essential oils, they play a role in stress relief and immune modulation.

Triterpene Acids: Compounds that protect the liver, calm inflammation, and may support the skin. Often found in adaptogenic and liver-supporting herbs.

Triterpene Glycosides: Compounds that combine a sugar molecule with a triterpene. They often boost stamina, regulate hormones, and support adrenal health.

Triterpenoids: Complex plant compounds with broad benefits, including antioxidant, skin-healing, and immune-supportive effects.

Triterpenoid Saponins: A foaming, sugar-linked compound that supports the endocrine system and helps the body cope with physical or emotional stress.

Volatile Oils: Highly aromatic oils that evaporate easily and carry a plant's medicinal essence. Used for digestion, relaxation, and immune defense.

References

Chapter 1: Defense Squad: Herbs for Immune Support

- Shah, S. A., Sander, S., White, C. M., Rinaldi, M., and Coleman, C. I. "Evaluation of Echinacea for the Prevention and Treatment of the Common Cold: A Meta-Analysis." *The Lancet Infectious Diseases* 7, no. 7 (2007), 473–80. https://doi.org/10.1016/S1473-3099(07)70160-3.

- Shah, S. A., Goel, V., Lovlin, R., Barton, R., Lyon, M. R., Bauer, R., Lee, T. D. G., and Basu, T. K. "Efficacy of a Standardized Echinacea Preparation (Echinilin™) for the Treatment of the Common Cold: A Randomized, Double-Blind, Placebo-Controlled Trial." *Journal of Clinical Pharmacy and Therapeutics* 29, no. 1 (2004), 75–83.

- Zakay-Rones, Z., Thom, E., Wollan, T., and Wadstein, J. "Randomized Study of the Efficacy and Safety of Oral Elderberry Extract in the Treatment of Influenza A and B Virus Infections." *The Journal of International Medical Research* 32, no. 2 (2004), 132–40. https://doi.org/10.1177/147323000403200205.

- Tiralongo, E., Wee, S. S., and Lea, R. A. "Elderberry Supplementation Reduces Cold Duration and Symptoms in Air-Travellers: A Randomized, Double-Blind Placebo-Controlled Clinical Trial." *Nutrients* 8, no. 4 (2016), 182. https://doi.org/10.3390/nu8040182.

- Josling, P. "Preventing the Common Cold with a Garlic Supplement: A Double-Blind, Placebo-Controlled Survey." *Advances in Therapy* 18, no. 4 (2001), 189–93. https://doi.org/10.1007/BF02850113.

- Ried, K. "Garlic Lowers Blood Pressure in Hypertensive Subjects, Improves Arterial Stiffness and Gut Microbiota: A Review and Meta-Analysis." *Experimental and Therapeutic Medicine* 19, no. 2 (2020), 1472–78. https://doi.org/10.3892/etm.2019.8374.

- Adiguna, S. B. P., Panggabean, J. A., Atikana, A., Untari, F., Izzati, F., Bayu, A., ... and Putra, M. Y. "Antiviral Activities of Andrographolide and Its Derivatives: Mechanism of Action and Delivery System." *Pharmaceuticals* 14, no. 11 (2021), 1102.

- Li, X., Yuan, W., Wu, J., Zhen, J., Sun, Q., and Yu, M. "Andrographolide, a Natural Anti-Inflammatory Agent: An Update." *Frontiers in Pharmacology* 13 (2022), 920435.

- Cáceres, D. D., Hancke, J. L., Burgos, R. A., Sandberg, F., and Wikman, G. K. "Use of Visual Analogue Scale Measurements (VAS) to Assess the Effectiveness of Standardized Andrographis Paniculata Extract SHA-10 in Reducing the Symptoms of Common Cold: A Randomized Double-Blind Placebo-Controlled Study." *Phytomedicine: International Journal of Phytotherapy and Phytopharmacology* 6, no. 4 (1999), 217–23. https://doi.org/10.1016/S0944-7113(99)80012-9.

Chapter 2: Breathe Easy: Herbs for the Respiratory System

- Blanco-Salas, J., Hortigón-Vinagre, M. P., Morales-Jadán, D., and Ruiz-Téllez, T. "Searching for Scientific Explanations for the Uses of Spanish Folk Medicine: A Review on the Case of Mullein (Verbascum, Scrophulariaceae)." *Biology*, 10, no. 7 (2021), 618. https://doi.org/10.3390/biology10070618.

- Nadeem, A., Ahmed, B., Shahzad, H., Craker, L. E., and Muntean, T. "*Verbascum Thapsus* (Mullein) Versatile Polarity Extracts: GC-MS Analysis, Phytochemical Profiling, Anti-Bacterial Potential and Anti-Oxidant Activity." *Pharmacognosy Journal* 13, no. 6 (2021).

- Kemmerich, B., Eberhardt, R., and Stammer, H. "Efficacy and Tolerability of a Fluid Extract Combination of Thyme Herb and Ivy Leaves and Matched Placebo in Adults Suffering from Acute Bronchitis with Productive Cough: A Prospective, Double-Blind, Placebo-Controlled Clinical Trial." *Arzneimittel-Forschung* 56, no. 9 (2021), 652–660. https://doi.org/10.1055/s-0031-1296767.

- Sim, J. X. F., Khazandi, M., Chan, W. Y., Trott, D. J., and Deo, P. "Antimicrobial Activity of Thyme Oil, Oregano Oil, Thymol and Carvacrol Against Sensitive and Resistant Microbial Isolates from Dogs with Otitis Externa." *Veterinary Dermatology* 30, no. 6 (2019), 524-e159.

- Jasemi, S. V., Khazaei, H., Morovati, M. R., Joshi, T., Aneva, I. Y., Farzaei, M. H., and Echeverría, J. "Phytochemicals as Treatment for Allergic Asthma: Therapeutic Effects and Mechanisms of Action." *Phytomdicine* 122 (2024), 155149.

- Kenny, C. R., Stojakowska, A., Furey, A., and Lucey, B. "From Monographs to Chromatograms: The Antimicrobial Potential of *Inula helenium* L. (Elecampane) Naturalised in Ireland." *Molecules* 27, no. 4 (2022), 1406. https://doi.org/10.3390/molecules27041406.

- Zhou, Y., Guo, Y., Wen, Z., Ci, X., Xia, L., Wang, Y., Deng, X., and Wang, J. "Isoalantolactone Enhances the Antimicrobial Activity of Penicillin G Against *Staphylococcus aureus* by Inactivating β-lactamase During Protein Translation." *Pathogens* 9, no. 3 (2020), 161. https://doi.org/10.3390/pathogens9030161.

- Awwad, A., Poucheret, P., Idres, A. Y., Bidel, L., and Tousch, D. "The Bitter Asteraceae: An Interesting Approach to Delay the Metabolic Syndrome Progression." *NFS Journal* 18 (2020), 29–38.

Chapter 3: Take Heart: Herbs for the Cardiovascular System

- Wu, M., Liu, L., Xing, Y., Yang, S., Li, H., and Cao, Y. "Roles and Mechanisms of Hawthorn and Its Extracts on Atherosclerosis: A Review." *Frontiers in Pharmacology* 11 (2020), 118.

- Pittler, M. H., Schmidt, K., and Ernst, E. "Hawthorn Extract for Treating Chronic Heart Failure: Meta-Analysis of Randomized Trials." *The American Journal of Medicine* 114, no. 8 (2003), 665–74. https://doi.org/10.1016/s0002-9343(03)00131-1.

- Pittler, M. H., Guo, R., and Ernst, E. "Hawthorn Extract for Treating Chronic Heart Failure." *The Cochrane Database of Systematic Reviews* 1 (2008), CD005312-CD005312.

- Shikov, A. N., Pozharitskaya, O. N., Makarov, V. G., Demchenko, D. V., and Shikh, E. V. "Effect of Leonurus Cardiaca Oil Extract in Patients with Arterial Hypertension Accompanied by Anxiety and Sleep Disorders." *Phytotherapy Research* 25, no. 4 (2011), 540–43.

- Dwivedi, S., and Agarwal, M. P. "Antianginal and Cardioprotective Effects of Terminalia Arjuna, an Indigenous Drug, in Coronary Artery Disease." *The Journal of the Association of Physicians of India* 42, no. 4 (1994), 287–89.

- Kaur, N., Shafiq, N., Negi, H., Pandey, A., Reddy, S., Kaur, H., ... and Malhotra, S. "Terminalia Arjuna in Chronic Stable Angina: Systematic Review and Meta-Analysis." *Cardiology Research and Practice* 1 (2014), 281483.

- Mojarradgandoukmolla, S., Nanakali, N. M. Q., and Abjabbar, A. "Hypolipidemic and Anti-Oxidative Activities of Terminalia Arjuna Barks Against Induced Hyperlipidemic Albino Rats." *Plant Archives* 21, no. 1 (2021), 2082–86.

- Shiyong, Y., Yijia, X., Peng, Z., Chong, L., Wuming, H., Linchun, L., and Chunlai, Z. "Ginkgo Biloba Extract Inhibits Platelet Activation via Inhibition of Akt." *Integrative Medicine International* 1, no. 4 (2015), 234–42.

- Singh, S. K., Srivastav, S., Castellani, R. J., Plascencia-Villa, G., and Perry, G. "Neuroprotective and Antioxidant Effect of Ginkgo Biloba Extract Against AD and Other Neurological Disorders." *Neurotherapeutics: The Journal of the American Society for Experimental NeuroTherapeutics* 16, no. 3 (2019), 666–74.

Chapter 4: Radiant Shield: Herbs for Skin Health

- Zournatzis, I., Liakos, V., Papadopoulos, S., and Wogiatzi, E. "*Calendula Officinalis*: A Comprehensive Review." *Pharmacological Research—Natural Products* (2024), 100140.

- Ejiohuo, O., Folami, S., and Maigoro, A. Y. "Calendula in Modern Medicine: Advancements in Wound Healing and Drug Delivery Applications." *European Journal of Medicinal Chemistry Reports* (2024), 100199.

- Wu, X. X., Law, S. K., Ma, H., Jiang, Z., Li, Y. F., Au, D. C. T., Wong, C. K., and Luo, D. X. "Bio-Active Metabolites from Chinese Medicinal Herbs for Treatment of Skin Diseases." *Natural Product Research* (2024), 1–23.

- Zhang, T., Guo, Q., Xin, Y., and Liu, Y. "Comprehensive Review in Moisture Retention Mechanism of Polysaccharides from Algae, Plants, Bacteria and Fungus." *Arabian Journal of Chemistry* 15, no. 10 (2022), 104163.

- Mahboub, M., Attari, A. M. A., Sheikhalipour, Z., Attari, M. M. A., Davami, B., Amidfar, A., and Lotfi, M. "A Comparative Study of the Impacts of Aloe Vera Gel and Silver Sulfadiazine Cream 1% on Healing, Itching and Pain of Burn Wounds: A Randomized Clinical Trial." *Journal of Caring Sciences* 11, no. 3 (2021), 132.

- Proença, A. C., Luis, A., and Duarte, A. P. "The Role of Herbal Medicine in the Treatment of Acne Vulgaris: A Systematic Review of Clinical Trials." *Evidence-Based Complementary and Alternative Medicine* 1 (2022), 2011945.

- Aghmiuni, A. I., and Khiavi, A. A. "Medicinal Plants to Calm and Treat Psoriasis Disease." *Aromatic and Medicinal Plants—Back to Nature* (2017), 1–28.

- Abers, M., Schroeder, S., Goelz, L., Sulser, A., St. Rose, T., Puchalski, K., and Langland, J. "Antimicrobial Activity of the Volatile Substances from Essential Oils." *BMC Complementary Medicine and Therapies* 21, no. 1 (2021), 124. https://doi.org/10.1186/s12906-021-03285-3.

- Swamy, M. K., Akhtar, M. S., and Sinniah, U. R. "Antimicrobial Properties of Plant Essential Oils against Human Pathogens." *Evidence-Based Complementary and Alternative Medicine* (2016), 3012462. https://doi.org/10.1155/2016/3012462.

- Enshaieh, S., Jooya, A., Siadat, A. H., and Iraji, F. "The Efficacy of 5% Topical Tea Tree Oil Gel in Mild to Moderate Acne Vulgaris: A Randomized, Double-Blind Placebo-Controlled Study." *The Journal of Dermatology* 44, no. 4 (2017), 415–22. https://doi.org/10.1111/j.1346-8138.2017.00205.x.

- Ettakifi, H., Abbassi, K., Maouni, S., Erbiai, E. H., Rahmouni, A., Legssyer, M., ... and Maouni, A. "Chemical Characterization and Antifungal Activity of Blue Tansy (*Tanacetum annuum*) Essential Oil and Crude Extracts against *Fusarium oxysporum* f. sp. *albedinis*, an Agent Causing Bayoud Disease of Date Palm." *Antibiotics* 12, no. 9 (2023), 1451.

- Goyal, A., Sharma, A., Kaur, J., Kumari, S., Garg, M., Sindhu, R. K., ... and Abdel-Daim, M. M. "Bioactive-Based Cosmeceuticals: An Update on Emerging Trends." *Molecules* 27, no. 3 (2022), 828.

Chapter 5: Roots of Vitality: Herbs for the Reproductive System

- Kronenberg, F., and Fugh-Berman, A. "Complementary and Alternative Medicine for Menopausal Symptoms: A Review of Randomized, Controlled Trials." *Annals of Internal Medicine* 137, no. 10 (2002), 805–13.

- Mohammad-Alizadeh-Charandabi, S., Shahnazi, M., Nahaee, J., and Bayatipayan, S. "Efficacy of Black Cohosh (*Cimicifuga racemosa* L.) in Treating Early Symptoms of Menopause: A Randomized Clinical Trial." *Chinese Medicine* 8, no. 1 (2013), 20. https://doi.org/10.1186/1749-8546-8-20.

- Simpson, M., Parsons, M., Greenwood, J., and Wade, K. "Raspberry Leaf in Pregnancy: Its Safety and Efficacy in Labor." *Journal of Midwifery & Women's Health* 46, no. 2 (2001), 51–59.

- Brooks, N. A., Wilcox, G., Walker, K. Z., Ashton, J. F., Cox, M. B., and Stojanovska, L. "Beneficial Effects of *Lepidium meyenii* (Maca) on Psychological Symptoms and Measures of Sexual Dysfunction in Postmenopausal Women Are Not Related to Estrogen or Androgen Content." *Menopause* 15, no. 6 (2008), 1157–62. https://doi.org/10.1097/gme.0b013e3181732953.

- Sommariva, D., Kleemann, J., Loleit, A., Abels, C., and Stute, P. "Use of *Vitex Agnus-Castus* in Patients with Menstrual Cycle Disorders: A Single-Center Retrospective Longitudinal Cohort Study." *Archives of Gynecology and Obstetrics* 309, no. 5 (2024), 2089–98. https://doi.org/10.1007/s00404-023-07363-4.

- Kenda, M., Glavač, N. K., Nagy, M., Sollner Dolenc, M., and Oemonom. "Herbal Products Used in Menopause and for Gynecological Disorders." *Molecules* 26, no. 24 (2021), 7421. https://doi.org/10.3390/molecules26247421.

- Romm, A., Ganora, L., Hoffmann, D., Yarnell, E., Abascal, K., and Coven, M. *Fundamental Principles of Herbal Medicine*. London: Churchill Livingstone, 2010, 27–74.

- Johnson, A., Roberts, L., and Elkins, G. "Complementary and Alternative Medicine for Menopause." *Journal of Evidence-Based Integrative Medicine* 24 (2019). https://doi.org/10.1177/2515690X19829380.

- Gonzales, G. F., Cordova, A., Gonzales, C., Chung, A., Vega, K., and Villena, A. "*Lepidium meyenii* (Maca) Improved Semen Parameters in Adult Men." *Asian Journal of Andrology* 3, no. 4 (2001), 301–304.

- Bower-Cargill, C., Yarandi, N., and Petróczi, A. "A Systematic Review of the Versatile Effects of the Peruvian Maca Root (*Lepidium meyenii*) on Sexual Dysfunction, Menopausal Symptoms and Related Conditions." *Phytomedicine Plus* 2, no. 4 (2022), 100326.

- Sellandi, T. M., Thakar, A. B., and Baghel, M. S. "Clinical Efficacy of *Tribulus terrestris* on Oligospermia: A Randomized, Double-Blind, Placebo-Controlled Trial." *Phytomedicine* 23, no. 9 (2016), 991–97.

- Shin, B. C., Lee, M. S., Yang, E. J., Lim, H. S., and Ernst, E. "Maca (*L. meyenii*) for Improving Sexual Function: A Systematic Review." *BMC Complementary and Alternative Medicine* 10 (2010), 1–6.

- Arentz, S., Abbott, J. A., Smith, C. A., and Bensoussan, A. "Herbal Medicine for the Management of Polycystic Ovary Syndrome (PCOS) and Associated Oligo/Amenorrhoea and Hyperandrogenism: A Review of the Laboratory Evidence for Effects with Corroborative Clinical Findings." *BMC Complementary and Alternative Medicine* 14 (2014), 511. https://doi.org/10.1186/1472-6882-14-511.

- GamalEl Din, S. F. "Role of *Tribulus terrestris* in Male Infertility: Is It Real or Fiction?" *Journal of Dietary Supplements* 15, no. 6 (2018), 1010–13. https://doi.org/10.1080/19390211.2017.1402843.

- Sirotkin, A. V., Harrath, A. H., Alwasel, S. H., and Skalicka-Woźniak, K. "*Tribulus terrestris* and Reproductive Function: A Review." *Phytomedicine* 81 (2021), 153462. https://doi.org/10.1016/j.phymed.2021.153462.

Chapter 6: Mind Matters: Herbs for Mental Health, Cognition, and Mood

- Choudhary, D., Bhattacharyya, S., and Bose, S. "Efficacy and Safety of Ashwagandha Root Extract in Improving Memory and Cognitive Functions." *The Journal of Dietary Supplements* 14, no. 6 (2017), 599–612.

- Sharma, A. K., Basu, I., and Singh, S. "Efficacy and Safety of Ashwagandha Root Extract in Subclinical Hypothyroid Patients: A Double-Blind, Randomized Placebo-Controlled Trial." *The Journal of Alternative and Complementary Medicine* 24, no. 3 (2018), 243–48.

- Wankhede, S., Langade, D., Joshi, K., Sinha, S. R., and Bhattacharyya, S. "Examining the Effect of *Withania somnifera* Supplementation on Muscle Strength and Recovery." *The Journal of the International Society of Sports Nutrition* 12, no. 1 (2015), 43.

- Linde, K., Berner, M. M., and Kriston, L. "St John's Wort for Major Depression." *The Cochrane Database of Systematic Reviews* 4 (2008), CD000448.

- Ng, Q. X., Venkatanarayanan, N., and Ho, C. Y. "Clinical Use of *Hypericum perforatum* (St. John's Wort) in Depression: A Meta-Analysis." *BMC Medicine* 14, no. 1 (2016), 192.

- Gray, N. E., Alcazar Magana, A., and Stevens, J. F. "*Centella asiatica*: Phytochemistry and Mechanisms of Neuroprotection and Cognitive Enhancement." *Evidence-Based Complementary and Alternative Medicine* (2016), 2143685.

- Orhan, I. E. "*Centella asiatica* (L.) *Urban*: From Traditional Medicine to Modern Medicine with Neuroprotective Potential." *Evidence-Based Complementary and Alternative Medicine* 1 (2012), 946259.

- Bylka, W., Znajdek Awiżeń, P., Studzińska Sroka, E., Dańczak Pazdrowska, A., and Brzezińska, M. "*Centella asiatica* in Dermatology: An Overview." *Phytotherapy Research* 28, no. 8 (2014), 1117–24.

- Capasso, F., Gaginella, T. S., Grandolini, G., Izzo, A. A., Capasso, F., Gaginella, T. S., ... and Izzo, A. A. "Plants and the Cardiovascular System." *Phytotherapy: A Quick Reference to Herbal Medicine* (2003), 109–133.

- Akhondzadeh, S., Naghavi, H. R., Vazirian, M., Shayeganpour, A., Rashidi, H., and Khani, M. "Passionflower in the Treatment of Generalized Anxiety: A Pilot Double-Blind Randomized Controlled Trial." *Phytomedicine* 18, nos. 8–9 (2011), 715–18.

- Movafegh, A., Alizadeh, R., Hajimohamadi, F., Esfehani, F., and Nejatfar, M. "Preoperative Oral *Passiflora Incarnata* Reduces Anxiety in Ambulatory Surgery Patients: A Double-Blind, Placebo-Controlled Study." *Anesthesia & Analgesia* 106, no. 6 (2008), 172–32.

- Ngan, A., and Conduit, R. "A Double-Blind, Placebo-Controlled Investigation of the Effects of *Passiflora incarnata* (Passionflower) Herbal Tea on Subjective Sleep Quality." *Sleep Science* 10, no. 3 (2017), 96–102.

- Bawazir, A. A., and Lafferty, L. "The Anxiolytic Effect of *Scutellaria lateriflora* (American Skullcap): A Literature Review." *Nutritional Perspectives: Journal of the Council on Nutrition* 47, no. 2 (2024).

- Awad, R., Arnason, J. T., Trudeau, V., Bergeron, C., Budzinski, J. W., Foster, B. C., and Merali, Z. "Phytochemical and Biological Analysis of Skullcap (*Scutellaria lateriflora* L.): A Medicinal Plant with Anxiolytic Properties." *Phytomedicine* 10, no. 8 (2003), 640–49.

- Brock, C., Whitehouse, J., Tewfik, I., and Towell, T. "American Skullcap (*Scutellaria lateriflora*): An Ancient Remedy for Today's Anxiety?" *British Journal of Wellbeing* 1, no. 4 (2010), 25–30.

- Sun, X. Z., Liao, Y., Li, W., and Guo, L. M. "Neuroprotective Effects of *Ganoderma Lucidum* Polysaccharides Against Oxidative Stress-Induced Neuronal Apoptosis." *Neural Regeneration Research* 12, no. 6 (2017), 953–58.

- Jin, H., Aquili, L., Heng, B. C., Strekalova, T., Fung, M. L., Tipoe, G. L., ... and Lim, L. W. "*Ganoderma lucidum*: An Emerging Nutritional Approach to Manage Depression." *Food Reviews International* (2025), 1–22.

Chapter 7: Good Bones: Herbs for the Skeletal and Muscular System

- Jugdaohsingh, R., Tucker, K. L., Qiao, N., Cupples, L. A., Kiel, D. P., and Powell, J. J. "Dietary Silicon Intake Is Positively Associated with Bone Mineral Density in Men and Premenopausal Women of the Framingham Offspring Cohort." *Journal of Bone and Mineral Research* 19, no. 2 (2004), 297–307.

- Klontzas, M. E., Kakkos, G. A., Papadakis, G. Z., Marias, K., and Karantanas, A. H. "Advanced Clinical Imaging for the Evaluation of Stem Cell-Based Therapies." *Expert Opinion on Biological Therapy* 21, no. 9 (2001), 1253–64.

- Anvari, M., Dortaj, H., Hashemibeni, B., and Pourentezari, M. "Application of Some Herbal Medicine Used for the Treatment of Osteoarthritis and Chondrogenesis." *Traditional and Integrative Medicine* 5, no. 3 (2020), 126–49.

- Min, K. H., Kim, D. H., Youn, S., and Pack, S. P. "Biomimetic Diatom Biosilica and Its Potential for Biomedical Applications and Prospects: A Review." *International Journal of Molecular Sciences* 25, no. 4 (2024), 2023.

- Drobnic, F., Riera, J., Appendino, G., Togni, S., Franceschi, F., Valle, X., ... and Tur, J. "Reduction of Delayed Onset Muscle Soreness by a Novel Curcumin Delivery System (Meriva®): A Randomised, Placebo-Controlled Trial." *Journal of the International Society of Sports Nutrition* 11 (2014), 1–10.

- Gupta, S. C., Patchva, S., and Aggarwal, B. B. "Therapeutic Roles of Curcumin: Lessons Learned from Clinical Trials." *Journal of Medicinal Food* 19, no. 2 (216), 123–38.

- Chrubasik, J. E., Roufogalis, B. D., Wagner, H., and Chrubasik, S. "A Comprehensive Review on the Stinging Nettle Effect and Efficacy Profiles." *Phytomedicine* 14, nos. 7–8 (2007), 568–79. https://doi.org/10.1016/j.phymed.2006.09.003.

- Bhusal, K. K., Magar, S. K., Thapa, R., Lamsal, A., Bhandari, S., Maharjan, R., Shrestha, S., and Shrestha, J. "Nutritional and Pharmacological Importance of Stinging Nettle (*Urtica dioica* L.): A Review." *Heliyon* 8, no. 6 (2022), e09717. https://doi.org/10.1016/j.heliyon.2022.e09717.

- Rathaur, H., Juyal, D., and Mukhopadhyay, S. "Arthritis Alleviation with *Urtica Dioica*: Unveiling the Latest Findings from Preclinical and Clinical Trials." *Biochemical and Cellular Archives* 24, no. 1 (2024).

- Majeed, M., Majeed, S., Narayanan, N. K., and Nagabhushanam, K. "A Pilot, Randomized, Double-Blind, Placebo-Controlled Trial to Assess the Safety and Efficacy of a Novel Boswellia serrata Extract in the Management of Osteoarthritis of the Knee." *Phytotherapy Research: PTR* 33, no. 5 (2019), 1457–68. https://doi.org/10.1002/ptr.6338.

- Kimmatkar, N., Thawani, V., Hingorani, L., and Khiyani, R. "Efficacy and Tolerability of *Boswellia serrata* Extract in Treatment of Osteoarthritis of Knee: A Randomized Double-Blind Placebo-Controlled Trial." *Phytomedicine* 10, no. 1 (2003), 3–7. https://doi.org/10.1078/094471103321648593.

Chapter 8: Hormonal Harmony: Herbs for the Endocrine System

- Jamshidi, N., and Cohen, M. M. "The Clinical Efficacy and Safety of Tulsi in Humans: A Systematic Review of the Literature." *Journal of Ayurveda and Integrative Medicine* 8, no. 2 (2017), 121–27. https://doi.org/10.1016/j.jaim.2017.05.008.

- Lopresti, A. L., Smith, S. J., Metse, A. P., and Drummond, P. D. "A Randomized, Double-Blind, Placebo-Controlled Trial Investigating the Effects of an *Ocimum tenuiflorum* (Holy Basil) Extract (Holixer™) on Stress, Mood, and Sleep in Adults Experiencing Stress." *Frontiers in Nutrition* 9 (2022), 965130. https://doi.org/10.3389/fnut.2022.965130

- Sampath, S., Mahapatra, S. C., Padhi, M. M., Sharma, R., and Talwar, A. "Holy Basil (*Ocimum-sanctum* Linn.) Leaf Extract Enhances Specific Cognitive Parameters in Healthy Adult Volunteers: A Placebo-Controlled Study." *Indian Journal of Physiology and Pharmacoly* 59, no. 1 (2015), 69–77.

- Gupta, A., Gupta, R., and Lal, B. "Effect of *Trigonella foenum-graecum* (Fenugreek) Seeds on Glycemic Control and Insulin Resistance in Type 2 Diabetes Mellitus: A Double-Blind Placebo-Controlled Study." *Journal of the Association of Physicians of India* 49 (2001), 1057–61.

- Sharma, M. M., Kumar, K., Kumari, P., and Katoch, N. K. "A Systematic Analysis on Antidiabetic Activity, of Medicinal Plants and Their Ethnobotanical Study with Special Reference to Udhampur District." *International Journal of All Research Education and Scientific Methods* (2024).

- Panossian, A., and Wikman, G. "Effects of Adaptogens on the Central Nervous System and the Molecular Mechanisms Associated with Their Stress–Protective Activity." *Journal of Ethnopharmacology* 155, no. 3 (2014), 1332–46.

- Addissouky, T. A., El Sayed, I. E. T., Ali, M. M., Alubiady, M. H. S., and Wang, Y. "*Schisandra chinensis* in Liver Disease: Exploring the Mechanisms and Therapeutic Promise of an Ancient Chinese Botanical." *Archives of Pharmacology and Therapeutics* 6, no. 1 (2024), 27–33.

- Chun, J. N., Cho, M., So, I., and Jeon, J. H. "The Protective Effects of *Schisandra chinensis* Fruit Extract and Its Lignans Against Cardiovascular Disease: A Review of the Molecular Mechanisms." *Fitoterapia* 97 (2014), 224–33.

- Tiwari, R., Latheef, S. K., Ahmed, I., Iqbal, H. M., Bule, M. H., Dhama, K., ... and Farag, M. R. "Herbal Immunomodulators—A Remedial Panacea for Designing and Developing Effective Drugs and Medicines: Current Scenario and Future Prospects." *Current Drug Metabolism* 19, no. 3 (2018), 264–301.

- Erten, F., Er, B., Ozmen, R., Tokmak, M., Gokdere, E., Orhan, C., ... and Sahin, K. "Effects of Integrated Extracts of *Trigonella foenum-graecum* and *Asparagus racemosus* on Hot Flash–Like Symptoms in Ovariectomized Rats." *Antioxidants* 14, no. 3 (2025), 355.

Chapter 9: Nature's Detox: Herbs for Liver Health and Detoxification

- Musazadeh, V., Karimi, A., Jafarzadeh, J., Sanaie, S., Vajdi, M., Karimi, M., and Niazkar, H. R. "The Favorable Impacts of Silibinin Polyphenols as Adjunctive Therapy in Reducing the Complications of COVID-19: A Review of Research Evidence and Underlying Mechanisms." *Biomedicine & Pharmacotherapy*, 154 (2022), 113593.

- Mirhashemi, S. H., Hakakzadeh, A., Yeganeh, F. E., Oshidari, B., and Rezaee, S. P. "Effect of 8 Weeks Milk Thistle Powder (Silymarin Extract) Supplementation on Fatty Liver Disease in Patient Candidates for Bariatric Surgery." *Metabolism Open* 14 (2022), 100190.

- Wadhwa, K., Pahwa, R., Kumar, M., Kumar, S., Sharma, P. C., Singh, G., ... and Jeandet, P. "Mechanistic Insights into the Pharmacological Significance of Silymarin." *Molecules* 27, no. 16 (2022), 5327.

- Tanasa, M. V., Negreanu-Pirjol, T., Olariu, L., Negreanu-Pirjol, B. S., Lepadatu, A. C., Anghel, L., and Rosoiu, N. "Bioactive Compounds from Vegetal Organs of Taraxacum Species (Dandelion) with Biomedical Applications: A Review." *International Journal of Molecular Sciences* 26, no. 2 (2025), 450.

- Chatterjee, S. J., Ovadje, P., Mousa, M., Hamm, C., and Pandey, S. "The Efficacy of Dandelion Root Extract in Inducing Apoptosis in Drug-Resistant Human Melanoma Cells." *Evidence-Based Complementary and Alternative Medicine* 1 (2011), 129045.

- Souad, E., Hassan, E. M., Farouk, H. A., Refaee, A. A., Mohammed, M. A., and Mossa, A. T. H. "Hepatoprotective of *Taraxacum officinale* Against Liver Damage Induced by Carbon Tetrachloride in Male Rats." *Journal of Chemical and Pharmaceutical Research* 8, no. 5 (2016), 538–45.

- Chan, Y. S., Cheng, L. N., Wu, J. H., Chan, E., Kwan, Y. W., Lee, S. M. Y., and Leung, G. P. H. "A Review of the Pharmacological Effects of *Arctium lappa* (Burdock)." *Phytotherapy Research* 24, no. 9 (2010), 1262–71.

- Ishii, T., Shimizu, T., Imai, M., Healy, J., Rouzard, K., Tamura, M., and Fitzgerald, C. "Arctigenin-Enriched Burdock Seed Oil (ABSO): A New Skin-Brightening Botanical Extract." *Cosmetics* 10, no. 1 (2023), 10.

- Lee, S. S., Kim, D. H., Yim, D. S., and Lee, S. Y. "Anti-Inflammatory, Analgesic and Hepatoprotective Effect of Semen of *Rumex Crispus*." *Korean Journal of Pharmacognosy* 38, no. 4 (2007), 334–38.

Chapter 10: Clean and Clear: Herbs for the Urinary System and Kidney Health

- Kreydiyyeh, S. I., and Usta, J. "Diuretic Effect and Mechanism of Action of Parsley." *Phytomedicine* 20, no. 13 (2013), 1080–83.

- Alobaidi, S. "Renal Health Benefits and Therapeutic Effects of Parsley (*Petroselinum crispum*): A Review." *Frontiers in Medicine* 11 (2024), 1494740.

- Farzaei, M. H., Abbasabadi, Z., Ardekani, M. R. S., Rahimi, R., and Farzaei, F. "Parsley: A Review of Ethnopharmacology, Phytochemistry and Biological Activities." *Journal of Traditional Chinese Medicine* 33, no. 6 (2013), 815–26.

- Singh, P., Singh, J., Rasane, P., Kaur, S., and Nanda, V. "Nephroprotective Effect of Corn Silk: A Review on Its Mechanism of Action and Safety Evaluation." *Journal of Food Chemistry and Nanotechnoly* 9, S1 (2023), S28–S35.

- Apampa, S. A., and Adedapo, D. A. "A Review of Phytochemicals Isolated from Corn Silk and Their Medicinal Applications." *International Journal of Science and Research Archive* 11, no. 2 (2024), 1726–34.

- Awad, R., and Haubrick, K. "Cranberries vs. Antibiotics: Impact on UTI Recurrence in Women." *Research Review* 5, no. 12 (2024), 2663–75.

- Komala, M., and Kumar, K. S. "Urinary Tract Infection: Causes, Symptoms, Diagnosis and Its Management." *Indian Journal of Research in Pharmacy and Biotechnology* 1, no. 2 (2013), 226.

- Garg, R., Dobhal, K., and Singh, A. "Utilization of Medicinal Herbal Plants in the Management of Respiratory Conditions." *Immunopathology of Chronic Respiratory Diseases* (2024).

- Vamenta-Morris, H., Dreisbach, A., Shoemaker-Moyle, M., and Abdel-Rahman, E. M. "Internet Claims on Dietary and Herbal Supplements in Advanced Nephropathy: Truth or Myth." *American Journal of Nephrology* 40, no. 5 (2014), 393–98.

Chapter 11: Gut Check: Herbs for the Digestive System

- Hu, M. L., Rayner, C. K., Wu, K. L., Chuah, S. K., Tai, W. C., Chou, Y. P., and Chiu, Y. C. "Effect of Ginger on Gastric Motility and Symptoms of Functional Dyspepsia: A Randomized, Double-Blind, Controlled Trial." *Phytotherapy Research* 32, no. 2 (2018), 228–34.

- Palatty, P. L., Haniadka, R., Valder, B., Arora, R., and Baliga, M. S. "Ginger in the Prevention of Nausea and Vomiting: A Review." *Critical Reviews in Food Science and Nutrition* 53, no. 7 (2013), 659–69.

- Viljoen, E., Visser, J., Koen, N., and Musekiwa, A. "A Systematic Review and Meta-Analysis of the Effect and Safety of Ginger in the Treatment of Pregnancy-Associated Nausea and Vomiting." *The American Journal of Obstetrics and Gynecology* 222, no. 5 (2020), 482–91.

- Samimi, S., Nimrouzi, M., Zarshenas, M. M., Fallahzadeh, E., Vardanjani, H. M., Sadeghi, E., and Salehi, Z. "The Efficacy of a Traditional Herbal Medicine Compound for Functional Dyspepsia: A Randomized, Double-Blind, Placebo-Controlled Trial." *Jundishapur Journal of Natural Pharmaceutical Products* 19, no. 4 (2024).

- Shahrahmani, H., Ghazanfarpour, M., Shahrahmani, N., Abdi, F., Sewell, R., and Rafieian-Kopaei, M. "Effect of Fennel on Primary Dysmenorrhea: A Systematic Review and Meta-Analysis." *Journal of Complementary and Integrative Medicine* 18, no. 2 (2021), 261–69. https://doi.org/10.1515/jcim-2019-0212.

- Savino, F., Cresi, F., Castagno, E., Silvestro, L., and Oggero, R. "A Randomized Double-Blind Placebo-Controlled Trial of a Standardized Extract of *Matricariae recutita, Foeniculum vulgare* and *Melissa officinalis* (ColiMil®) in the Treatment of Breastfed Colicky Infants." *Phytotherapy Research: An International Journal Devoted to Pharmacological and Toxicological Evaluation of Natural Product Derivatives* 19, no. 4 (2005), 335–40.

- Kumar, S., Narwal, S., Kumar, V., and Prakash, O. "α-glucosidase Inhibitors from Plants: A Natural Approach to Treat Diabetes." *Pharmacognosy Reviews* 5, no. 9 (2011), 19.

- Leach, M. J. "*Gymnema sylvestre* for Diabetes Mellitus: A Systematic Review." *The Journal of Alternative and Complementary Medicine* 13, no. 9 (2007), 977–83.

- Ibrahim, A., Babandi, A., Tijjani, A. A., Murtala, Y., Yakasai, H. M., Shehu, D., ... and Umar, I. A. "In Vitro Antioxidant and Anti-Diabetic Potential of *Gymnema sylvestre* Methanol Leaf Extract." *European Scientific Journal* 13 (2017), 218–38.

- Godard, M. P., Johnson, B. A., and Richmond, S. R. "Body Composition and Hormonal Adaptations Associated with Forskolin Consumption in Overweight and Obese Men." *Obesity Research* 13, no. 8 (2005), 1335–43.

- Henderson, S., Magu, B., Rasmussen, C., Lancaster, S., Kerksick, C., Smith, P., ... and Kreider, R. B. "Effects of *Coleus forskohlii* Supplementation on Body Composition and Hematological Profiles in Mildly Overweight Women." *Journal of the International Society of Sports Nutrition* 2 (2005), 1–9.

- Alasbahi, R. H., and Melzig, M. F. "Forskolin and Derivatives as Tools for Studying the Role of cAMP." *Die Pharmazie-An International Journal of Pharmaceutical Sciences* 67, no. 1 (2012), 5–13.

- Bhardwaj, N., Chavez, M., Fleeks, J., Ondari, A., and Payne, S. "Does Peppermint Essential Oil Relieve Headache Pain in Adults with Tension Headaches?" *Evidence-Based Practice* 26, no. 1 (2023), 16–17.

- Ertürk, N. E., and Taşcı, S. "The Effects of Peppermint Oil on Nausea, Vomiting and Retching in Cancer Patients Undergoing Chemotherapy: An Open Label Quasi–Randomized Controlled Pilot Study." *Complementary Therapies in Medicine* 56 (2021), 102587.

- Reay, J. L., Kennedy, D. O., and Scholey, A. B. "Single Doses of *Panax Ginseng* (G115) Reduce Blood Glucose Levels and Improve Cognitive Performance During Sustained Mental Activity." *Journal of Psychopharmacology* 19, no. 4 (2005), 357–65.

- Barton, D. L., Soori, G. S., Bauer, B. A., et al. "Pilot Study of *Panax Quinquefolius* (American Ginseng) to Improve Cancer-Related Fatigue: A Randomized, Double-Blind Trial." *Journal of Clinical Oncology* 31, no. 29 (2013), 3415–23.

- Lu, G., Liu, Z., Wang, X., and Wang, C. "Recent Advances in *Panax ginseng* CA Meyer as an Herb for Anti-Fatigue: An Effects and Mechanisms Review." *Foods* 10, no. 5 (2021), 1030.

- Kim, H. G., Cho, J. H., Yoo, S. R., Lee, J. S., Han, J. M., Lee, N. H., ... and Son, C. G. "Antifatigue Effects of *Panax Ginseng* CA Meyer: A Randomised, Double-Blind, Placebo-Controlled Trial." *PLOS One* 8, no. 4 (2013), e61271.

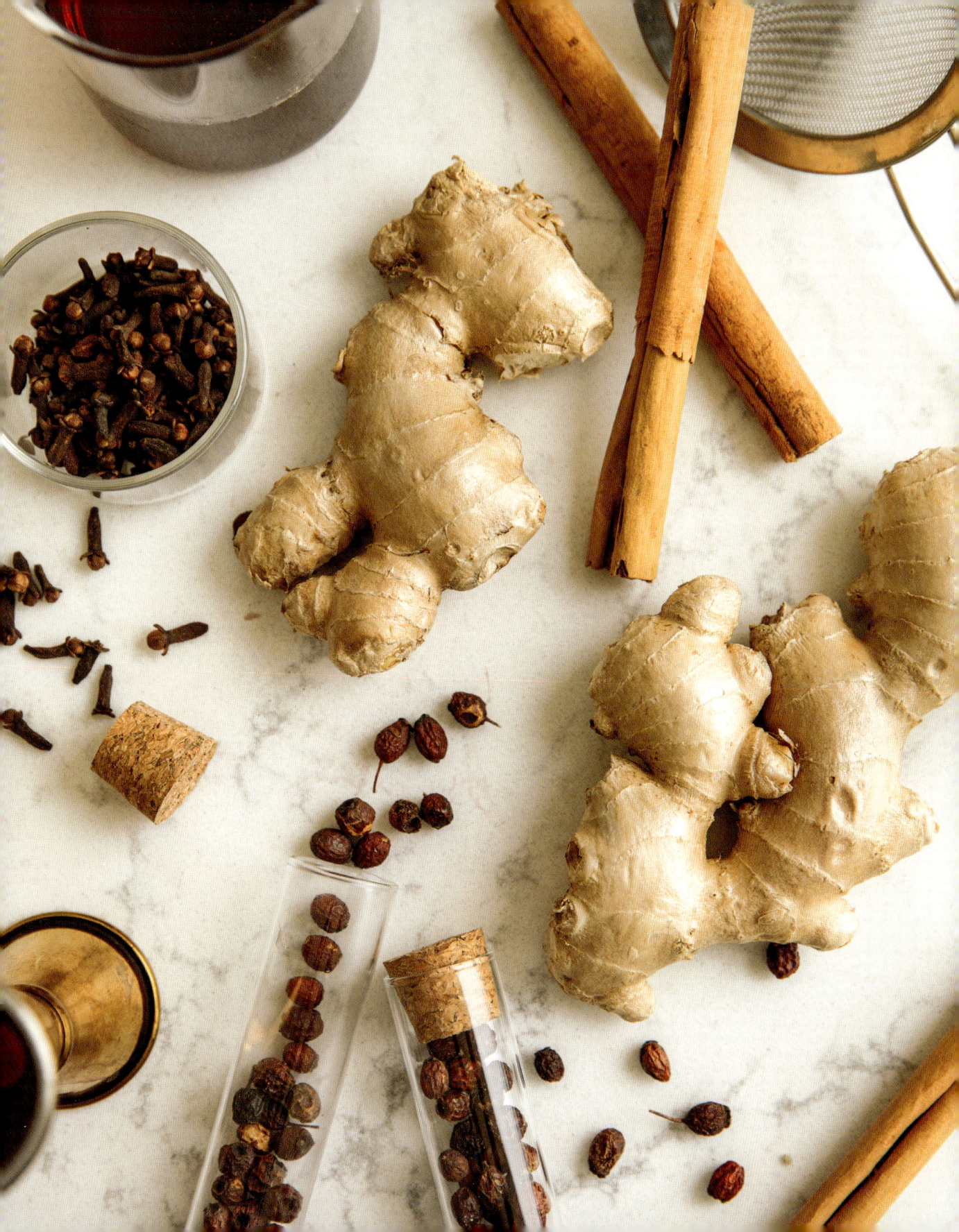

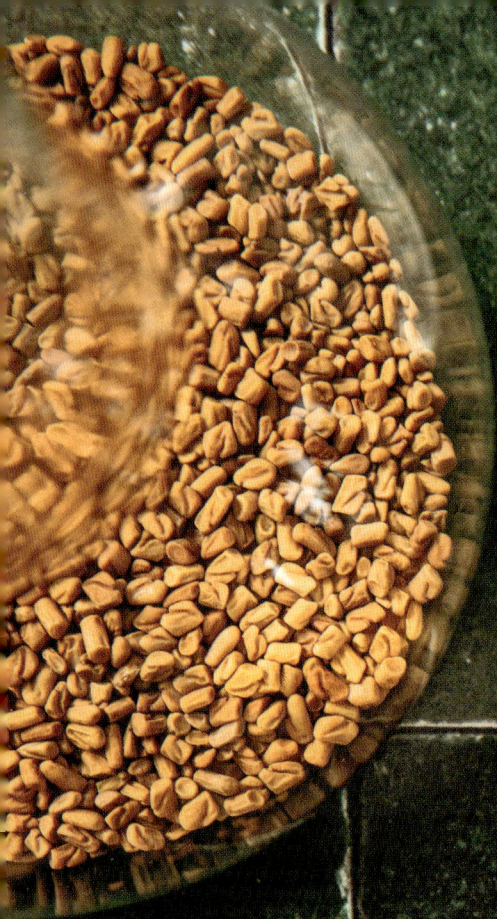

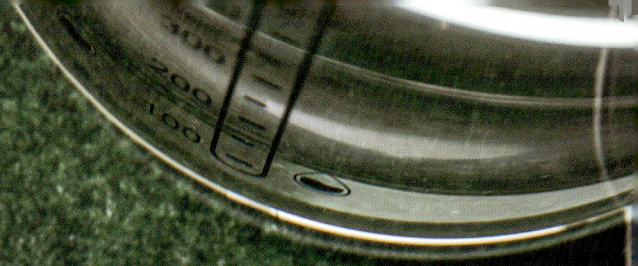

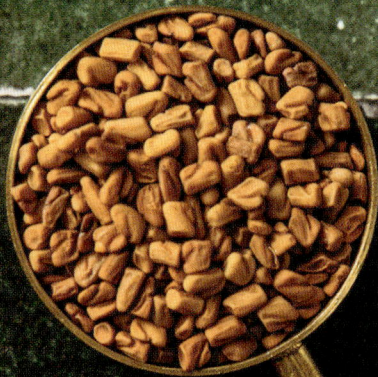

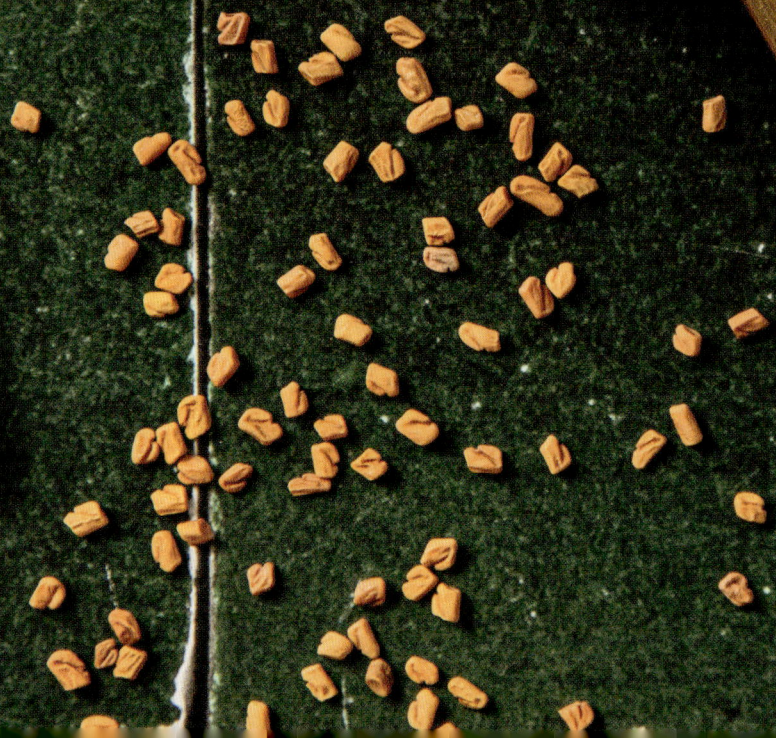

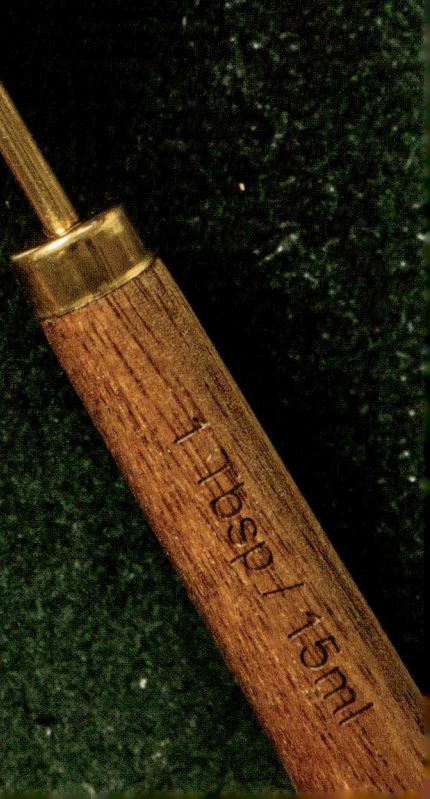

Acknowledgments

This book grew the way herbs do—slowly, stubbornly, and with the right kind of light.

Sheldon, you already know. Every page has your fingerprints. Every chapter—your patience. Thank you for being the soft wind at my back and the quiet magic that steadies me when I forget my own rhythm. You make everything I dream feel possible.

Justin, you've always been my built-in compass. Thank you for the sarcasm, the real talk, and the way you protect what matters. You remind me who I am when I start to forget.

Dear Mom (Vickie) and Dad (Claude), thank you for letting your daughter wander far but never feel lost. You gave me wonder, work ethic, and permission to be a little wild. That's everything.

To my in-laws, Mr. Sam and Mrs. Faye, thank you for loving me fully and freely, and for letting this herb-obsessed, science-loving dreamer feel right at home in your world.

Blake, little one, you made "Apple" sound like a whole universe. I'll never hear it the same way again. You're already teaching me about joy, about presence, about magic.

Michele, you helped me gather myself—quietly, powerfully. Thank you for helping me make room for softness in the middle of becoming.

To the leaves that leaned toward me. To the roots that held. To the water that waited. Nature, thank you for every lesson, every metaphor, every medicine. You've been the most consistent teacher of them all.

And to those who came before (the scientists, the storytellers, the medicine makers), I carry your legacy in every line.

To my friends and this beautiful The Active Herb community: Your curiosity, encouragement, and plant nerd enthusiasm kept me going when I was running on flower fumes.

This is for every girl who crushed herbs with a spoon, who wrote spells in the margins of her science notes, who knew healing could be both evidence-based *and* enchanted.

Thank you for finding me here.

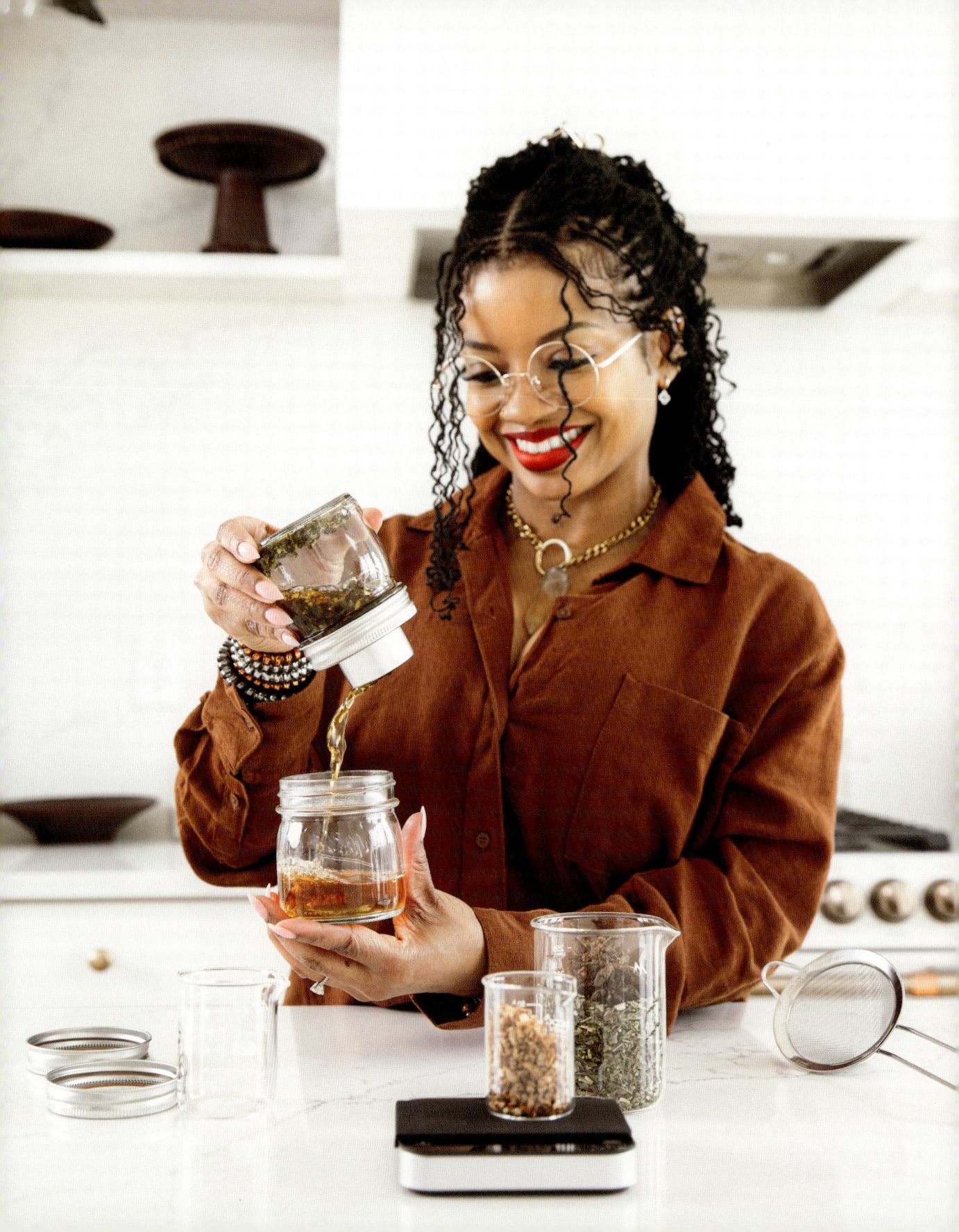

About the Author

Dr. Aisha Hill-Hart is a scientist, herbalist, and published epidemiologist who makes herbal wisdom accessible without watering down the science. With a PhD in epidemiology, a master's in biotechnology, and a deep-rooted love for medicinal plants, she brings together lab precision and ancestral intuition to help others reconnect with the healing power of nature.

Her work spans biomedical research, plant biotechnology, and public health. She has authored numerous peer-reviewed articles and spent years investigating the science behind what truly nourishes us.

When she's not deep in the data or crafting a tincture, you can find her outside on a run, experimenting with herbal lattes as a self-taught barista, wine tasting with her husband, or vibing to old-school tracks that make everything feel just right.

She's the voice behind The Active Herb, where she teaches the beauty of botanical medicine with equal parts grit, grace, and groove.

Index

The Practical Science of Herbs